Principles and Practice of Therapeutic Massage

Principles and Practice of Therapeutic Massage

Third Edition

Akhoury Gourang Sinha
BPT MSPT PhD (Sports Medicine and Physiotherapy)
Professor
Department of Physiotherapy
Ex-Dean Faculty of Medicine
Punjabi University
Patiala, Punjab, India

Foreword
Bharati Bellare

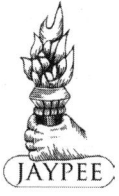

JAYPEE BROTHERS MEDICAL PUBLISHERS
The Health Sciences Publisher
New Delhi | London

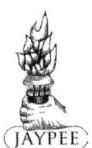 **Jaypee Brothers Medical Publishers (P) Ltd**

Headquarters
Jaypee Brothers Medical Publishers (P) Ltd
EMCA House
23/23-B, Ansari Road, Daryaganj
New Delhi - 110 002, India
Landline: +91-11-23272143, +91-11-23272703
+91-11-23282021, +91-11-23245672
Email: jaypee@jaypeebrothers.com

Corporate Office
Jaypee Brothers Medical Publishers (P) Ltd
4838/24, Ansari Road, Daryaganj
New Delhi 110 002, India
Phone: +91-11-43574357
Fax: +91-11-43574314
Email: jaypee@jaypeebrothers.com

Overseas Office
J.P. Medical Ltd
83 Victoria Street, London
SW1H 0HW (UK)
Phone: +44 20 3170 8910
Fax: +44 (0)20 3008 6180
Email: info@jpmedpub.com

Website: www.jaypeebrothers.com
Website: www.jaypeedigital.com

© 2021, Jaypee Brothers Medical Publishers

The views and opinions expressed in this book are solely those of the original contributor(s)/author(s) and do not necessarily represent those of editor(s) of the book.

All rights reserved. No part of this publication may be reproduced, stored or transmitted in any form or by any means, electronic, mechanical, photocopying, recording or otherwise, without the prior permission in writing of the publishers.

All brand names and product names used in this book are trade names, service marks, trademarks or registered trademarks of their respective owners. The publisher is not associated with any product or vendor mentioned in this book.

Medical knowledge and practice change constantly. This book is designed to provide accurate, authoritative information about the subject matter in question. However, readers are advised to check the most current information available on procedures included and check information from the manufacturer of each product to be administered, to verify the recommended dose, formula, method and duration of administration, adverse effects and contraindications. It is the responsibility of the practitioner to take all appropriate safety precautions. Neither the publisher nor the author(s)/editor(s) assume any liability for any injury and/or damage to persons or property arising from or related to use of material in this book.

This book is sold on the understanding that the publisher is not engaged in providing professional medical services. If such advice or services are required, the services of a competent medical professional should be sought.

Every effort has been made where necessary to contact holders of copyright to obtain permission to reproduce copyright material. If any have been inadvertently overlooked, the publisher will be pleased to make the necessary arrangements at the first opportunity. The **CD/DVD-ROM** (if any) provided in the sealed envelope with this book is complimentary and free of cost. **Not meant for sale.**

Inquiries for bulk sales may be solicited at: jaypee@jaypeebrothers.com

Principles and Practice of Therapeutic Massage

First Edition: 2001
  Reprint: 2002
  Reprint: 2004
Second Edition: 2010
Third Edition: 2021

Reprint **2023**
ISBN 978-93-89776-89-8

Printed at: Sterling Graphics Pvt. Ltd.

*To
Ma, Papa, Uru Didi
and
Babuji*

FOREWORD TO THE THIRD EDITION

When Prof (Dr) Akhoury Gourang Sinha approached me for writing foreword for the third edition of his textbook *Principles and Practice of Therapeutic Massage*, my first reaction was—"why have you used the term Massage?". I believe most of senior therapists confronted with a similar situation would have reacted in the similar stereotypical manner. I belong to the era when physiotherapists were considered as masseurs and were treated like technicians rather than clinicians. It is with painstaking efforts and sheer perseverance, that today we have established ourselves, as independent healthcare professionals. However, the repulsion against the term *massage* still persists. Though the term *massage* is substituted in most places by the term *soft tissue manipulations* and even though the subject is an integral part of the undergraduate curriculum, the Indian physiotherapist simply to avoid "humiliation" of being addressed as masseurs, hardly uses any typical massage techniques during clinical practice, despite the proven clinical efficacy of healing human touch.

However, all my apprehensions and misgivings about the term *massage* were proven ill-founded, when I screened the chapters, particularly those which included comprehensive description of, how "Massage", the ancient traditional method of "Healing" by using "touch" as a mode in different forms.

Dr Sinha has not only elaborated various techniques of massage, their physiological and therapeutic effects, indications and contraindication in a simplified manner for the benefit of undergraduate students of physiotherapy but his extensive research on the evolution of massage with most recent citations deserves to serve as a textbook for postgraduate students too.

Dr Sinha has beautifully explained about how this component of ancient traditional medicine got evolved into a wide spectrum of massage practices based on various concepts which represents countries across the globe, viz. "Abhyanga" of India, "Tuina" of China, "Shiatsu" of Japan or *Nuad phaen boran*—the traditional Thai massage to name a few. Dr Sinha has also explained the latest evidence, as to how the typical techniques of massage included in physiotherapeutics have evolved into globally popular methods termed as "trigger point mobilization", "physiological movements and manual therapy", "myofascial release", etc. Inclusion of latest references in this book justifies, that these methods with fancy nomenclature are not different but are the newly evolved styles of massage since all of them involve healing with "Touch".

I congratulate Dr Sinha for his wonderful work on the subject and highly appreciate his sincere efforts taken to highlight the concept of "healing touch" without any prejudice about the term "massage", which is indeed a very bold step as mentioned by Dr Dandapani in his foreword in the earlier edition of this book.

The prior editions of the book have been well received, having been through several reprints. Now, years later since its inception, Dr Sinha has carefully updated the art and science of massage in physiotherapy in this third edition, enriching it with clinical reasoning. I am absolutely delighted and honored to write a foreword for the third edition of this textbook, which I believe, would go a long way in not just resurrecting but strengthening the conceptual model of massage in physiotherapy practice.

I am well aware of the exam-centric reading practice adopted by young students today, where reading of foreword is considered redundant, nevertheless I urge the students and fellow professionals to read this current creation as a "story book" instead of textbook and discern the difference in our understanding of the genuine concept behind *Massage*.

Best Wishes !!

Bharati Bellare
Ex-Professor and Head, Department of Physiotherapy
LTM Medical College
Sion, Mumbai, Maharashtra, India
Ex-Dean, Faculty of Allied Health Sciences
Maharashtra University of Health Science
Ex-Associate Dean
Kasturba Medical College
In-Charge, Allied Health Faculty
Manipal Academy of Higher Education (MAHE)
Manipal, Karnataka, India

FOREWORD TO THE FIRST EDITION

It is my proud privilege to write the foreword to *Principles and Practices of Therapeutic Massage* by AG Sinha.

Massage or manipulation of soft tissues is the oldest form of physical therapy mentioned in ancient medical records. Of late due to several reasons physiotherapists started paying it least attention. However, learning the skills of massage is the basic step to achieve success in specialised manual therapy techniques, as this is one of the main techniques that helps physiotherapists to develop the palpatory skills and sensory awareness.

Most of the books available for physiotherapists are by the overseas authors and often present diversified explanation of techniques, uses and applications. This always confuses a learner as well as teacher and Mr Sinha, after performing an extensive search of literature, has written this comprehensive book. I strongly feel that this would help very much not only to the students but also to the teachers.

This book is a great boon for everyone concerned, as this is the first book on massage written by an Indian physiotherapist. In a situation, where massage as a therapeutic modality is neglected or given least priority, I appreciate the author for his boldness to bring out this book. This may catalyse others to write books on physiotherapy field.

I pray Almighty for the success of Mr Sinha in this endeavor.

AG Dhandapani
Additional Professor
Department of Physiotherapy
Sri Ramachandra Institute of Higher Education
and Research (Deemed University)
Chennai, Tamil Nadu, India
Formerly
Head, Department of Physiotherapy
National Institute of Rehabilitation Training and Research
Cuttack, Odisha, India

PREFACE TO THE THIRD EDITION

The purpose of this revised third edition of the *Principles and Practice of Therapeutic Massage* is same as that of the original text, to bring together the scattered knowledge of the diverse aspects of therapeutic massage in a manner that is comprehensive to all those who are interested in the scientific use of this ancient mode of treatment. Last decade witnessed the massage therapy being the subject of intense scientific investigations and popularization of several new evolving approaches that use the basic principles of classical massage though are essentially different from it.

The revised third edition of this text assimilates the scientific advancement occurring in the field and includes a gist of several new approaches, such as myofascial release, instrument-assisted massage, craniosacral therapy, manual lymphatic drainage, etc. The resurgent emergence of massage in therapeutics in recent times has generated an interest in the ancient massage systems worldwide. The newly added chapter on ancient massage systems presents a brief description of the theoretical foundation and technical aspects of the massage approaches originated from India, China, Japan, and Thailand.

Basic structure of the book has not been altered and like previous editions each chapter can be read as complete entity relatively independent from rest of the book. I believe this revised edition would serve to stimulate the appreciation of the role of massage in health and disease and would receive the same support from academicians and researchers of not only physiotherapy but also of the disciplines like physical education, ayurveda, sports medicine that use massage as a part of the study and practice.

Akhoury Gourang Sinha

PREFACE TO THE FIRST EDITION

This book has been written for all those who are interested in the scientific use of massage—an ancient mode of treatment for painful muscles. Information on various aspects of massage is scattered throughout the literature. The available texts on massage, mostly written by western authors, focus usually on specific dimension of massage. In those places where enough books are not available, it often becomes a problem for a new teacher to collect the teaching material. As a result of this the teaching of massage is often neglected. These problems, which I experienced both as a student and a teacher, have stimulated me to work on this text. In nutshell, it is an attempt to collect the scattered knowledge and present it in a form of systematic and comprehensive exposition of principles, techniques and clinical uses of massage.

Divided into 11 chapters, this book attempts to critically evaluate the different aspects of massage. It includes detailed discussions on the general physiological effects of massage, its uses in different conditions and the contraindications.

The chapter on Definition and Classification of Massage assimilates the similarity and dissimilarity of different techniques and classify them accordingly. Different techniques of massage are described in detail along with their specific effects on the body tissue.

A chapter on the Practical Aspect of Massage explains the rationales behind the use of different sequence of techniques and mentions the points to be considered while administering massage. This intends to cater to the practical examination requirement of the students. These two chapters contain several photographs/illustrations to simplify the subject.

The essential features of the application of massage in different pathological conditions are explained in a chapter, which intends to serve as guideline for the beginners.

The features of lymphatic system, quite essential for the scientific practice of massage have been presented in a separate chapter. This chapter includes four charts showing schematically the distribution of lymph node and the direction of lymphatic flow in the different parts of body.

The important landmarks and milestones in the development of this modality are described under the history of massage, while the chapter on New Systems of Massage gives a brief introduction of some specific forms of massage which are widely used in different parts of the world.

Sports massage has emerged as an important modality in the field of athletic and sports world. A separate chapter presents a detailed account of the various theoretical and practical aspects of this advancing area of massage.

While working on this text, I came across a volume of literature on the topic. Out of which, however, I could refer only a portion. These titles are listed out in References. The remaining titles which are not quoted in this book, but I feel, can be of immense help to anyone who wishes to know more about this modality, are listed in Bibliography.

Given at the end, these up-to-date lists might help those who are interested to take up this modality as a special interest subject in postgraduate classes and research.

The main aim of this book is to make the subject matter more meaningful and realistic from the academic point of view. I am aware, that curriculum in many physiotherapy program may not permit as comprehensive a study on massage as this book may entail. For this reason each chapter has been written as a fairly independent entity relatively independent from rest of the book.

Although, primarily written for physiotherapy undergraduate students who have to study this subject as part of the curriculum, I earnestly hope that it would also serve as a useful reference to the members and students of other disciplines like naturopathy, ayurveda, physical education, sports medicine, etc.

Every attempt has been made to avoid errors though some might have crept in inadvertently. I shall be obliged if any such error is brought to my notice. I further solicit suggestions and criticism from learned teachers for further improvement.

Akhoury Gourang Sinha

ACKNOWLEDGMENTS

I take this opportunity to express my gratitude to all those who have helped me in the preparation of this book. In particular my thanks are due to my *Guru* Mr AG Dhandapani, Additional Professor, Department of Physiotherapy, Sri Ramachandra Medical College and Research Institute, Chennai, Tamil Nadu; India, who not only read my manuscript and gave valuable suggestions? I express my sincere thanks to Dr PK Nishank (PT), Dr Saibal Bose (PT), Dr Anupam Bhunia (PT), all my former colleagues at Srinivas College of Physiotherapy, Mangaluru, Karnataka, India and my friends Dr Shiv Kumar (PT) and Dr Raju Sharma (PT), whose constructive criticism helped me a lot in drafting this book in its present form. I am also thankful to Dr GS Kang, Dr S Koley and Dr Amarjeet Singh (PT) my colleagues at Guru Nanak Dev University (GNDU), Amritsar, Punjab, India, for their help in many ways in preparation of the manuscript.

I fall short of words to express my feeling to Prof JS Sandhu MS (Ortho) DSM, Dean Faculty of Sports Medicine and Physiotherapy, GNDU, who not only encouraged me to go ahead with all my endeavors, but also stood behind me like a rock on the occasions when I was sinking deep into solitude and dejection.

I am also indebted to my friends Dr Deepak Kumar, for sparing his valuable hours to take photographs and Mr Digvijay Srivastava of Indian National Trust for Art and Cultural Heritage (INTACH), Lucknow, Uttar Pradesh, India, for drawing all the diagrams of this book. I am also thankful to my friends Dr Jitender Sharma (PT) and Dr R Thangaraj, for helping me with the manuscript. I express my gratitude to Ms S Kalai Selvi and Miss Suman Makkar, for converting my illegible handwriting into beautiful letters.

I would be failing in my duties if I do not acknowledge my thanks to all those authors whose works have been consulted and quoted in this book.

I am also thankful to my publisher M/s Jaypee Brothers Medical Publishers (P) Ltd, New Delhi, India, especially Shri Jitendar P Vij (Group Chairman), Mr Ankit Vij (Managing Director), Mr MS Mani (Group President), Dr Madhu Chaudhary (Publishing Head–Education), Ms Pooja Bhandari (Production Head), Ms Sunita Katla (Executive Assistant to Group Chairman and Publishing Manager), Dr Akanksha Singh (Development Editor), Ms Seema Dogra (Cover Visualizer), Mr Rajesh Sharma (Production Coordinator), Mr Akshay Thakur (Typesetter), Ms Ritika Ahuja (Proofreader), and Mr Sharvan Kumar (Graphic Designer), for making efforts in bringing out this book.

Last but not the least, I wish to put on record my deep sense of gratitude to my brother Hemant Sinha (Munnu) without whose support and encouragement, it would not have been possible for me to reach at this destination.

CONTENTS

1. **DEFINITION AND CLASSIFICATION OF MASSAGE** — 1
   - Features of Massage Technique 2
   - Classification of Techniques 2
   - Classification of Massage 3

2. **PHYSIOLOGICAL EFFECTS** — 7
   - Effects of Massage on the Circulatory System 8
   - Effects on Blood 11
   - Effects on the Exchange of Metabolites 12
   - Effects on Metabolism 12
   - Effects on the Nervous System 15
   - Effects on the Soft Tissue 20
   - Effects on the Respiratory System 21
   - Effects on the Skin 22
   - Effects on the Adipose Tissue 22
   - Psychological Effects 22
   - Immunological Effects of Massage 22

3. **THERAPEUTIC USES** — 25
   - Mobility of Soft Tissues 25
   - Muscle Spasm and Pain 26
   - Reduction of Edema 27
   - Enhancement of Circulation 27
   - Mobilize Secretions in the Lungs 28
   - General and Local Relaxations 28
   - Massage and Obesity 29
   - Massage and AIDS 29
   - Massage and Cancer 30
   - Massage and Hypertension 32

4. **CONTRAINDICATIONS** — 35
   - General Contraindications 36
   - Local Contraindications 38

5. **TECHNIQUES** — 41
   - Stroking Group of Manipulation 41
   - Pressure Manipulations 48
   - Percussion or Tapotement 60
   - Vibratory Manipulations 64

6. **PRACTICAL ASPECTS OF MASSAGE** — 68
   - Positioning of the Patient 68
   - Draping 72
   - Stance of the Therapist 73

- Attitude of the Therapist *75*
- Appearance of the Therapist *75*
- Contact and Continuity *75*
- Selection of a Technique *76*
- Lubricant *76*
- Accessories *78*
- Sequence of the Massage *79*

7. **THERAPEUTIC APPLICATIONS OF MASSAGE** 83
   - Edema *83*
   - Radical Mastectomy *84*
   - Venous Ulcer *85*
   - Lower Motor Neuron Lesion *86*
   - Bell's Palsy *86*
   - Sprain *87*
   - Tenosynovitis *88*
   - Tendonitis *88*
   - Muscle Injury/Strain *89*
   - Traumatic Periostitis *90*
   - Fibrositis *90*
   - Painful Neuroma *91*
   - Adherent Skin *91*
   - Engorged Breast *92*
   - Flatulence *93*
   - Relaxation *93*
   - Removal of Secretion *94*

8. **HISTORY OF MASSAGE** 95

9. **NEW SYSTEMS OF MASSAGE** 99
   - Connective Tissue Massage *99*
   - Tread Massage *101*
   - Periosteal Massage *101*
   - Stripping Massage *101*
   - Hoffa Massage *102*
   - Rolfing *102*
   - Mechanical Devices of Massage *103*
   - Digital Ischemic Pressure *104*
   - Vacuum Cupping *105*
   - Stylus Massage *105*
   - Acupressure Massage *106*
   - External Cardiac Massage *106*
   - Underwater Massage *108*
   - Manual Lymphatic Drainage *110*
   - Craniosacral Therapy *111*
   - Instrument-assisted Soft Tissue Mobilization *113*
   - Roller Massage *114*
   - Myofascial Release *115*

10. SPORTS MASSAGE — 118
- Historical Perspective *118*
- Role of Massage in Athletic World *119*
- Categories of Sports Massage *136*

11. ANCIENT MASSAGE SYSTEMS — 141
- Ayurvedic Massage *141*
  - Gua Sha
  - Tuina
  - Shiatsu
- Traditional Thai Massage *147*

12. OUTLINES OF THE LYMPHATIC SYSTEM — 150
- General Considerations *150*
- Lymphatic Drainage of the Upper Limb *150*
- Lymphatic Drainage of the Lower Limb *152*
- Lymphatic Drainage of Trunk *154*
- Lymphatic Drainage of the Head *156*

Glossary — 159
References — 161
Bibliography — 175
Index — 179

CHAPTER 1

Definition and Classification of Massage

DEFINITION

What is massage? No uniform answer seems to exist to this question. Massage is one of those terms which are easily understood than expressed. People find it difficult to define massage, although they are confident of its meaning. Many definitions of massage have been offered from time-to-time. Given below are some of the definitions:

- Massage is the scientific mode of curing certain forms of disease by systematic manipulations.
  —*Murrell*
- Massage refers to all mechanical procedures that can cure illness. —*Hoffa*
- Massage signifies a group of procedures, which are usually done with hand on the external tissue of the body in a variety of ways either with a curative, palliative, or hygienic point in view. —*Graham*
- Massage is the scientific manipulation of the soft tissues of body with the palmar aspect of hand(s) and/or fingers.
- Massage can be defined as the hand motions practiced on the surface of body with a therapeutic goal.
- Massage is the application of force to the soft tissue without producing any movement or change in the position of joints.
- Massage is a term applied to certain manipulations of the soft tissues. These manipulations are most efficiently performed with the palmar aspect of hand and administered for the purpose of producing effects on the nervous system, muscular system as well as on the local and general circulation of the blood and lymph. —*Beard*
- Massage is the mechanical stimulation of soft tissues of the body by rhythmically applied pressure and stretching.
- Massage is a healing art.

Most of these definitions are inadequate because neither do they include the complete dimension of massage nor do they offer any criteria to decide whether a given technique can be included in massage or not.

Definitions of Murrell and Hoffa restrict the application of massage to sick people. Though, throughout the history, massage has been used not only by sick, but also by the healthy people for therapeutic, restorative as well as preventive purposes. Moreover, these definitions do not address the technical specifications of massage.

Few definitions emphasize that manipulation of soft tissue should be performed by hand. While this is true for most of the techniques, it cannot be considered as a criteria for defining massage because in some methods of massage parts of body other than the hands are also being used during manipulation. For example, in tread massage, there is predominance of leg work. Besides, according to these criteria, several mechanical devices like vibrator, percussor, pneumatic massage, etc. which essentially have the similar mechanism of action and physiological effects cannot be included in massage, despite the fact that these machines were primarily devised to save the time and energy of the therapist.

If the techniques of massage are analyzed carefully, it becomes obvious that mere rubbing or handling of the skin by hand does not produce the desired effects. Rather it is the variable amount of mechanical energy imparted to the body tissue during various maneuvers which accounts for the effects of massage. These mechanical forces may be generated by hand or by any other mechanical device and can be a criteria for defining massage and classifying its various techniques.

This concept has been dealt within the definitions of massage given by Graham and Beard. These definitions while acknowledging the predominance of hand works in massage also hint at the possibilities of other ways of manipulating the tissues.

However, transmission of mechanical energy is also involved in the various joint mobilization and manipulative procedures which also use the therapist's hand as a major tool. Therefore, it is imperative that these two major categories of manual therapy should be distinguished from each other. While the joint mobilization and manipulation procedures achieve their aim by producing movement (either physiological or accessory) of the joint, massage manipulates the soft tissue and essentially does not produce any change in the position of the joint during manipulations.

These facts can be assimilated to outline the essential features of massage technique which may then form the criteria to decide whether a given technique can be included in the category of massage or not.

FEATURES OF MASSAGE TECHNIQUE

Essential features of massage technique can be listed as follows:
1. Technique should apply mechanical force to the soft tissue of the body.
2. These forces must not produce any change in the position of the joint.
3. The technique must evoke some physiological and/or psychological effect which serve to achieve the therapeutic, restorative, or the preventive goal.

Considering these features, any technique, be it manual or mechanical which imparts mechanical energy to the soft tissue of body through the skin without producing any change in the position of joint, in order to elicit certain physiological or psychological effect which can be utilized for therapeutic, restorative, or preventive purposes either on sick or a healthy individual can be defined as massage.

CLASSIFICATION OF TECHNIQUES

Basis of Classification

Application of touch and pressure in various manners constitutes the maneuvers of massage. The effects produced by a technique entirely depend upon the type of tissue approached during a particular technique and the character of the technique governs this. Any given technique can be analyzed and compared with other techniques of massage in terms of:
- Magnitude of applied force
- Direction of force
- Duration of force
- Means of application of force.

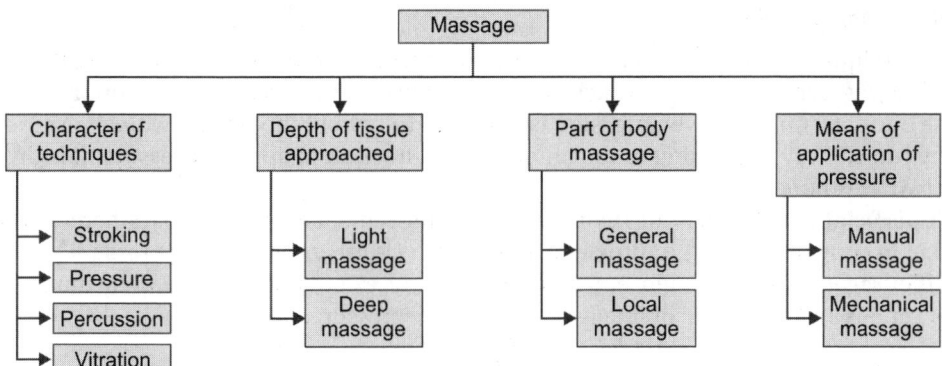

Fig. 1.1: Basis of classification of massage.

So, the characters of technique could be one of the basis of classification. Massage can also be classified on the basis of depth of tissue approached during a technique. The region of body, to which massage is given, has also been used to classify massage. Massage maneuvers can be done either by hands of the therapist or by various mechanical devices. This can be another basis of classifying massage **(Fig. 1.1)**.

CLASSIFICATION OF MASSAGE

On the Basis of Character of Technique

According to the nature of character of technique, classical/manual massage techniques are classified into following 4 basic groups. Each group has more than one subgroup **(Fig. 1.2)**:
1. Stroking manipulations: Superficial stroking, effleurage
2. Pressure manipulations: Kneading, petrissage, and friction
3. Tapotement/percussion manipulations
4. Vibratory manipulations

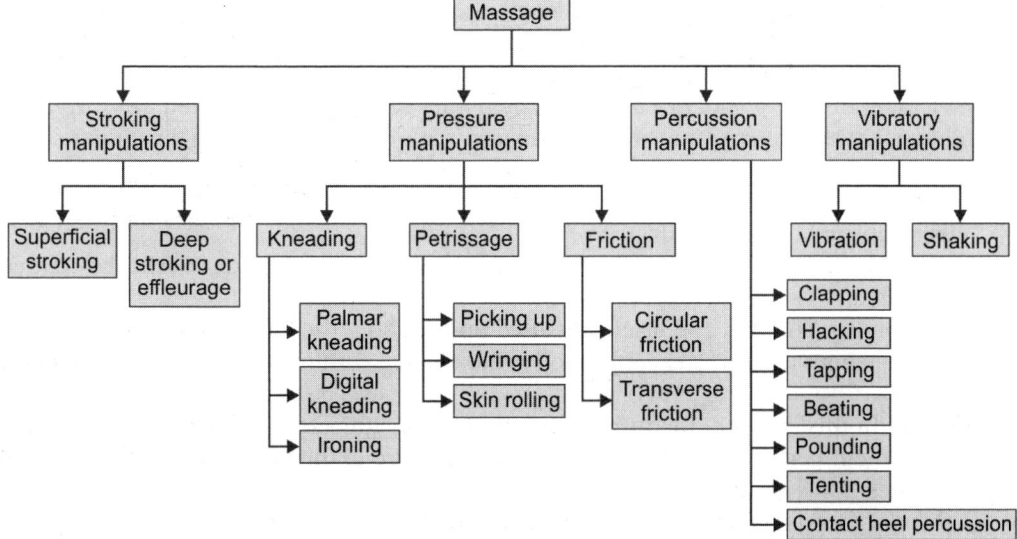

Fig. 1.2: Classification of massage techniques on the basis of character of techniques.

Stroking Manipulations

The technique of this group consists of linear movements of relaxed hand along the whole length of segment known as "strokes" which usually cover one aspect of the entire segment of the body at a time. An even pressure is applied throughout the strokes which are repeated in rhythmical way. According to the amount and direction of applied pressure, it is divided into two techniques:
1. **Superficial stroking:** It is the rhythmical linear movement of hand or a part thereof over the skin in either direction, i.e., proximal to distal or *vice versa*, without any pressure.
2. **Effleurage:** It is the linear movement of hand over the external surface of body in the direction of venous and lymphatic drainage with moderate pressure.

Pressure Manipulations

In this group of techniques, the hand of the therapist and skin of the patient move together as one and fairly deep localized pressure is applied to the body. The techniques are directed toward the deeper tissue. The aim is to achieve the maximal mechanical movement of different fibers with the application of that maximum pressure which a patient/subject can tolerate comfortably.

Depending upon the type and direction of applied pressure, it can be divided into following three major subgroups. Each subgroup consists of more than one technique:
1. Kneading
2. Petrissage
3. Friction

- **Kneading:** In this group of techniques, the tissues are pressed down onto the underlying firm structure and intermittent pressure is applied in circular direction, parallel to the long axis of bone. The applied pressure increases and decreases in a gradual manner, but the contact of the therapist's hand(s) with the patient's body is never interrupted. Different techniques of this group are:
    - *Digital kneading:* Pressure is applied with the fingers (finger kneading) or thumb (thumb kneading).
    - *Palmar kneading:* Pressure is applied with the palm.
    - *Reinforced kneading/ironing:* Both the hands placed over one another are used to apply pressure. The lower hand which is in contact with the patient's skin, receives reinforcement from the other hand.
- **Petrissage:** In this category of massage, the tissues are grasped and lifted away from the underlying structures and intermittent pressure is applied to the tissue in the direction that is perpendicular to the long axis of bone. Different techniques of this group are:
    i. *Picking up:* Tissues are lifted away from underlying structures, squeezed, and then released using one or both the hands.
    ii. *Wringing:* Using both the hands, tissues are lifted away from the underlying structures, squeezed, twisted, and then released.
    iii. *Skin rolling:* The skin and fascia are lifted up with both the hands and moved over the subcutaneous tissues by keeping a roll of lifted tissue continuously ahead of the moving thumb.
- **Friction:** In this group of technique, the tissues are subjected to small range of to and fro movement performed with constant deep pressure of the finger or thumb. Different techniques of this group are:
    - *Circular friction:* Direction of movement is circular.
    - *Transverse friction* to and fro movement is performed across the length of structure. It is also called cross-fiber massage.

Tapotement/Percussion Manipulations

In this group of techniques, the mechanical energy is transmitted to the body by the vibrations of the distal part of upper limb, i.e. hand and/or fingers, which are in constant contact with the subject's skin using the body weight and generalized cocontraction of the upper limb muscles. This technique is mainly directed toward the lung and other hollow cavities.

The different parts of hand are used to strike the subject's skin and accordingly the techniques are named:

Techniques	Administered with
Clapping	Cupped palm
Hacking	Ulnar border of the 5th, 4th, and 3rd digits
Beating	Anterior aspect of the clenched fist
Tapping	Pulp of the fingers
Pounding	Medial aspect of the clenched fist

The features of various techniques of classical massage are given in **Table 1.1**.

Vibratory Manipulations

In this group of techniques, a succession of soft, gentle blows are applied over the body which produce a characteristic sound. The striking hands are not in constant contact with the skin and strike the body part at regular interval. This results in the application of an intermittent touch and pressure to the body during these manipulations.

Depending upon the direction and frequency of vibration, it is divided into two techniques:
1. **Vibration:** In this technique, the fine vibrations are produced which tend to produce fine movement of hand in upward and downward direction.
2. **Shaking:** In this technique, coarse vibrations are produced which tend to produce fine movement of hand in sideways direction.

Table 1.1: Features of various techniques of classical massage.

Techniques	Salient features
Stroking	Linear movements of hand or parts thereof, along the entire length of segment with the lightest pressure and constant touch
Effleurage	Linear movements of hand or a part thereof, along the entire length of segment with moderate pressure and constant touch
Kneading	Circular movements of soft tissue parallel to the long axis of underlying bone with constant touch and intermittent pressure
Petrissage	Circular movements of soft tissue, perpendicular to the long axis of underlying bone with constant touch and intermittent pressure
Friction	Small range, to and fro movement of soft tissue with constant touch and constant deep pressure
Percussion	Oscillatory movement of hand or a part thereof with intermittent touch and pressure
Vibration	Small range, oscillatory movement of hand in upward, downward directions with constant touch
Shaking	Small range, oscillatory movement of hands in sideways direction with constant touch

On the Basis of Depth of Tissue Approached

Depending upon the depth of tissue approached during manipulations, massage techniques can be classified as:

1. Light Massage Techniques

The forces applied during the maneuver are light, so that the effect of massage is confined to the superficial tissue only, e.g., stroking, tapping, etc.

2. Deep Massage Techniques

The forces applied during the massage are moderate to deep, so that the effect of massage reaches to the deeper tissues like muscle, e.g., friction, kneading, etc.

On the Basis of Region Massaged

Massage can also be classified as below according to the region to which it is given:

1. General Massage

Massage applied to the entire body is usually termed as general massage. However, massage administered to a large body segment like back, lower limb, etc., can also be included in this category. It is usually administered in debilitated persons following prolonged recumbency and on athletes after exhaustive physical work to bring a sense of well-being and comfort.

2. Local Massage

When massage is administered in a particular area of the body segment, it is termed as local massage. This is used in the treatment of the local pathological conditions. For example, massage of wrist in tenosynovitis, friction to lateral ligament of ankle following sprain, etc. can be considered as local massage.

On the Basis of Means of Administration of Technique

On this basis, the massage can be classified into the following two categories:

1. Manual Massage

The word "manual" refers to the "lying on" of hand over the subject's body. The massage administered with the hand or other body part of the therapist is called manual massage, e.g., technique of classical massage, connective tissue massage, trigger point massage, acupressure massage, myofascial release, etc.

2. Mechanical Massage

When the mechanical devices based on the principles of massage, administer the mechanical energy to the patient's body, in order to manipulate soft tissue, it may be termed as mechanical massage, e.g., vibrator, compression devices, pneumatic massage, etc. In the recent years, the practice of instrument-assisted soft tissue manipulation through foam roller and stainless steel equipment has gained some popularity. These can also be included in this category. Some information on these methods is included in Chapter 9.

CHAPTER 2

Physiological Effects

As a therapeutic modality, massage is being used for the relief of pain, swelling, muscle sprain, restricted movement, tension and anxiety associated with a large number of disorders, and afflicting muscular, nervous, cardiorespiratory and other systems.

The therapeutic value of massage lies in its numerous and combined physiological effects. The effect of massage of the body is very much technique dependent. Massage, be it manual or mechanical, imparts pressure and stimulates mechanically the various tissue approached at the time of application of a particular technique. It is the magnitude, duration, and the direction of force applied during a particular technique that determines the effects produced by that technique on the body.

Various authors have described the effects of massage in various ways. Hollis (1987) classified the effects of massage into two groups—mechanical and physiological, whereas Lehn and Prentice (1994) talked about reflex and mechanical effects of massage. However, during massage treatment, the effects produced are the combination of various mechanical, physiological, reflex, and psychological consequences of massage and in one way or the other are pronounced on some tissue system of the body. Thus, it is much rational to study the effects of this modality in reference to a specific system. This chapter discusses the effects of massage on the body as a whole. The effects associated with specific individual techniques are listed in Chapter 5, which presents a complete discussion on the individual techniques.

This chapter presents physiological effects of this modality on different systems of the body. The effect of massage on respiratory system is the specific effect of percussion and vibration, though they are included in this chapter in order to complete the discussion.

The physiological effects of massage can be discussed under the following headings:
- Effects on the circulatory system:
  - On the venous and the lymphatic flow
  - On the arterial flow.
- Effects on blood
- Effects on the exchange of nutritive elements
- Effects on metabolism
- Effects on the nervous system:
  - On sensory nervous system
  - On motor nervous system
  - On autonomic nervous system.
- Effects on the mobility of the soft tissue
- Effects on the respiratory system
- Effects on the skin

- Effects on the adipose tissue
- Psychological effects
- Effects on immune system.

EFFECTS OF MASSAGE ON THE CIRCULATORY SYSTEM

On the Venous and the Lymphatic Flow

Massage aids in the mechanical emptying of the veins and the lymphatics. It facilitates the forward movement of the venous blood and the lymph and thereby reduces the chance of stagnation of the blood and the lymph in the tissue space.

The flow of the venous and the lymphatic channels from the extremities mainly depends on the activity of the smooth muscles present in the walls of the vessels. The contraction of these small muscles in conjunction with the valves present in the vessels acts as a strong pumping mechanism which keeps the tissue space clear from the free fluid. Other factors, such as the skeletal muscle pump, thoracic pump (i.e., aspiration of the lymph into the thorax during the inspiration), arterial pulsation adjacent to the lymphatics, and the force of gravity have a minor role in the normal circumstances but under the conditions where the normal lymph mechanism does not function properly, these factors become more important.

The contraction of the skeletal muscles compresses the blood vessels and exerts a pressure on the fluid present inside. This increase in intravascular pressure, which stimulates the contraction of the smooth muscles present in the wall of the vessels. Contraction of smooth muscles further increases the pressure inside the vessels. When this pressure increases beyond the threshold, the valves open up and the fluid moves onto the next segments. As the valves provide only unidirectional flow, the fluid cannot come back to the empty segment. When the muscles relax, the segment is refilled by the fluid from the distal segments. This way the venous and the lymphatic fluids are allowed to move only in one direction.

The mechanical action of massage resembles with that of normal muscular contraction. The different techniques of massage alternately compress and release the soft tissue. This facilitates the venous and lymphatic flow. The effleurage, kneading, and petrissage squeeze the veins and the lymphatic vessels and force the venous blood and the lymph toward the heart, causing an increased drainage of the blood and lymph from the massaged part/segment.

In case of fluid stagnation due to mechanical factors, the flow of venous and lymphatic fluid is obstructed. Massage facilitates the drainage, and reduces the stagnation of fluids and also speeds up the removal of waste products. According to Paikov (1986), the body contains 1,200–1,500 mL of lymph moving at the speed of 4 mm/sec and massage increases the speed to eight-folds.

On the Arterial Flow

Massage improves the blood supply of the area being massaged. A definite vasodilation along with an increase in the peripheral blood flow is usually observed after massage. This moderate, consistent, and definite increase in the arterial flow may be attributed to the following events happening during massage:
- Release of vasodilators
- Activation of axon reflex
- Decrease of venous congestion.

Release of Vasodilators

Massage acts as a succession of mild traumatization. It provokes and brings about the release of histamine and other substances by the stimulation of mast cells. This liberation of histamine plays an important role in the vasodilation produced during massage (Hollis, 1987). These substances increase the arterial diameter and are partially responsible for the axon reflex. The patent capillaries open up under the influence of these chemicals and bring about an increase in the blood flow to the part massaged.

Activation of Axon Reflex

Massage activates the axon reflex which produces cutaneous vasodilation. When an area of the skin is firmly stroked, the sensory nerve ending is stimulated. The impulse is carried to the spinal cord by the peripheral nerves. In the way itself, a branch of the nerves may be stimulated and instead of going to the spinal cord, impulses return back to the periphery to produce its effects on the cutaneous vessels which are supplied by the branch of the same peripheral nerve **(Fig. 2.1)**. The effect is the relaxation of the smooth muscles of the arterial wall and the vasodilation (Chatterjee, 1985).

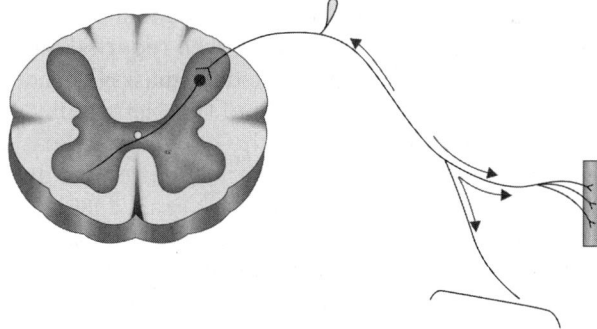

Fig. 2.1: Axon reflex.

So, the reflex arc of the axon reflex is completed by the two branches of the same sensory fibers. Through one branch, the impulse is received and through the other, it is transmitted back of the peripheral vessels causing vasodilation. This type of impulse is known as antidromic impulse. In fact, axon reflex is the only reflex that does not involve the central nervous system (CNS) (Choudhary, 1993).

Decrease of Venous Congestion

If any portion of the vessel is dilated, then the neighboring vessels also become constricted (axon reflex) (Chatterjee, 1985). The arterioles become compressed if the venous congestion is increased. The congested venous and lymphatic fluid exerts a compressive force on the arterioles. The lumen of the arterioles becomes narrow and so the blood supply to the part is reduced. It is a physiological process which the body adopts in order to relieve the congestion. As a result of this, the outflow from the veins exceeds the inflow to the constricted arterioles and the congestion is reduced.

Massage promotes the forward movement of lymph and blood and indirectly helps in restoring the arterial flow.

Research on the Circulatory Effects of Massage

Wolfson (1931) examined the effect of deep kneading massage on the venous blood on an animal model (dog). The venous blood flow was measured by anesthetizing the dog and by cannulation of the femoral vein. He found that massage caused a great initial increase with a fairly rapid decrease in the flow of blood to a rate less than normal. Immediately following massage, blood flow is slowly returned to normal. He concluded that the decrease in the blood flow is due to a more complete emptying of venous blood for a short period of time. Wakim (1949) used plethysmography technique to measure the flow of blood, and observed that deep stroking and kneading produced a consistent increase in the flow of blood of extremities in the subjects with flaccid paralysis. No such increase was found in the normal subjects, patients of rheumatoid arthritis, and subjects with spastic paralysis.

With the advent of new techniques of measuring the blood flow, several studies have been carried out to determine the efficacy of massage on the blood flow. The results of these reports are at best conflicting at the moment.

Dubrovsky (1982) and Hensen and Kristensen (1973) used radioisotope of Xe^{133} to determine the flow of blood, reported an increased clearance rate of Xe^{133} after massage, and attributed it to the increase in the blood flow. However, Hovind and Nielsen (1974) founded that no net increase in the blood flow though the increase clearance rate of Xe^{133} was observed in their study which they attributed to the mechanical emptying and refilling of vascular bed.

Bell (1964) conducted plethysmographic studies and reported that the rate of blood flow was doubled during massage, which lasted for about 40 minutes after the termination of massage. Sereveni and Venerando (1967) even reported an increased blood flow in the nontreated homologous limb in response to deep massage in adults.

Recent studies with ultrasound Dopplerography, however, do not support the notion that massage leads to increase in the blood flow. Harichaux and Viel (1987) noted that slower massage was more beneficial for venous return than massage repeated at high frequency. Though the studies performed by Ek et al. (1985), Linde (1986), Shoemaker et al. (1997), and Tiidus and Shoemaker (1995) could not demonstrate any increase in blood flow of muscle and skin following massage. However, Ek et al. (1985) noted the individual and sexual variation in the effect of massage and reported that woman, more than men, increased their skin blood flow bilaterally after massage.

Hinds et al. (2004) compared the effects of massage against a resting control condition upon femoral artery blood flow, skin blood flow, and skin and muscle temperature after dynamic quadriceps exercise. Thirteen male volunteers were participated in 3 × 2 minutes bouts of concentric quadriceps exercise followed by 2 × 6 minutes bouts of deep effleurage and petrissage massage or a control (rest) period of similar duration in a counterbalanced fashion. Blood flow and temperature, blood lactate concentration, heart rate, and blood pressure were taken at baseline, immediately after exercise, as well as at the midpoint and end of the massage/rest periods. They observed that massage to the quadriceps did not significantly elevate femoral artery blood flow, but the skin blood flow and temperature were found elevated which was not accompanied by any significant deviation of other parameters as compared to the resting control. Similar increase in the skin blood flow confined to the local massaged area has also been reported by Mori et al. (2004).

In an elegant study, Wiltshire et al. (2010) reported that contrary to common believe, massage impairs postexercise muscle blood flow and impairs the lactate removal. Using Doppler and echo ultrasound of the brachial artery, they measured forearm blood flow (FBF) every minute for 10 minutes and after 2 minutes of strenuous isometric handgrip exercise under three conditions: Passive rest, active recovery (rhythmic exercise at 10% maximum voluntary contraction), and massage. Massage maneuvers consisted of firm effleurage for the first and the last 2.5 minute intervals with petrissage during the 5 minute period in between. They reported that during passive rest, pulsatile flow of brachial artery was uninterrupted, whereas during active recovery and massage, rhythmic retrograde brachial artery blood velocity (negative velocity) was observed which was consistent with compression produced by muscle contraction and passive compression of massage strokes. With petrissage and effleurage, consistent retrograde flow with each massage stroke was followed by increase in blood flow velocity during brief pauses. They concluded that massage results in severe impairment to blood flow during the massage stroke, and this impairment has a net effect of decreasing muscle blood flow early in the recovery period after strenuous exercise. They also reported a reduced lactic acid efflux during massage which they viewed as a direct consequence of impairment to blood flow.

On the other hand, Franklin et al. (2014) reported that lower extremity massage enhances brachial artery flow-mediated dilation (FMD) both in presence and in absence of exercise-induced muscle injury to lower limb. 30 minutes massage was performed on the bilateral lower extremity muscle groups using Swedish massage techniques of superficial stroking, effleurage, and petrissage varying in depth from superficial to deep. Brachial artery FMD and flow were measured at 90 minutes, 24 hours, 48 hours, and 72 hours after the intervention. They reported that 90 minutes after the intervention, FMD increased from baseline and remaining elevated until 72 hours.

Definitely, more well-controlled and defined studies are required before we approve or disapprove the circulatory effects of massage. For the time being, clinical as well as experimental result in terms of decrease in edema and increased muscle clearance rate following massage are beyond doubt (Kresge, 1988). Though much needs to be done to pinpoint whether these are due to increased blood flow, increased lymphatic drainage, or due to more complete emptying and refilling of the vessels.

EFFECTS ON BLOOD

Few studies are available on the effect of massage on the blood cells. Wood and Becker (1981) quoted Mitchell to state that RBC count increased after massage both in health and in anemia. Schneider and Havens (1915) also reported an increase in red blood cells and hemoglobin count following abdominal massage. This increase in RBC and hemoglobin count may increase the oxygen carrying capacity of blood.

Increase in the platelets count after massage has been reported in an animal model (Lucia and Rickards, 1933). They performed massage on the ear of 5 rabbits in gentle, but firm manner for 5 minutes. The ear was then punctured and the first drop of blood was studied. They found an increase in the blood platelets count of the massaged ear, but found no change on the opposite unmassaged ear.

Smith et al. (1994) have demonstrated an increase in the neutrophil count following 30 minutes of massage performed 2 hours after intense exercise. However, Viitasalo et al. (1995) found no effects of 20 minutes underwater water-jet massage, after exercises, on the circulating lymphocytes, neutrophils, or monocytes.

Hilbert et al. (2003) also did not observe any change in the neutrophil count following 20 minutes of massage. Though of late, a number of studies have reported alteration in the leukocyte counts following massage in patients afflicted with AIDS and cancer patients (Hernandez-Reif et al., 2005; Zeitlin et al., 2000).

No satisfactory explanation is available in the literature as to why these changes occur after massage. According to Kresge (1989), massage raises the RBC count by mobilizing stagnant blood cells in the splanchnic circulation rather than by increased production. Malone (1990) is of opinion that secondary to mechanical stimulation, the body reacts by increasing the cellular component in the blood. Smith et al. (1994) have postulated that increase in neutrophil count may have the potential to retard the inflammatory changes associated with strenuous exercises which may be of some use in the management of delayed-onset muscle soreness.

Studies have also reported beneficial effects of massage on inflammatory markers. Crane et al. (2012) in a novel study reported that massage attenuated the production of the inflammatory cytokines like tumor necrosis factor-a (TNF-a) and interleukin-6 (IL-6) and reduced heat shock protein 27 (HSP27) phosphorylation, though it had no effect on muscle metabolites (glycogen, lactate). Further, they observed that massage activated the mechanotransduction signaling pathways, such as focal adhesion kinase (FAK) and extracellular signal-regulated kinase 1/2 (ERK1/2), potentiated mitochondrial biogenesis signaling [nuclear peroxisome proliferator-activated receptor-gamma coactivator 1alpha (PGC-1α)], and mitigated the rise in nuclear factor-kappa beta p65 (NF-kB p65) nuclear accumulation caused by exercise-induced muscle trauma. These observations made them to conclude that massage therapy appears to be clinically beneficial by reducing inflammation and promoting mitochondrial biogenesis. Objective of this study was to assess the influence of massage within muscle that had performed a bout of intense exercise. The acute aerobic cycling exercise (where subject after completing 30 minutes at 60% of their predetermined VO_2 peak, intermittently increased the speed to reach 85% VO_2 peak, and continued till exhaustion) in unconditioned individuals (eleven healthy, recreationally active males) was used to cause contraction-induced muscle damage. Immediately after exercise, subjects were allowed to recover for 10 minutes while massage oil was lightly applied to both quadriceps. Thereafter, a single leg was randomized to receive massage treatment for 10 minutes from a registered massage therapist. The massage treatment was composed of effleurage, petrissage, and slow muscle to knee extensor muscles. The muscle biopsies were obtained at rest, immediately after administration of massage and after a 2.5 hours period of recovery and targeted real-time reverse transcription-polymerase chain reaction (RT-PCR), protein signaling analysis, and metabolite quantification were performed to characterize the processes within skeletal muscle that are influenced by massage.

Rapaport et al. (2010) reported that a single session of Swedish massage of 45 minutes duration increased the number of circulating lymphocytes, CD25P lymphocytes, CD56P lymphocytes, CD4P lymphocytes, and CD8P lymphocytes. The same research group in a subsequent publication (Rapaport et al., 2012) observed that twice-weekly massage was associated with increased production of proinflammatory cytokines.

More studies with proper design and statistical analysis are required to explore the effect of massage on blood cells in both healthy and diseased subjects.

EFFECTS ON THE EXCHANGE OF METABOLITES

Massage promotes rapid disposal of waste products and the replenishment of the nutritive elements. Massage also increases the movement of liquids and gases in the body (Hollis, 1987). The increased arterial blood flow following massage brings more oxygen and nutritive elements and also causes more rapid oxygenation of the blood. Massage speeds up the lymphatic and venous flow which promotes rapid disposal of the waste products of metabolism. These changes make the exchange of waste products between the blood and the tissue at cellular level more efficiently. This may overall improve the trophic condition of the part being massaged. However, Gupta et al. (1996) did not find any difference in the rate of lactate removal between massage-assisted recovery and simple passive recovery from a supramaximal exercise bout in 10 male athletes. Their subject received 10 minutes of massage consisting of kneading and stroking of upper and lower limbs. They concluded that short-term massage is ineffective in enhancing lactate removal following supramaximal exercise.

Detailed discussion on the effect of massage on lactate removal is presented in the Chapter 10.

EFFECTS ON METABOLISM

Traditionally, massage has been applied for the purpose of promoting the general status of well-being. By virtue of increasing arterial blood flow and venous lymphatic drainage, theoretically massage may accelerate the various metabolic processes of the body. However, very little research has been done in this area with conflicting reports. Some 70 years ago, Cuthbertson (1933) in a review article summarized the various studies and reported an increase in the output of urine, increase rate of excretion of nitrogen, inorganic phosphorus, and sodium chloride following massage. He reported no effect either on the acid-base balance of the blood, or on the basal consumption of O_2.

Recently, Boone and Cooper (1995), while investigating the effect of massage on oxygen consumption at rest on 10 healthy adult males, also observed no significant change in O_2 consumption, heart rate, stroke volume, cardiac output, and a-VO_2 during the massage.

Zelikovski (1993) using a pneumatic sequential device found no difference in the blood level of lactate, pyruvate, ammonia, bicarbonate, and pH before and after massage. However, Flore et al. (1998) reported a slight increase in maximum O_2 consumption after a special massage protocol called biokingeriga (BK).

Danneskiold et al. (1983) stated that massage performed in the area of regional muscle tension and pain increased muscle myoglobin and this increase is proportional to the degree of muscle tension. They suggested that this could be related to the loss of oxidative metabolic capacity within the muscle. The increase in serum myoglobin was also reported by Viitasalo et al. (1995). However, Rodenburg et al. (1994) could not find any change in the myoglobin concentration in the blood of the subjects who received massage after an extensive eccentric exercise program, although they have found a significant change in the creatine kinase (CK) activity in the blood.

Smith et al. (1994) also reported a significant decrease in the rise of plasma creatine in massaged subject compared to the control group.

Reduction of blood CK concentration is considered as a marker for reduction in muscle damage and a faster recovery after exercise (Clarkson and Hubal, 2002; Sorichter et al., 2007; Bishop et al., 2008). Of late, several studies (Bakar et al., 2015; Kargarfard et al., 2016; Zainuddin et al., 2005) have reported a significant reduction in serum creatine kinase level in subjects who received massage therapy after intense exercise. Bakar et al. (2015) reported a more rapid fall of the lactate dehydrogenase (LDH), CK and myoglobin (Mb), muscular enzymes of LDH, CK, and myoglobin in participants who received manual lymph drainage massage for 30 minutes after strenuous exercise. These enzymes are the biochemical markers of muscle damage and manual lymph drainage (MLD) is a massage technique that involves the skin surface only and follows the anatomic lymphatic pathways of the body. Kargarfard et al. (2016) examined the effect of massage on the performance of bodybuilder . After five repetition sets at 75–77% of 1 RM of knee extensor and flexor muscle groups, the experimental group received 30 minutes massage, whereas the control group underwent normal passive recovery. Plasma CK level was measured over 6 time periods: Baseline, immediately after the delayed-onset muscle soreness (DOMS) inducing protocol right after the massage, and 24 hours, 48 hours, and 72 hours after the massage. They reported that massage decreased the CK level at 48 hours and 72 hours in male bodybuilders after intense exercise.

In a meta-analysis of eleven articles involving 504 participants, Guo et al. (2017) noted that the serum CK level was reduced when participants received massage intervention after intense exercise. Dupuy et al. (2018) in a meta-analysis aimed at comparing the effects of the most commonly used recovery techniques (active recovery, massage, compression garments, immersion, contrast water therapy, and cryotherapy) observed that massage was the most effective recovery technique for reducing the concentrations of circulating CK and IL-6 in the blood after exercise. However, Behringer et al. (2018) observed that CK response after 30 minutes of massage was no different than simple rest. They assessed CK along with h-FABP, neutrophil granulocytes, and the perceived muscle soreness before, immediately after, and 1 hour, 4 hours, and 24 hours after the exercise and reported that the time course of these parameters did not differ between the treatments. In this experiment, 30 minutes of manual lymphatic drainage type massage was compared with local cryotherapy and rest of same duration.

Several studies, of late, have reported that infant massage resulted in significant reduction in bilirubin level of neonates suffering from hyperbilirubinemia and ameliorates neonatal jaundice (Chen et al., 2011; Moghadam et al., 2012; Lin et al., 2015; Basiri-Moghadam et al., 2015; Dalili et al., 2016; Eghbalian et al., 2017).

Chen et al. (2011) in a controlled clinical trial examined the effects of gentle baby massage on neonatal jaundice in 42 full-term breastfed newborns who were not receiving phototherapy. 20 infants included in the massage group received 15–20 minutes of baby massage, twice daily 1 hour after the morning mid-day feeds from day 1 to day 5 after birth. Baby massage consisted of gentle massage of face, chest, abdomen, upper and lower limbs, and back. They reported that mean stool frequency of the massaged infants on day 1 and day 2 (4.6 and 4.3) was significantly ($p < 0.05$) higher than that of the control group (3.3 and 2.6). The transcutaneous bilirubin levels on the second to fifth day and serum total bilirubin levels on fourth day were significantly decreased in the massage group (11.7 = 2.8) in comparison to control group (13.7 = 1.7).

Using the similar technique of massage, Basiri-Moghadam et al. (2015) in a study of 40 newborns (20 in each group) observed a significant difference in the number of times of defecation ($p = 0.002$) and in the level of bilirubin ($p = 0.003$) between the groups with those in the massage group having a higher number of defecations as well as a lower level of transcutaneous bilirubin. The mean difference in bilirubin between the first day and fourth day was 7.56 ± 1.36 mg/dL and 4.79 ± 1.84 mg/dL for the control and the massage groups, respectively.

Lin et al. (2015) in randomized clinical trial of 56 full-term neonates with jaundice, admitted for phototherapy at a regional teaching hospital reported that on the third day, the massage group showed significantly higher defecation frequency (4.6 ± 1.3 vs 3.9 ± 1.3) and significantly lower bilirubin levels (10.8 ± 0.9 mg/dL) compared with the control group (12.2 ± 1.8 mg/dL). Each massage therapy session started on the first day of phototherapy lasted for 15–20 minutes per session, and was conducted twice daily (between meals) for 3 consecutive days. Phototherapy was stopped for the 15–20 minutes during which neonates received massage therapy. The leg and foot were massaged first before progressing to the abdomen, hands, and finally, the back.

Dalili et al. (2016) evaluated the effects of baby massage on transcutaneous bilirubin levels and stool frequency on 50 healthy term newborns. The massage group received massage therapy for 4 days from the first day postnatal. They reported significant difference in the TCB levels between two groups with those in the massage group having lower bilirubin levels; however, they did not observe any difference in the defecation frequency between the group.

In a randomized double-blind clinical trial involving 134 patients, Eghbalian et al. (2017) concluded that massage therapy combined with phototherapy is an effective method for reducing serum total bilirubin in infants with neonatal jaundice. They reported significant differences between the groups in serum total bilirubin levels and frequency of daily bowel movements.

On the other hand, Seyyedrasooli et al. (2014) have not observed any significant reduction in skin bilirubin of massaged infant when compared with control group. However, with respect to the defecation frequency, they reported significant difference between two groups on the 4th day with the frequency of defecation in the massage group was higher. In this study, 43 healthy term infants, with 1st day bilirubin levels of less than 5 mg/dL were randomly allotted to two groups. Control group received routine care, whereas the massage group received 4 days of Vimala massage which is a combination of Indian and Swedish massages techniques. This massage is performed on term infants from head to toe and from center to periphery.

In a meta-analysis of six randomized clinical trials (RCTs) involving 357 patients, Zhang et al. (2018) reported that massage therapy can significantly reduce serum bilirubin level and transcutaneous bilirubin level.

It is proposed that massage leads to stimulation of vagus nerve and intestinal movement that contributes to increased defecation frequency resulting in expulsion of greater amounts of bilirubin containing meconium (Lin et al., 2015; Chen et al., 2011). Diminished the enterohepatic circulation due to vagal stimulation (Seyyedrasooli et al., 2014) and increased in the flow of blood and lymph following massage are also proposed as some of mechanism by which massage may reduce the bilirubin.

Although these studies are preliminary, yet they offer a new dimension for use of massage in these conditions.

EFFECTS ON THE NERVOUS SYSTEM

The nervous system consists of sensory, motor, and autonomic components. Different techniques of massage produce effects on all these components.

Sensory System

Massage has a sedative effect on the central nervous system which can be easily demonstrated if applied monotonously with slow rhythm (Knapp, 1990). The use of massage for the relief of pain of various origins is an age-old practice. However, exact mechanism by which massage brings about pain relief was not understood until Melzack and Wall (1965) put forward their famous theory of pain gate. The cognizance that the various sensory inputs that are carried over by afferent fibers can significantly affect the perception of pain has provided a rationalized scientific basis to the use of massage as a therapeutic modality for pain relief.

The different maneuvers of massage imparts an array of sensory experience by stimulating the peripheral sensory receptor mainly touch and pressure receptors present in the skin and soft tissue. These sensations are carried by the large diameter A β (beta) fibers which play an important role in inhibition of the perception of pain carried by A δ (delta) and C fibers.

The stimulation of low threshold mechanoreceptor blocks the pathway of pain sensation by presynaptic inhibition at the level of substantia gelatinosa of spinal cord. This could be the mechanism by which light pressure maneuvers massage like effleurage, stroking, hacking, tapping, beating, etc. that reduce the pain.

Some massage maneuvers also produces mild-to-moderate pain by stimulation of painful areas of the body. It is said to facilitate the secretion of certain antipain substances, such as β-endorphin and enkephalin, in the periaqueductal gray (PAG) matter at the level of midbrain. From there, these substances descend to the dorsal horn of spinal cord, and suppress the release of substance P (neurotransmitter of pain). This blocks the transmission of pain impulses to the higher pain perception area of brain.

This effect is, otherwise, also known as counterirritant effect. It is attributed to the pain relief obtained by acupuncture and acupressure which also relieve pain by producing localized pain. This could be one of the mechanisms responsible for the pain relief obtained by heavy pressure maneuvers like kneading, friction, petrissage, connective tissue massage, etc.

Kaada and Tersteinbo (1989) have reported a moderate mean increase of 10% in β-endorphin level, lasting for about 1 hour with a maximum effect after 5 minutes, after termination of connective tissue massage in 12 volunteers. They linked the release of β-endorphin with the pain relief, feeling of warmth, and well-being associated with massage.

On the other hand Morhenn et al [2012] reported that massage was associated with reductions in beta-endorphin (BE). They examined the effect of touch on oxytocin (OT) release and other associated physiologic factors, such as adrenocorticotropin hormone (ACTH), nitric oxide (NO), and BE. 15 minutes of moderate-pressure Swedish massage of the upper back were given to 65 participants in prone position whereas control group rested quietly for 15 minutes. They concluded that massage was associated with an increase in OT and reductions in ACTH, NO, and BE and the intergroup differences were significant.

According to Bender et al. (2007), publications on the potential stimulating effect of manual therapy and massage on β-endorphin release are controversial as the efficacy of analgesia and the improvement of general well-being do not necessarily correlate with β-endorphin level.

Motor System

According to Kuprian (1982), the physiological effects of classical massage lie primarily in its ability to exert regulatory influences on the muscle tone. It is generally agreed that massage can elicit facilitating and inhibiting responses in neuromuscular excitability (Hollis, 1987; Wood and Becker, 1981). This seemingly paradoxical claim may be attributable to the difference in the rate of application and the degree of pressure applied during various massage maneuvers (Sullivan, 1993).

Facilitatory Effects of Massage on Motor System

It is said that massage can reflexly increase the muscle tone by stimulation of the skin receptor or stretch of the muscle spindle (Hollis, 1987). Superficial stroking, taping, hacking, etc. are commonly used for this purpose.

The tone of muscle is maintained by the activity of muscle spindle. Muscle spindle contains the intrafusal fibers supplied by gamma motor neuron and lies parallel to the extrafusal fibers of the muscles that are supplied by alpha motor neuron. The capsule of muscle spindle is attached with the extrafusal fibers. Any stretch to the muscle spindle, either by activation of gamma motor neuron or by passive mechanical procedures, activates the reflex arc. The impulse travels via the afferent nerve fibers and propagates toward the spinal cord. Some impulses are monosynaptically transmitted to the alpha motor neuron of the same muscle. The activation of alpha motor neuron produces contraction of the extrafusal fibers of the muscle.

Various massage maneuvers stretch the muscle fiber which may facilitate the muscle contraction. However, according to Lehn and Prentice (1994), massage does not increase muscle tone. Wood and Becker (1981) also commented that the notion that massage causes increase in muscle tone has not been substantiated by experimental scientific research.

Nevertheless, in various facilitation techniques, different massage maneuvers are used for the purpose of increasing the tone of hypotonic muscles, the mechanism of which is not yet understood. It is claimed that most facilitation techniques are directed at stretch reflex with a view of controlling them more efficiently by having an inhibitory or excitatory effect on motor neuron pool. The basis of this assumption is the observation that factors creating abnormalities in the stretch reflex mechanism have devastating effects on the production of normal movement (Atkinson, 1986).

Following are the few of the facilitation techniques which utilize massage maneuvers:
- Touch applied over the working muscles and/or the surface against which the movement has to occur, supplies skin stimulation which acts as a guidance to the movement and facilitates the activities in the motor neuron pool.
- Pressure over the muscle belly has the effect of activating the muscle spindle probably by distorting the shape of muscle fibers and creating a stretch stimulus.
- Cutaneous stimulation by quick light brushing, stroking, clapping, and pressure over the relevant dermatome is being used as a preparatory facilitation to increase the excitability of motor neurons which supply the inhibited muscle.
    a. For the skin supplied by anterior primary rami, the excitatory effect is local and is mainly confined to superficial muscles.
    b. For the skin supplied by posterior primary rami, the excitatory effect is on deep muscles.

It is postulated that cutaneous stimulation causes rapid and large modulation of muscle spindle sensitivity presumably through complex gamma motor neuron fibers (Atkinson, 1986).

Inhibitory Effects of Massage on Motor System

Massage techniques can also reduce the tone of muscle. It has been claimed that petrissage or massage in which muscles are kneaded can exert an inhibitory effect on motor neuron (Hollis, 1987; Tapan, 1988). It is said that effleurage is capable of producing both stimulating and relaxing effects (Wood and Becker, 1981; Hollis, 1987).

According to Rood, slow stroking if carried out from neck to sacrum over the center of back will reduce fluctuating muscle tone. Deep rhythmic massage with pressure over the insertion of muscle has been proved effective in some cases of spasticity.

Activation of tension-dependent Golgi tendon organ which has an inhibitory effect on the stretch reflex mechanism, has been postulated as a mechanism of these effects.

Recently, studies have been conducted to substantiate these claims by providing scientifically documented evidence. These rigorously designed experiments have shown that some techniques of massage (petrissage, kneading, and effleurage) exert an inhibitory effect on the spinal alpha motor neuronal excitability. This inhibitory effect is transient (Sullivan et al., 1992), directly related to the pressure applied during massage (Goldberg et al., 1992) and is not only restricted to homonymous motor neuron pool (Sullivan, 1991), but could also be demonstrated for a close synergistic muscle uninvolved in the massage (Morelli et al., 1998).

Efficacy of massage on motor neuronal excitability was objectively examined in all these studies using the amplitude of H (Hoffmann) reflex which is an indirect, but reliable measure of motor neuron excitability.

Sullivan et al. (1992) recorded H-reflex from the distal aspect of right triceps surae muscle in a controlled experiment where 4 minutes massage of ipsilateral and contralateral triceps surae, and hamstrings muscle group was used as the technique of intervention. They observed that massage of ipsilateral triceps surae resulted in a reduction of H-reflex amplitude (0.83 mV) in comparison with the pretest control condition and remaining experimental condition (range 1.77–2.33 mV). They concluded that the stimulus and receptor activated during massage are specific to the muscle being massaged.

Similar reduction in H-reflex amplitude has also been reported during 3 minutes petrissage (Morelli et al., 1990) and 6 minutes petrissage (Morelli et al., 1991) who concluded that reduction of H-reflex amplitude was observed only during the period of tissue manipulation, regardless of the duration of massage.

Sullivan et al. (1993) reported a mean reduction of 25% in amplitude of H-reflex recorded from ipsilateral triceps surae of 16 healthy subjects during 3 minutes of effleurage. In all these studies, the reduction was sustained only for the duration of massage. Immediately after the massage, H-reflex returned to the pretreatment control level with a tendency for the amplitude to increase with each successive trial.

Goldberg et al. (1992) compared the effects of two intensities of massage [light massage (5 mm H_2O) and deep massage (10 mm H_2O)] and found that though the H-reflex was reduced in both intensities of massage, the deep massage produced greater reduction than the light massage procedure.

It is suggested that H-reflex modulation results under the influence of rapidly adopting receptors or centrally-mediated pathways via polysynaptic and nonsegmental projections specific to the motor neuron pool (Morelli et al., 1991).

The attenuation in motor neuron excitability is manifested in the reduction of muscle tone and can form the plausible explanation of the efficacy of massage in the treatment of spasm and other conditions associated with increased muscle tone, such as psychological stress, precompetition anxiety, etc. in neurologically healthy individual.

However, these results cannot be extrapolated to the neurologically impaired people as these were obtained with neurologically healthy subjects (Sullivan, 1991). There is a need to examine the application of massage on the neurological disorders especially on the upper motor neuron lesion.

In an attempt to investigate the effect of massage in person with neurological impairment, Goldberg et al. (1994) examined the effect of 3 minutes petrissage on 10 spinal cord injured individuals and observed a 27% mean group decrease in the peak-to-peak amplitude of H-reflex during the 3 minutes massage (petrissage) as compared to premassage and postmassage conditions. However, the response was not uniform in all the subjects. In some subjects, the H-reflex amplitude increased by 20%, whereas in some, it decreased up to 80%. Moreover, the response was not associated with any long-term effects.

Of late, some studies have appeared in literature where the beneficial effects of massage were demonstrated in some clinical conditions where spasticity is a predominant feature. These studies have used nonconventional Ayurvedic massage (Sankaran et al., 2018), Chinese massage (Yang et al., 2017; Malila et al., 2015; Thanakiatpinyo et al., 2014), and also classical Swedish massage (Backus et al., 2016; Negahban et al., 2013).

Yang et al. (2017) suggested that a Chinese massage therapy (Tui Na) might be a safe and effective treatment to reduce poststroke spasticity of several muscle groups. Tui Na—pronounced as *"Twee Nah"*—is a Chinese massage system based on the principles of traditional Chinese medicine (TCM), which intends to develop a balance in vital energy (Qi) and a smooth flow of energy in the body (Al-Bedah et al., 2017). In a prospective, multicenter, blinded, randomized, and placebo-controlled intervention trial, 90 patients with poststroke spasticity were randomly assigned to two equal groups. The experimental group in addition to conventional rehabilitation received Tui Na therapy, whereas those in the control group received placebo Tui Na for 20–25 minutes per limb, once per day, 5 days per week for a total of 4 weeks. Modified Ashworth scale (MAS), the Fugl-Meyer assessment, and the Modified Barthel index were used to assess the severity of spasticity, motor function of limbs, and activities of daily living, respectively. It was reported that modified Ashworth scale score of elbow flexors, wrist flexors, knee flexors, and knee extensors showed significantly greater reduction at 4 weeks and the reduction was sustained at 3 months follow-up. However, the Fugl-Meyer assessment and modified Barthel index scores did not show significant intergroup difference.

Sankaran et al. (2018) in a prospective case–control study involving 52 patients undergoing acute inpatient rehabilitation concluded that utilizing Ayurvedic massage in poststroke patients with flaccidity can promote faster standing with minimal assistance and lead to less need for antispastic drugs at discharge. The study was conducted during 2014–2017. Twenty five received Ayurvedic massage (Abhyanga) with physiotherapy and 27 received only physiotherapy. Massage followed by steam application was delivered daily for a total of 10 sessions. For Abhyanga (Ayurvedic massage), the patient was first assessed by the Ayurvedic physician to determine their predominant constitution (prakriti) and to select oils to be used during massage. For *Vata*, predominant *Prakriti Dhanwantharam* oil was used, whereas in for *Pitha and* Kapha prakriti, Pinda Thailam oil, and Karpasasthyadi oil were used, respectively. Oil was warmed and rubbed with gentle pressure from the neck down by two massage therapists simultaneously, from the upper limbs to trunk, then lower limbs for 30 minutes while on a wooden table. Following this, the patient was exposed to steam for 15 minutes either via a chamber or hose. Patients of both groups received at least 6 hours of therapy in a week. Therapy consisted of passive and active range of motion (ROM), tilt tabling, gait training in parallel bars, and a variety of therapist guided, self/bystander-assisted exercises. Brunnstrom leg progression, spasticity using the MAS, time to achieve stand with minimal assistance, functional independence measure (FIM) score for walking at discharge, and use of antispastic drugs at discharge were the main outcome measures. They reported that patients who received Ayurvedic massage had lower MAS and lesser need for antispastic drugs. They achieved standing with minimal assistance sooner, and had better locomotion at discharge.

Backus et al. (2016) examined the effects of massage therapy on fatigue, pain, spasticity, perception of health, and quality of life in people with multiple sclerosis (MS) in a nonrandomized, prepost pilot study where 24 individuals with MS (age = 47.38 + 13.05 years) male received standardized massage therapy routine one time a week for 6 weeks. Massage therapy routine consisted of a combination of effleurage, petrissage, friction, and static compression strokes applied to back, head, neck, shoulder and both upper and lower limbs for minimum of 30 minutes and maximum for 1 hour. Modified fatigue index scale (MFIS), MOS pain effects scale (MOS pain), MAS, mental health inventory (MHI), and health status questionnaire were the outcome measures. A significant improvement with a large effect size in MFIS, MOS Pain (MHI and HSQ) was reported. The authors concluded that massage therapy is a safe and beneficial intervention for management of fatigue and pain in people with MS.

Malila et al. (2015) concluded that Thai massage decreased muscle spasticity. Thai massage (called Nuad Bo'Rarn) is based on a combination of Indian and Chinese traditions of medicine. It is a deep, full-body massage consisting of pressing and stretching techniques progressing from the feet up and focusing on sen (energy lines) throughout the body, with the aim of clearing blockages in these lines, and facilitating the smooth and constant flow of bioenergy (Chi, Qi, and Prana) throughout the body and mind (Gold, 2007). Malila et al. (2015) determined the effects of Thai massage on muscle spasticity in young people with spastic diplegia cerebral palsy. Spasticity of right quadriceps femoris muscles was measured by using MAS at pre- and immediately post 30-minute session of Thai massage. Thai massage was applied on the lower back and lower limbs. A significant difference of MAS was observed between pre- and post-treatment without any adverse events.

Thanakiatpinyo et al. (2014) indicated that Thai massage may relieve spasticity, but its effect was no superior than that of physiotherapy. In their study conducted on 50 elderly stroke patients, both Thai massage and physical therapy (PT) reduced spasticity by at least one grade, increase functional ability, and improve QoL. Both groups received treatment (either TTM or PT) twice a week for 6 weeks.

Negahban et al. (2013) in a randomized controlled pilot trial with repeated measurements suggested that massage therapy could be more effective than exercise therapy in multiple sclerosis. The objective of this study was to investigate the comparative effects of massage therapy and exercise therapy on patients with multiple sclerosis. 48 patients with multiple sclerosis were randomly assigned to four equal subgroups, i.e., massage therapy, exercise therapy, combined massage-exercise therapy, and control group. The massage therapy group received a standard Swedish massage. The exercise therapy group was given a combined set of strength, stretch, endurance, and balance exercises. Patients in the massage-exercise therapy group received a combined set of massage and exercise treatments. Patients in the control group were asked to continue their standard medical care. All groups received the 15 sessions of supervised intervention for 5 weeks. They observed that massage therapy resulted in significantly larger improvement in pain reduction, dynamic balance, and walking speed than exercise therapy. Patients involved in the combined massage-exercise therapy showed significantly larger improvement in pain reduction than those in the exercise therapy.

These studies call for relook into the use of massage therapy in spasticity.

On Autonomic Nervous System

Several authors have hypothesized that massage has definite reflex effect and it can influence the functioning of visceral organ by modulating the autonomic nervous system through peripheral sensory stimulation (Ebner, 1975; Mennell, 1945; Hollis, 1987; Lehn and Prentice, 1994).

Physiological responses associated with autonomic nervous system, such as heart rate, cardiac output, blood pressure, respiratory rate, skin temperature, skin conductance, activity of sweat gland, etc. are claimed to be influenced by massage. However, in the absence of conclusive experimental evidence, it becomes difficult to substantiate or refute these claims. In general, it is accepted that massage increases the temperature of skin, activates the sweat gland, and increases the skin conductance (electrodermal response). The reports on the effect of massage on other parameters, such as cardiac output, blood pressure, respiratory rate, etc. are conflicting. Some studies reported an increase in all these parameters whereas other reported either decrease or no change.

Ebner (1975) reported the investigation of skin temperature of three patients after connective tissue massage. An increase in skin temperature (1–2°C) of the foot was observed following 20 minutes of connective tissue massage on lumbosacral segment of back.

Connective tissue massage improves the blood supply of target organ by balancing the sympathetic and parasympathetic component of autonomic nervous system (Thompson et al., 1991). It is claimed that when soft tissue mobilization is performed for autonomic or reflex effects, sensory receptors in skin and superficial fascia are stimulated. The stimulus passes through afferent pathways to the spinal cord and may be channeled through autonomic pathways producing effects in the area corresponding to the dermatomal zone being massaged.

Barr and Taslitz (1970) examined the effect of back massage on autonomic function on 10 normal female subjects. They reported that an increase in sympathetic activity occurred during the massaged period in experimental group as evident by a delayed increase in systolic blood pressure, increased heart rate, increased sweat gland activity, and increased body temperature. However, they had not subjected their data to statistical analysis. Peshkov (1981) also found a marked increase in the electrodermal response (EDR)/galvanic skin response (GSR) in young gymnasts following massage.

The electrodermal response (or GSR) is a reflection of variation of the sweat gland activity and pore size, both of which are controlled by the sympathetic nervous system. Barr and Taslitz (1970) reported an increase in heart rate after 20 minutes of back massage. However, Boone and Cooper (1998) could not found any change in heart rate after 30 minutes massage of lower extremity.

In a single subject study, Resnick (2016) compared the effects of massage recovery and resting recovery on a subject's heart rate variability and selected metabolic effects following a submaximal treadmill exercise session and reported massage restored the heart rate recovery more quickly than rest alone. It took 60 minutes of resting recovery to reach similar heart rate variability levels (1.216 LF/HF) found after 30 minutes of massage. The author attributed this to a more immediate shift to the parasympathetic state.

EFFECTS ON THE SOFT TISSUE

Massage has significant effect on certain properties of the soft tissues like elasticity, plasticity, and mobility. The tissues which can be affected by massage include muscles, sheath, ligaments, tendons, aponeurosis, joint capsules, and superficial as well as deep fascia. Different maneuvers of massage stretches the constituent collagen fibers of these tissues in different directions. The adhesions present between fibers are broken and maximum mobility between fibers and adjacent structures is ensured. Cyriax (1998) stated that transverse friction restores the mobility of muscles in the same way as mobilization frees the joint.

The main function of a muscle is to contract. When a muscle contracts, not only its length reduces, but the width of muscle also increases. Cyriax refers this phenomenon as the broadening out of muscle and states that the full mobility of muscle in broadening out must be maintained in order to achieve adequate shortening of muscles. Different massage maneuvers especially transverse friction mechanically separates the glued muscle fibers and restores the mobility.

The fibrin formed within the chronic indurated structures following chronic or subacute inflammation can effectively be stretched and mobilized during pressure manipulations. This way massage maintains and restores the mobility of soft tissues as well as prevents adhesion formation, joint stiffness, contracture, etc.

Muscle Strength

Massage is capable of increasing muscular strength, which is one of the most persistent and widespread belief in both professional and lay medical circle (Kuprian, 1982). Most authorities on the subjects are of unanimous opinion that massage does not increase the strength of muscle (Lehn and Prentice, 1994; Wood and Becker, 1981; Knapp, 1990). Strengthening of a muscle can only be achieved by the active contraction of a muscle. Massage, at best, can prepare the muscle for contraction by increasing the circulation and facilitating the removal of metabolic waste.

Massage is used for facilitating the recovery of muscle function following exhaustive exercises. The experimental evidences with regards to this use of massage are equivocal. A detailed discussion on this topic is presented in Chapter 10.

EFFECTS ON THE RESPIRATORY SYSTEM

Percussion and vibration techniques of massage assist the removal of secretion from the larger airways, though their effect on the smaller airway is controversial (Imle, 1989). Increased secretion clearance after chest physiotherapy both in adult and in pediatric group can be the result of percussion and vibration loosening and advancing secretions from the airways more centrally. After the removal of secretion, gas exchange becomes more efficient. An increase in PaO_2 has been frequently reported after respiratory massage maneuvers in patients suffering from chronic obstructive pulmonary disease (Bateman et al., 1981), postoperative and post-traumatic patients (Ciesla et al., 1981; Mackenzie et al., 1978), and in neonatal patients suffering with respiratory distress (Finer et al., 1979). Significant decrease in partial pressure of oxygen has been reported in critically ill patients receiving chest physiotherapy in the form of postural drainage and percussion. However, percussion and vibration alone not proven to contribute to hypoxemia, though postural drainage which is often employed with these techniques does cause alteration in cardiorespiratory functions.

Efficacy of each treatment method is difficult to assess as in most of the chest physiotherapy research along with these manual techniques. Postural drainage, cough, suction, and breathing exercises are also included. The attempts to evaluate the specific contribution of percussion or vibration to the total therapy program are both rare and conflicting. Percussion is shown to effect intrathoracic pressure change of 5–15 cm of H_2O (Imle, 1989).

Percussion is thought to cause bronchospasm, which is evident by a fall in FEV_1 in some patients of chronic lung disease (Campbell *et al,* 1975) which is small and short-lived in most of these cases. However, other studies have either reported no change or increase in FEV_1. It is often stated that vibration dislodges the most stubborn secretion in larger as well as in smaller airways. Hyperinflation with vibration is associated with significant and deleterious increase in intracranial pressure (Garradd and Bullock, 1986) and fluctuation in cardiac output (Laws and McIntyre, 1969).

Efficacy of these techniques is dependent on the skill of the clinician and complications have been reported mostly due to poor technique administration.

EFFECTS ON THE SKIN

Massage, in general, improves the nutritive status of skin. Following massage, the temperature of skin rises. Massage facilitates the movement of skin over the subcutaneous structures. As a result, skin becomes soften, more supple, and finer. Furthermore, after prolonged massage, the skin also becomes tough, more flexible, elastic, and its sensitivity is reduced, so that it can be handled fairly, roughly without causing much discomfort. It has a soothing effect on the highly sensitive and vascular papillae over which deeper layers of the cuticle fits.

The dead cells are removed by the constant contact of the hand over the skin. The sweat glands, hair follicles, and the sebaceous glands, thus, become free from obstruction and can function more effectively (Hollis, 1987). Massage, by activating the sweat glands, increases perspiration, so that the heat dissipation is increased. It also facilitates the sebaceous secretions from exocrine glands of skin and thus, improves the lubrication and appearance of skin.

EFFECTS ON THE ADIPOSE TISSUE

Massage was found responsible for activation of lipolysis. The release of catecholamine by the tissue nerve ending was particularly stressed as the cause. This was confirmed when activation of lipolysis was depressed by beta-blockers (Wakim, 1985).

Similar claims have been made that massage can remove the deposits of adipose tissue in the various layers of the body.

However, experimental studies by Wright (1946), Kalb (1944), etc. do not support this notion. Knapp (1990) has also stated that massage is ineffective in weight reduction. Though massage is widely used in various obesity reduction programs, both manually and in the form of vibratory belt, lack of literature on this topic makes it difficult to justify this claim. However, it may be hypothesized that since massage improves the function of muscle and helps in reduction of fatigue, the subject may perform vigorous exercises with little more intensity after massage which ultimately burns the calories. So, at the best, massage can work only as an adjunct to weight reduction programs.

PSYCHOLOGICAL EFFECTS

Massage can lower the psychoemotional and somatic arousal, such as anxiety and tension.

During massage treatment, a close contact is established between therapist and patient which help to overcome the feeling of strangeness and anxiety. The surrounding equipment, treatment area, and the assured way in which therapist handles the patient, all exert a strong placebo effect. It helps to reduce tension and anxiety and induces relaxation. This effect is more pronounced when massage is used for the purpose of general relaxation.

IMMUNOLOGICAL EFFECTS OF MASSAGE

In recent times, several research groups started postulating that massage as a useful stress-reduction tool may be capable of inhibiting, or even reversing, potentially detrimental immunological effects associated with AIDS and cancers. On the basis of this postulation lies the studies that showed associations between stress and immune suppression (Glaser, 1984), and between stress-reduction interventions and immune enhancement (Kiecolt-Glaser, 1985). Since ages, the role of massage in inducing relaxation and combating the stress-related symptoms has been advocated. It is now believed that massage may exert some effect in modifying the immune system activities. Recent research focus is directed toward the investigation into the immunological effects of massage therapy in an attempt to provide rationales for its use in combating some late stage complications associated with AIDS and cancer.

Ironson et al. (1996) reported significant increases in natural killer (NK) cell number and function with HIV positive and HIV negative men following massage. Similar finding on the normal subjects undergoing a stressful situation has also been reported by Zeitlin et al. (2000) who examined the immunological effects of massage therapy as a stress-reduction intervention in a sample of nine medically healthy subjects. All the subjects were first and second-year female medical students (age range 21–25 years) who received a 1 hour full body massage 1 day before an academic examination that was causing them considerable anxiety. The massage protocol was developed to encourage relaxation and increase circulation and included the application of effleurage, petrissage, and friction strokes of Swedish massage. Blood samples, self-report psychosocial data, and vital signs were obtained immediately before and immediately after the massage treatment. Cell phenotypes of the major cells of the immune system, natural killer cell activity (NKCA), and mitogen-induced lymphocyte stimulation were also assessed. The results showed a significant reduction in respiratory rate, stress scores, and a decrease in the percentage of T-cells postmassage. Though no significant differences between pre- and postmeasures of blood pressure, pulse, or temperature were found. An increase in the total number of peripheral WBCs postmassage was observed which was not associated with the increase in the absolute number of T cells. Analysis of NKCA data revealed a significant time (prepost) effect indicating a significant increase in killing activity after the massage. The authors suggested that massage may have health benefits beyond and unrelated to its stress-reduction potential.

However Birk et al. (2000) could not observe any significant ($p < 0.05$) changes in peripheral blood levels of CD4+ lymphocytes, CD8+ lymphocytes, CD4+/CD8+ lymphocyte ratio, and natural killer cells following a 45-minute overall body massage once per week on a sample of 42 subjects with HIV infection.

Hernandez-Reif et al. (2004) reported that 30 minutes massage consisted of stroking, squeezing, and stretching techniques to the head, arms, legs/feet, and back three times per week for 5 weeks resulted in reduced depression and increased urinary dopamine, serotonin values, NK cell number, and lymphocytes in women diagnosed with stage 1 or 2 breast cancer postsurgery.

Goodfellow (2003) examined influences of 20 minutes therapeutic back massage on psychosocial, physiologic, and immune function variables in spouses of patients with cancer. Natural killer cell activity (NKCA), heart rate, systolic and diastolic blood pressures, mood, and perceived stress were measured before, immediately after and 20 minutes after massage. They suggested that back massage may enhance mood and reduce perceived stress in this population.

Field et al. (2004) reported that two sessions of 20 minutes therapy each week for 16 weeks during the second trimester of pregnancy resulted in higher dopamine and serotonin levels and lower levels of cortisol and norepinephrine in depressed pregnant women. They compared the massage therapy with progressive muscle relaxation and with a control group that received standard prenatal care alone. Those receiving massage therapy also reported lower levels of anxiety and depressed mood as well as less leg and back pain.

On the other hand, Moyer et al. (2004) in a meta-analysis observed that single applications of massage therapy did not lead to reduced cortisol level, although it reduced state of anxiety, blood pressure, and heart rate.

The purpose of the study of Rapaport et al. (2010) was to determine effects of a single session of Swedish massage on neuroendocrine and immune functions. They hypothesized that Swedish massage therapy would increase oxytocin (OT) levels which would lead to a decrease in hypothalamic–pituitary–adrenal (HPA) activity and enhanced immune function. OT, arginine vasopressin (AVP), ACTH, cortisol, circulating phenotypic lymphocytes markers, and mitogen-stimulated cytokine production were measured. They reported that when compared to light touch, 45 minutes of Swedish massage therapy caused a large effect size decrease in AVP, and a small effect size decrease in cortisol. Massage increased the number of circulating lymphocytes, CD25P lymphocytes, CD56P lymphocytes, CD4P lymphocytes, and CD8P lymphocytes, mitogen-stimulated levels of interleukin (IL)–1β, IL-2, IL-4, IL-5, IL-6, IL-10, IL-13, and decreased IFN-γ for subjects receiving Swedish massage therapy. Swedish massage therapy decreased IL-4, IL-5, IL-10, and IL-13 levels relative to baseline measures. They suggested that a single session of Swedish massage therapy produces measurable biologic effects.

Two years later, the same research group (Rapaport et al., 2012) examined the effects of repeated massage on the similar parameters and observed that weekly Swedish massage stimulated a sustained pattern of increased circulating phenotypic lymphocyte markers and decreased mitogen-stimulated cytokine production. Twice-weekly massage produced a different response pattern with increased OT levels, decreased AVP, and decreased cortisol, but had little effect on circulating lymphocyte phenotypic markers and a slight increase in mitogen-stimulated interferon-c, tumor necrosis factor-a, interleukin (IL)-1b and IL-2 levels, implicating increased production of proinflammatory cytokines. They suggested that massage and touch interventions produces cumulative biologic actions. These effects of massage depend on the dosage (frequency) of sessions and persist for several days.

Morhenn et al. (2012) examined the effect of massage on oxytocin and ACTH, NO and β-endorphin (BE). After drawing participants' blood, 15 minutes of moderate-pressure massage of the upper back were given to 65 participants, whereas control group rested quietly for 15 minutes. They reported that massage was associated with an increase in OT and reductions in ACTH, NO, and BE. **Box 2.1** shows physiological effects of message at a glance.

Box 2.1: Physiological effects of massage at a glance.

- ↑Venous and lymphatic flow[1]
- ↑Arterial blood flow to the muscle and skin[2]
- ↓Stagnation of fluid in tissue space[1]
- ↑Removal of waste products of metabolism[2]
- ↑WBC, RBC, and platelets count in circulating blood[2]
- ↑Nutritive exchange between blood and cells[3]
- ↑Trophic status of the part massaged[3]
- Induce sedation
- ↓Pain[3]
- Facilitate contraction in hypotonic muscle[3]
- ↓Excitability of motor neuronal pool in neurologically healthy person[1]
- Modulate autonomic response[2]
- ↑Electrodermal response or GSR[1]
- ↑Removal of secretion from lung[1]
- ↑Gaseous exchanges across pulmonary capillaries[1]
- ↑Removal of dead cells from skin[3]
- ↑Activity of sweat and sebaceous glands[1]
- Modulate psychosomatic arousal[1]
- Mobilize soft tissue[1]
- Break the soft tissue adhesions[1]
- Accelerate various metabolic processes[2]
- Promote lipolysis[3]

1 = Experimentally proved   2 = Conflicting claims   3 = No experimental evidence

CHAPTER 3

Therapeutic Uses

Massage is one of the oldest forms of treatment for human ills. It has been used as a therapeutic modality in various conditions since ancient times. However, often without rationalization and scientific evidence. In ancient Syria, massage was believed to be capable of expelling spirits from a person's body. It was also advocated in conditions like syphilis and intestinal obstructions (Kellogg, 1919). In ancient Rome and China, it was used extensively. It continues to be used in most of the traditional Indian systems of medicine till today, where its utility is claimed in almost every clinical condition. However, like any other form of treatment, massage cannot be beneficial in all the diseases or injuries (Wood and Becker, 1981). Rather, if the physiological effect of massage is analyzed carefully, it becomes clear that quite a few conditions are amenable to massage. In physiotherapy, massage is used for the following purposes:

- To improve the mobility of the soft tissues
- To reduce muscle spasm and pain
- To reduce edema
- To increase circulation
- To mobilize secretions in the lung
- To induce local and general relaxations.

MOBILITY OF SOFT TISSUES

The skin, fat, fascia, muscle, and the ligament are the soft tissues of the body. Any injury or inflammation to these soft tissues leads to adhesion formation which decreases their mobility and causes pain. After inflammation, the new granulation tissue formed during the process of healing is usually edematous. This is due to the presence of a protein-rich fluid which leaks into the tissue space from the capillaries in the process of neovascularization. This edema in the soft tissue persists long after the inflammatory response is over. It consolidates and binds the newly laid collagen fibers to each other and to the surrounding structures. This causes adhesion formation, extensive scarring, soft tissue tightness, and contracture which are the common causes of pain and dysfunction of the moving part of the body, i.e., the musculoskeletal system.

The to and fro movement of massage mechanically breaks down the adhesion and facilitates the free movement of the adherent structure. The aim of massage is to prevent the adherence of recently formed soft tissue and also to break the adherent scar tissue established in the long-standing cases. The different massage maneuvers roll the individual fibers of the soft tissue. This breaks the adhesion and aids in the facilitation of movement. Increased scar pliability and decreased scar bonding with the use of massage have been reported. Bodian (1969) founded that massage is useful in treating thick scar and keloid formation around eyelid. In an animal model (rat), Gahlsen et al. (1999) induced tendinitis in Achilles tendon using the enzyme collagenase and treated it with soft tissue mobilization of various pressure. They reported a statistically significant increase in the number of fibroblasts, determined by the use of light microscope and electron microscope, in cases treated with heavy pressure mobilization. They observed that the application of heavy pressure promotes the healing process to a greater degree than the light or moderate pressure.

However, Patino et al. (1999) failed to demonstrate any appreciable effect of massage therapy on the vascularity, pliability, and height of hypertrophic scar in 30 pediatric patients. Nevertheless, world over the scar massage is used in burn units to improve functional and cosmetic outcomes of hypertrophic scarring following a burn. In a systematic review, Ault et al. (2018) observed that preliminary evidence suggests that scar massage may be effective to decrease scar height, vascularity, pliability, pain, pruritus, and depression in hypertrophic burns scarring. They included eight publications with 258 human participants and 15 animals who received scar massage following a thermal injury resulting in hypertrophic scarring. However, in view of poor quality of evidence and lack of consistent and valid scar assessment tools, they expressed the need for controlled, clinical trials to develop evidence-based guidelines for scar massage in hypertrophic burns scarring.

Nonetheless, massage has an important role in the mobilization of soft tissue and its uses are advocated in conditions where adhesion and restricted mobility are the causative factors of pain and limitation of motion. Its role in prevention of the adherent tendon and skin, a common complication in all microsurgical procedures has now gained universal acceptance. The various conditions in which massage is used for mobilization of soft tissue are listed below:
- Tendinitis
- Tenosynovitis
- Fibrositis
- Muscular injury
- Ligament sprain
- Postsurgical scar
- Postburn contracture
- Pre- and postoperative cases in plastic, and reconstructive surgery.

MUSCLE SPASM AND PAIN

Spasm is the increased muscle tone in a localized area. It is one of the primary responses of body to pain or injury. The increase in muscle tone is a protective mechanism which helps to prevent further damage by restricting the movement. Often, this contracted state of the muscle is maintained for long periods and itself becomes the cause for pain. Physiologically, in presence of spasm, there occurs capillary constriction which reduces the blood flow. Circulatory restriction results in limitation of the flow of nutrients and oxygen to the area and retention of waste product. More spasm leads to more ischemic pain and less flexible tissue. This vicious cycle of pain-spasm-pain is advanced and spasm persists. This vicious cycle can be broken by massage (Liston, 1997). Massage interferes with this cycle by reducing the pain. It, thus, prevents the further occurrence of spasm.

Pain is reduced or minimized following massage which can be explained by following hypothesis:
1. By the stimulation of sensory nerve endings and production of mild pain, massage blocks the pathway of pain in accordance with the Melzack and Wall's theory of pain gate.
2. The mechanical movement of massage stretches the individual fibers of soft tissue and reduces their tension.

3. Removal of metabolic waste products results due to increased drainage of the massaged area. This results in reduction of pain, as these substances are noxious to the tissue and irritate the free nerve endings.
4. Increased blood flow following massage reduces the anoxic condition present in the tissue due to the compression of the blood vessels produced by the sustained muscular contraction. Thus, it reduces the danger of increased tissue damage.
5. The stimulation of the peripheral sensory receptors is said to have an effect on the general level of excitation and inhibition in the region of the anterior horn cells. This effect is utilized in massage to reduce the tone of muscles in neurologically healthy individuals.

All these factors together aid to reduce the spasm. For this purpose, massage is employed in the following conditions:
- Unspecified back pain
- Fibrositis
- Postexercise muscle soreness, etc.

In a Cochrane review of 25 RCTs examining effect of massage on low back pain, Furlan et al. (2015) observed that massage was better than passive controls for pain and function in the short term, but not in the long-term follow-up. However, on account of a high-risk of performance and measurement bias in the reviewed studies, they judged the quality of the evidence as "low" to "very low". Patel et al. (2012) in a Cochrane review of 15 trials commented that as a stand-alone treatment, massage for mechanical neck disorders was found to provide an immediate or short-term effectiveness or both in pain and tenderness.

REDUCTION OF EDEMA

Edema is the accumulation of tissue fluid in the extracellular space. Untreated edema is an established causative factor for delayed healing, pain, as well as for decreased mobility with subsequent compromised functional use of the afflicted part. Massage is an important aspect of edema reduction program (Mager and McCue, 1995). Massage reduces edema utilizing its mechanical effect of forcing the fluid into the drainage channels. When the edema is due to mechanical factors, such as muscle inactivity as in paralysis, valve insufficiency, lymph node blockage, etc. massage procedures are helpful in the reduction of swelling. For the same purpose, it is also used in the management of venous ulcer, lymphedema following radical mastectomy, etc. However, it should be supplemented with active exercises, elastic bandages, and elevation to offer better and sustained effects.

ENHANCEMENT OF CIRCULATION

Massage has been used throughout the ages as a treatment for cold extremities where the blood supply is decreased due to the vasoconstriction in response to the cold. The rubbing activity causes vasodilation and thus increases the temperature of the affected part of the body.

Massage is prescribed in nerve palsies, and in various lower motor neuron lesions. The purpose of this is to maintain the trophic condition of the paralyzed part, utilizing the circulatory effects of massage.

Massage becomes an important substitute for muscle activity in conditions when the body parts cannot be moved due to various reasons including severe exhaustion following intense physical works, old age, prolonged recumbency, generalized paresis, etc. The mechanical compression and relaxation of massage creates a pumping effect and improves the lymphatic and venous drainage. This hastens absorption of fluid and reduces stagnation. The improved arterial circulation following massage facilitates the exchange of nutritive elements into the paralyzed extremities. In this way, the nourishment of the paralyzed muscle is maintained to a certain extent.

For this effect, only massage is advised in all type of flaccid paralyses, i.e., Bell's palsy, poliomyelitis, neurotmesis, Guillain-Barré syndrome, etc.

In these cases, however, the purpose of massage is only to maintain the nutrition of the muscle. It does not have any effect on the strength of the muscle which can only be increased by active exercises.

The increased circulation following massage is also utilized in the management of sports-specific conditions. Preactivity massage brings more blood and oxygen to the massaged part and thus helps in warming up of the muscles. Postactivity massage removes excess of lactic acid and other metabolites accumulated in the muscle and is said to decrease the severity of delayed-onset muscle soreness. However, massage cannot increase strength of the muscle; nevertheless it can prepare the muscle for high-intensity activity/exercise for a longer duration, which ultimately leads to increase in muscle strength.

MOBILIZE SECRETIONS IN THE LUNGS

Certain techniques of massage (i.e., clapping, vibration, and shaking) are exclusively used for the management of chest disorders. Massage finds a major role in the treatment of those chest disorders where increased and viscid secretions are the source of problem. In diseases like chronic bronchitis, emphysema, cystic fibrosis, bronchiectasis, etc. there occurs an increased production of sputum which accumulates, stagnates, dries up, and blocks the small respiratory pathways.

The gaseous exchange of the part distal to the block becomes restricted and gradually that segment of lung collapses. Similar increase of sputum production is seen in postoperative periods of cardiothoracic and abdominal operations. The various manual and mechanical respiratory techniques of massage, i.e., vibration, shaking, percussion, etc. produce a jarring effect on the lung tissue. The mechanical energy transmitted to the lung tissue through the chest walls leads to the loosening up of the viscid secretions. Massage also moves the sputum up in the bronchial tree. Drainage of the sputum is facilitated by postural drainage. Once the secretions loosen up and go up in the upper respiratory tract, they can be removed by coughing.

Doering et al. (1999) examined the influence of manual vibratory massage on the pulmonary function of postoperative patients of heart and lung transplants. The vibratory massage was performed with a frequency of 8–10 vibrations per second for 7.5 minutes on each side of thorax, starting from the lower costal arch and progressing to the upper thoracic aperture. They found that during the vibratory massage, a significant increase ($p < 0.05$) in mean tidal volume by 30% and in the percutaneous oxygen saturation. Significant decrements were observed in the central venous pressure (by 11%), and the pulmonary vessels resistance (by 18.3%). They found no change in cerebral blood flow velocity. They observed that vibratory massage by reducing ventilation-perfusion mismatch and by increasing oxygen saturation, could be a helpful method for improving pulmonary mechanism and perfusion.

GENERAL AND LOCAL RELAXATIONS

The importance of touch as a means of communication and its importance in imparting a sense of well-being and confidence cannot be underestimated. Psychologically and emotionally, massage has been used since ages to enhance a feeling of well-being and relaxation. Tiredness after prolonged work, anxiety of a feverish child as well as pain, and apprehension of an arthritic elderly responding well to massage are a common man's experience. Therefore, the use of massage for ensuring comfort and relaxation has remained one of the most common practices in all cultures and civilizations throughout the world.

Massage has been shown to have a beneficial influence on development, attitudes, and emotional status of a baby (Schneider, 1992). Psychological parameters associated with tension and anxiety have been shown to decrease significantly with massage (Makechnic et al., 1983). Crompton and Fox (1987) also observed that massage techniques promote two-three times faster recovery of psychological and physiological status of athletes.

Recently several studies have appeared in literature where the efficacy of massage in reducing anxiety and stress associated with several clinical conditions has been examined scientifically. Richards (1998) compared the efficacy of 6 minutes of back massage with psychological relaxation technique (muscle relaxation, mental imagery, and music) on the sleep of elderly cardiovascular patients admitted in critical care unit. He observed that the quality of sleep was improved among the back massage group whose patients slept 1 hour longer than the other groups.

Field et al. (1998) reported that asthmatic children treated with 20 minutes massage before bedtime for 30 days showed immediate decrease in behavioral anxiety. Their attitude toward asthma also improved along with other pulmonary functions over the period of 1 month. Similar decrease in anxiety, improved mood, and pulmonary function with massage have also been reported in children with cystic fibrosis (Hernandez-Reif et al., 1999). Massage was shown to decrease fidgeting in adolescent with attention deficit hyperactivity disorder (Field et al., 1998). On their study on pregnant women, Field et al. (1999) founded that 20 minutes massage session twice a week for 5 weeks resulted in reduced anxiety, improved mood, better sleep, and less low back pain in addition to fewer complications during labor and postnatal period.

In an interesting study, Hernandez-Reif et al. (1999) taught hand or ear self-massage to smokers (mean age 32.6 years), during 3 cravings per day for 1 month and found that self-massage group smoked few cigarettes by the last week of the study. They suggested that self-massage may be an effective adjunct to the treatment for the adults attempting smoking cessation to alleviate smoking-related anxiety, reduce craving and withdrawal symptoms, improve mood, and to reduce the number of cigarettes smoked per day.

Though the role of massage in reducing anxiety and improving mood has long been accepted, these studies provide an insight into the newer application of this therapy.

In the recent times, the use of massage as a form of complementary therapy has increased. The following paragraphs present a brief discussion on these recent trends on the use of massage.

MASSAGE AND OBESITY

Deep mechanical massage has been advocated as an alternative or adjunctive therapy for the contouring of subcutaneous fat and as a treatment for cellulite (Adcock, 2001). However, experimental evidence with regard to this effect is scarce and contradictory. Till today, no controlled clinical trial has established the role of massage in the reduction of obesity. Though several equipment based on the principles of vibratory massage is being marketed for this purpose.

MASSAGE AND AIDS

Of late, a number of studies have appeared in the literature reporting the increasing use of massage by the AIDS patients (Williams et al., 2005; Mills and Ernst, 2005; Gore-Felton, 2003; Toups, 1999). Several articles have also appeared in the literature that examined the role of massage in the management of AIDS-related problems (Siegel et al., 2004; Toups, 1999).

These reports are to be read with caution. Some studies reported increase in natural killer cell activity after massage in both AIDS as well as in normal individual under stressful condition. In an extensive review on the use of complementary therapies on the AIDS, Mills and Ernst (2005) found only four clinical trials on massage and commented that available data are insufficient for demonstrating effectiveness of massage therapy in the management of AIDS. They further commented that notwithstanding the widespread use of complementary and alternative medicine by people living with HIV/AIDS, the paucity of clinical trials and their low methodological quality are a matter of concern.

However, the most important role of massage in the management of these patient groups may exist in the area of stress reduction. Massage therapy is proposed to have a positive effect on quality of life and may also have a positive effect on immune function through stress mediation. Several studies have documented that massage or touch helps allay the anxiety, depression, and the other stress-related symptoms in this patient group. According to Müller-Oerlinghausen (2004) slow-stroke massage is suitable for additional acute treatment of patients with depression which was very readily accepted also by very ill patients. Birk et al. (2003) in a controlled clinical trial observed that massage administered once per week to HIV-infected persons does not enhance immune measures, though massage combined with stress management favorably alters health perceptions and leads to less utilization of healthcare resources.

Shor-Posner et al. (2006) evaluated the effectiveness of massage therapy on immune parameters in 54 young HIV-positive children who did not have access to antiretroviral therapies. 22 children randomized to receive massage treatment whereas the rest of them constituted the control group who received only a friendly visit twice weekly. The total period of study was 12 weeks. The authors observed a significant reduction in both CD4+ and CD8+ cell counts in control group whereas massage-treated older children remained stable or showed immune improvement. A significant increase in CD4+ and CD25+ cells in the massage-treated older children was also observed. In 2–4 years old massage-treated children, a significant increase in natural killer cells was also reported. The authors opined that massage therapy may have some role in immune preservation in HIV-positive children.

Hillier et al. (2010) in a systematic review examined the safety and effectiveness of massage therapy on quality of life, pain, and immune system parameters in people living with HIV/AIDS. They found some evidence to support the use of massage therapy to improve quality of life for people living with HIV/AIDS, particularly in combination with other stress-management modalities. They also commented that massage therapy may have a positive effect on immunological function.

Reychler et al. (2017) reported a significant improvement in anxiety and hyperventilation in HIV-infected patients after 4 weeks of massage. They examined the effect of massage therapy on anxiety, depression, hyperventilation, and quality of life in 29 HIV-infected patients.

On the basis of current evidences, it can be suggested that as far management of stress and fatigue-related symptoms associated with AIDS, the use of massage may have some role which needs to examined further. However, claims with regards to its role in the cure of the diseases should be dismissed.

MASSAGE AND CANCER

Many people with cancer experience pain, anxiety, and mood disturbance. Conventional treatments do not always satisfactorily relieve these symptoms, and some patients may not be able to tolerate their side effects. Complementary therapies, such as acupuncture, mind-body techniques, massage, and other methods are now increasing being used in providing palliative care to the terminally ill cancer patients in order to relieve symptoms and improve physical and mental well-being (Deng and Cassileth, 2005). It is suggested that patients who receive massage have less procedural pain, nausea, and anxiety and report improved quality of life. Increase in the level of dopamine levels, natural killer cells, and lymphocytes following massage in women diagnosed with breast cancer has been reported by Hernandez-Reif et al. (2005). However, the strongest evidence for benefits of massage is for stress and anxiety reduction, although research for pain control and management of other symptoms common to patients with cancer including pain is also promising (Corbin, 2005).

Manual lymph drainage is a specialized form of massage used in patients with lymphedema. Two small trials (Johansson et al., 1998; Johansson et al., 1997) founded that manual lymph drainage to be an effective adjunct to compression bandaging or sleeves in patients with arm lymphedema after surgery for breast cancer.

Cassileth and Vickers (2004) studied that the patients reported symptom severity before and after the application of massage therapy in 1,290 patients over 3 years period using 0–10 rating scales of pain, fatigue, stress/anxiety, nausea, depression, etc. They observed that symptom scores were reduced by approximately 50%, even for patients reporting high baseline scores. These data indicate that massage therapy is associated with substantive improvement in cancer patients' symptom scores.

In a quasi-experimental design on a sample of 41 patients admitted to the oncology unit at a large urban medical center in the United States for chemotherapy or radiation, Smith et al. (2002) examined the effects of therapeutic massage on perception of pain, subjective sleep quality, symptom distress, and anxiety in patients hospitalized for treatment of cancer. Twenty participants received therapeutic massage and 21 received the control therapy of nurse interaction. It was observed that mean scores for pain, sleep quality, symptom distress, and anxiety improved from baseline for the subjects who received therapeutic massage; only anxiety improved from baseline for participants in the comparison group. Similar findings have also been reported by Cassileth and Vickers (2004) who in a randomized clinical trial involving 1,290 patients reported about 50% reduction in symptoms scores of pain, fatigue, stress/anxiety, nausea, depression, etc. In patients receiving massage therapy, the benefits of massage persisted throughout the duration of 48-hour follow-up.

Gensic et al. (2017) reported that effleurage hand massages performed by trained volunteers effectively reduced anxiety and pain in patients receiving chemotherapy. 24 patients received 10 minutes hand massages at the beginning of their chemotherapy session. Significant reductions were noted in systolic BP, heart rate, visual analog scale for anxiety, and visual analog scale for pain after the chemotherapy session. Cutshall et al. (2017) also reported the similar observations.

In a case report, Cunningham et al. (2013) reported that a course of manual therapy effleurage and petrissage was associated with almost complete resolution of the tingling and numbness and pain of a patient with grade 2 chemotherapy-induced peripheral neuropathy subsequent to prior treatment with docetaxel and cisplatin for stage III esophageal adenocarcinoma. Improvements in superficial temperature as monitored using infrared thermistry were also observed in fingers and toes.

Shin et al. (2015) in a Cochrane review commented that "While we accept that aromatherapy and massage may be a positive experience for some people, we found no evidence to support the use of this intervention for clinical benefit". They expressed the need for well-designed studies to give some definitive answer to the question of effectiveness both in terms of clinical results and cost-effectiveness.

These studies indicate that massage therapy has the potential to bring about improvement in the symptoms of the patients afflicted with cancer and it can be used as a palliative therapeutic aid in the overall care of cancer patients, especially at the end of life in an attempt to improve the quality of life. However, the massage therapy is not entirely risk-free and it can also be associated with increased risks in the oncology population (Corbin, 2005). Thus, it is important that the adverse effects and the contraindications of massage be kept in mind while using this therapy in terminally ill patients.

The contraindications of the massage which have high degree of possibility of presence in the cancer patients include thrombosis, and bleeding tendencies owing to reduced platelets counts. Further care must be taken to avoid injury to tissues damaged by surgery or radiation therapy. Weiger et al. (2002) in a review article on the use of complementary therapies in cancer observed that though no evidence indicates that massage promotes tumor metastasis, it is prudent to avoid massage directly over known tumors or even predictable metastasis and special caution should be exercised in patients with bony metastases as they are prone to fracture. Likewise, massage should also be avoided over stents or other prosthetic devices because of obvious danger of displacement (Kerr, 1997).

According to Weiger et al. (2002), if the described precautions are observed, available evidence suggests that it is reasonable to accept the use of massage for relief of anxiety and as adjunct therapy for lymphedema.

MASSAGE AND HYPERTENSION

Long-term unchecked, stress response is implicated as a causative factor for hypertension. The relaxation response elicited by the massage has been suggested to aid in the reduction of hypertension. This hypothesis was investigated by Olney (2005) who examined the effects of a regularly applied back massage on the blood pressure of patients with clinically diagnosed hypertension. A 10-minute back massage was given to the experimental group (n = 8) three times a week for 10 sessions. The control group (n = 6) relaxed in the same environment for 10 minutes, three times a week for 10 sessions. Statistical analysis showed reduction of both systolic and diastolic blood pressure in the massage group with effect size 2.25 for systolic pressure and 1.56 for diastolic pressure (alpha of 0.05 and power at 0.80). This preliminary study suggests that regular massage may lower blood pressure in hypertensive persons. Holland and Pokorny (2003) also reported a significant decrease in systolic and diastolic blood pressure after slow stroking back massage in the adults patients admitted in a rehabilitation setting. In this study, a statistically significant decrease in mean heart rate and mean respiratory rate was also observed.

Reduction in BP following massage has also been reported in subsequent studies (Aourell et al., 2005; Cambron et al., 2006; Basler, 2011; Moeini et al., 2011; Givi, 2013; Supa'at et al., 2013; Mohebbi et al., 2014; Walaszek, 2015).

Cambron et al. (2006) compared the effect of Swedish massage, trigger point therapy, and sports massage on 150 current adults with BP lower than 150/95 mm Hg and reported that while Swedish massage resulted in BP reduction, the trigger point therapy and sports massage increased the systolic BP. They suggested that type of massage was the main factor affecting change in BP with potentially painful massage techniques tends to increase the BP.

Basler (2011) reported a similar reduction in BP in prehypertensive individual after a 1 hour of Abhyanga—the classic Ayurvedic oil massage. He also reported a reduction of HR and clinically significant reduction in subjective stress experience.

Givi (2013) conducted a single-blind clinical trial on fifty prehypertensive women to evaluate the effect of Swedish massage (face, neck, shoulders, and chest) on BP in comparison to simple rest. The massage group received Swedish massage for 10–15 minutes, 3 times a week for 10 sessions and the control groups were relaxed at the same environment without receiving massage. BP was measured before and after each session and 72 hours after finishing the massage therapy. They reported that in comparison with the control group, mean systolic and diastolic BP in the massage group was significantly lower, and significant difference between the test and control groups in systolic and diastolic BP persisted at 72 hours after finishing the study. Moeini et al. (2011) reported the similar observations.

Supa'at et al. (2013) in a randomized control trial compared the effects of whole body SMT (massage group) with simple resting (control group) for an hour per week for four weeks on hypertensive women. The massage protocol was an hour of Swedish massage therapy to the whole body, once a week for 4 weeks. The massage techniques used were a combination of *petrissage* or kneading, *tapotement* or beating/hacking/cupping, and *effleurage* applied at medium pressure. Olive oil was used as the lubricant. Along with blood pressure (BP) and heart rate (HR), the researchers also measured endothelial inflammatory markers: Vascular endothelial adhesion molecule-1 (VCAM-1) and intracellular adhesion molecule-1 (ICAM-1). They hypothesized that increased blood flow following massage would increases shear stress on the blood vessel wall, which, in turn, would reduces the expression of VCAM-1 and increases ICAM-1. They reported that after four sessions, massage group showed significant systolic BP reduction of 12 mm Hg and diastolic BP reduction of 5 mm Hg. VCAM-1 showed significant reduction after four sessions, but there were no changes in ICAM-1. However, in any of the studied parameter, significant difference between the massage and rest group was not observed.

Mohebbi et al. (2014) reported the similar reduction in hypertension after a 10-minute Swedish back massage. They observed that after back massage, systolic and diastolic blood pressure decreased to 6.44 mm Hg and 4.77 mm Hg, respectively.

Walaszek (2015) suggested that classic massage might provide a safe supportive measure in pharmacologic treatment of hypertension. In this study, the impact of 10 sessions of classic massage on blood pressure alteration was assessed in women aged 60–68 years with previously diagnosed hypertension. Ten sessions of classic massage of the lower limbs were performed on the subjects and blood pressure was measured 1 minute before the massage, as well as 1 minute and 5 minutes after each session. In massage of the lower limbs, the following techniques were used in sequence: Stroking (10% of the total time of the massage session; 5% at the beginning of the session and the other 5% at the end), rubbing (30% of the total time of the massage session), kneading (40%), vibration (10%), and skin rolling (10%). The author reported that for ten consecutive days, the blood pressure values in the examined women were found decreasing.

However, Walaszek et al. (2013) *observed that* classic back massage made no significant difference to blood pressure of the male subjects, though the patient felt more relaxed after ten classic back massage sessions.

In a systematic review, Xiong et al. (2015) reported that meta-analysis of twenty four articles involving 1,962 patients with essential hypertension (EH) demonstrated that massage combined with antihypertensive drugs may be more effective than antihypertensive drugs alone in lowering both systolic BP and diastolic BP.

Liao et al. (2016) performed a meta-analysis to evaluate the evidence concerning the effect of massage on blood pressure in patients with hypertension or prehypertension where they assessed the methodological quality of nine randomized controlled trials using the Cochrane Collaboration tool. They observed a medium effect of massage on SBP and a small effect on DBP in patients with hypertension or prehypertension. The data suggested that massage contributes to significantly enhanced reduction in both systolic blood pressure (SBP) (7.39 mm Hg) and diastolic blood pressure (DBP) (5.04 mm Hg) as compared with control treatments. They expressed the need of the high-quality randomized controlled trials to confirm these results.

There is no clear explanation in literature with regard to the mechanism through which massage may reduce blood pressure. Nelson (2015) in a thematic analysis of 27 publications identified six potential BP-mediating pathways through which massage therapy may exerts its effects on hypertension. According to this study, massage exerts sympatholytic effects through physiological and psychological mechanisms, improves hypothalamus-pituitary-adrenocortical axis function, and increases in blood flow, which, in turn, may improve endothelial function.

It is postulated that massage helps in reducing anxiety and stress which may decrease sympathetic activity and increase parasympathetic activity which may contribute to blood pressure reduction. It is important to note that none of studies so far have reported any adverse effect of massage on hypertensive persons. This suggests that the classic massage could be a safe supportive measure in pharmacologic treatment of hypertension (Walaszek et al., 2015). However, in view of available medium quality evidence, better designed trials are needed to establish classical massage as therapeutic adjunct for hypertension.

CHAPTER 4

Contraindications

Contraindications are the conditions in which one should not administer a particular therapeutic modality. Before the application of any therapeutic agent, its contraindications must be ruled out scrupulously, otherwise the treatment may not only be ineffective, it may also be harmful.

Generally, massage is considered as a safe treatment modality. Quite often, laymen who do not have much knowledge of body structure and function practice it. However, treatment by massage as such is not completely in free from risk. There are several conditions where application of massage may prove to be counterproductive. Myositis ossificans after vigorous massage to the fracture around elbow is a very common occurrence in those areas where traditionally massage is used in each and every condition of pain and locomotor dysfunction.

In a literature review, Ernst (2003) observed that even though the occurrence of serious adverse events with massage is not very common, this modality cannot be considered as entirely risk-free. The review listed about 23 papers that recorded the adverse events occurred during the execution of massage. These events include cerebrovascular accidents, displacement of a ureteral stent, embolization of a kidney, hematoma, leg ulcers, nerve damage, posterior interosseous syndrome, pseudoaneurysm, pulmonary embolism, ruptured uterus, strangulation of neck, thyrotoxicosis, and various pain syndromes. Serious adverse effects were associated mostly with exotic types of manual massage techniques rather than "Swedish" massage. The massage delivered by the laymen was also found associated with majority of the complications.

Tak et al. (2012) reported an incidence of peripheral embolization after an abdominal massage. A 65-year-old man developed acute-onset pain in toes of the right foot immediately after an abdominal massage by a "local healer". The patient had dyspepsia for 5 days and consulted a local healer. The healer gave him a vigorous and deep abdominal massage for 5 minutes in the epigastric and umbilical areas with the heel of his hand. The patient developed pain and a burning sensation in the right foot within a few minutes. This case highlights the risk of an apparently safe, and harmless-looking abdominal massage.

Ryu et al. (2018) reported a case of epidural hematoma that occurred in the anterior spinal cord after receiving a cervical spine massage. A 38-year-old male patient was admitted to the emergency department for sudden weakness in the lower extremity. There was no fracture but in cervical magnetic resonance imaging, an acute epidural hematoma was observed in the anterior spinal cord from the C6 and C7 vertebrae to the T1 vertebra, compressing the spinal cord. Patient recovered on its own after 7 days.

In a systematic review, Yin et al. (2014) observed that massage therapies are not totally devoid of risks, but the incidence of such events is low. Disk herniation, soft tissue trauma, neurologic compromise, spinal cord injury, and dissection of the vertebral arteries were the main complications of massage.

Therefore, ascertaining that patient/subject is free from any such condition, where massage may provoke adverse effects should be the first and foremost step for massage treatment. Several of these contraindications are present in even otherwise normal adult and babies. So, not only in ailing people but also in normal persons, the contraindications should be ruled out meticulously.

The contraindications of massage can be divided into two broad categories—(1) general and (2) local. In general contraindications, those conditions are included in which massage must not be given to any part of the body whereas in the local contraindications, those conditions are included in which a particular area of the body affected by a condition must not be massaged, but massage can be done to other unaffected parts of the body.

This chapter presents a detailed discussion on each contraindication. Most of these contraindications are based on theoretical assumptions and personal experience of clinicians. The nature of exact harm caused by application of massage in many of these conditions cannot precisely be proved for want of scientific literature on this topic. Many experienced clinicians may opt to administer massage in several conditions described as contraindication in this chapter. However, the purpose of this chapter is not to challenge them, but only to rationalize the practice of massage and safeguard the interest of newcomers to the profession.

GENERAL CONTRAINDICATIONS

These are the conditions where the application of massage to any part of the body is not without risk. Therefore, even before physical examination and positioning of patients, one should ensure that he/she is not afflicted with any general contraindication of massage **(Table 4.1)**.

High Fever

Fever is the generalized rise of body temperature. It is one of the systemic manifestations of the inflammation. Massage is not indicated in high fever as it may increase the overall body temperature (Liston, 1995). This will further increase the metabolic rate which is already elevated due to fever.

It is, however, seen that during fever, light massage of the hip, back, and lower limbs in the form of squeezing, gentle kneading, and superficial stroking has a relaxing effect and in India, this is regularly used in the household practice.

Nevertheless, there are certain conditions associated with high fever where the application of massage produces damage to the underlying tissues. In the acute stage of poliomyelitis,

Table 4.1: Contraindications of massage.

General contraindications	Local contraindications
High fever	Acute inflammation
Severe renal or cardiac diseases	Skin diseases
Deep X-ray therapy	Recent fractures
Osteoporosis	Severe varicose veins
Severe spasticity	Atherosclerosis
Very hairy skin	Thrombosis
Patient's preference	Myositis ossificans Malignancy Open wound Poisonous foci Other conditions

characterized by high fever and acute tenderness of joints and muscles, complete rest is required as any trauma to the tender muscle may result in the complete loss of function in that muscle.

Acute flare-up of systemic arthropathies is also characterized by high fever where massage may accentuate the inflammatory response and leads to exaggeration of the symptoms.

Therefore, the application of massage in the presence of fever should be judged meticulously and if at all administered, it should be done very carefully, so that it does not compromise the tissue function.

Severe Renal and Cardiac Diseases

Edema is a feature of renal and cardiac conditions as evident in cardiac failure (peripheral edema) and in nephrotic syndrome (generalized edema).

Generalized increase in venous pressure is a feature of cardiac failure where the raised pressure at the venous end of capillaries counteracts the osmotic pressure of the plasma protein, and impedes the reabsorption of the tissue fluid leading to the production of edema. In renal failure, there occurs an increase in the concentration of sodium ions in tissue fluid owing to increased salt retention by distal tubules of kidney which increases its osmotic pressure. This interferes with the reabsorption of fluid and edema results. Unlike gravitational edema or paralytic edema, in the abovementioned conditions, massage will not be of much help to decrease the edema as the cause of edema is not mechanical, but the individual pathology of the involved systems.

Further, in terminal stages of these disorders, patient may present with vascular disorders like thrombosis, atherosclerosis, etc. where massage may provoke serious consequences like pulmonary embolism. Chest percussion has adverse effects, as it may provoke the onset of cardiac arrhythmia and subsequent fall in cardiac output and partial pressure of oxygen in blood. These effects may prove to be fatal in severe cardiac diseases. Moreover, the different positionings adopted during the massage treatment may also not be suitable for these patients. Therefore, it is not wise to practice the massage techniques for patients suffering from severe renal and cardiac disorders.

Deep X-ray Therapy

Deep radiotherapy has a devitalizing effect on the body tissues. In all irradiated tissues, be it normal or abnormal, the vascular changes are prominent. During immediate postirradiation period, vessels may show only dilation. Later on or with higher dose immediately after sometime, a variety of regressive changes appears which range from endothelial cell swelling to the total necrosis of the wall of the small vessels (capillary and venules). Affected vessels may thrombose or even rupture leading to hemorrhage (Robbins and Kumar, 1987).

In this stage, tissues will not sustain any kind of mechanical trauma. Since massage is mechanical in nature, tissues may react abnormally during manipulations leading to more harmful effects. Therefore, massage should not be given to a patient who underwent deep X-ray therapy.

Osteoporosis

Osteoporosis is a bone disease characterized by a decrease in the absolute amount of bone mass sufficient to render the skeleton vulnerable to fractures. The skeleton becomes fragile and may not tolerate the pressure and force (whatever minimal it may be to a normal skeleton) applied to body during maneuvers like kneading, vibration, tapotement, etc. Due to lack of structural stability of bone, even a minimal trauma can produce fracture. One must be very cautious while applying massage to the suspected cases of osteoporosis (e.g., old age group, postmenopausal women, patient on prolonged steroid therapy, etc.).

In fact, all passive procedures of physiotherapy (mobilization, massage, or manipulation) should be administered with caution in all the other conditions also where the bones become fragile (e.g., osteomalacia, Paget's diseases, osteogenesis imperfecta, etc.).

Severe Spasticity

Spasticity is the abnormal increased tone of muscles due to lesion of upper motor neuron. This is the characteristic feature of all upper motor neuron lesion (UMNL) including hemiplegia, cerebral palsy, spinal cord injury, multiple sclerosis, etc. Massage should not be used in these conditions.

The muscle tone is maintained by muscle spindles. The sensitivity of muscle spindles is maintained by alpha and gamma fibers which keep them sensitive to stretch. In UMNL, the fusimotor activity is increased and therefore, the threshold of intrafusal muscle fiber to stretch stimulus is decreased. Even a minimal amount of stretch (exerted by massage or otherwise) can activate the myotatic reflex arc and provoke hypertonicity, spasm, and flexor withdrawal.

Further, the abnormal handling, pain, and discomfort have all been found to increase the spasticity. Massage may provoke all these factors and may increase the tone of the spastic muscles. Though the studies have shown that massage can decrease the activity of alpha motor neurons leading to decrease in muscle tone in healthy subjects (*see* Chapter 2), these findings cannot be generalized to neurological patient as the behavior of neural tissue changes drastically in diseased state and is not yet properly understood.

The only study that investigated the effect of deep massage on the neurologically impaired individuals reported an average decrease in the amplitude of H-reflex, though this response was not uniform (Goldberg et al., 1994). In some subjects, the H-reflex was increased even up to 80%. This highlights the need of further investigation before the massage is considered in the management of UMNL.

Very Hairy Skin

Rubbing the hairy skin especially opposite to the direction of the hair follicle is painful. Usually, massage is not administered to a very hairy skin, but it is a relative contraindication as the excessive hair can be shaved off and the part can be massaged. Heavy oil lubrication of the area prior to massage can also reduce the chance of hair pulling.

Patient's Preference

On account of social, religious, cultural, and personal reasons, some people do not like massage. They also feel embarrassed while exposing the body part during the massage especially if the therapist is of the opposite sex. In these situations, as far as possible, the people's wish must be respected and they should not be forced to undertake massage until it is very essential like in tendon adherence, etc.

LOCAL CONTRAINDICATIONS

In presence of these conditions, the affected body part should not be massaged. However, if required, the techniques can be administered to the other parts of the body. For example, in acute sprain, the ankle should not be approached for massage immediately after the injury, but the thigh and the knee of the athlete can be massaged to promote relaxation, and recovery. These contraindications should be ruled out during pretreatment physical examination of the patient.

Acute Inflammation

Acute inflammation is an absolute local contraindication of massage. The reasons are following:
1. Massage exacerbates the vascular changes taking place during acute inflammatory period, i.e., increased blood flow, vasodilatation as well as increase in vascular permeability and makes the condition worse. As the effect of massage on vasculature is very similar to that occurring during acute inflammation, massage during inflammation (acute phase) will further increase swelling, pain, tenderness, and may lead to more tissue damage.
2. Granulation tissue (formed 48–72 hours after the injury) has a very delicate blood supply which can easily be damaged by movements and shearing forces of massage maneuvers. This interferes with the repair process and delays the healing.

Therefore, massage must not be administered during acute inflammation of tissues by any means.

Skin Diseases

Massage is contraindicated in the presence of infectious skin diseases (Knapp, 1990) like eczema and other weeping conditions characterized by pruritus, edematous vesicle, pustules, and papules for the following reasons:
1. Infection may spread from one part to other
2. Therapist may get cross-infection
3. Massage is painful to the patient.

In an interesting study, Donoyama et al. (2004) demonstrated that bacteria from the client's skin were transferred to the therapist's hands during massage therapy. They obtained medium cultures from the therapist's palms and the client's skin before, during, and after the massage session.

After each massage session, the therapist washed his or her hands and a bacterial sample was again taken. It was observed that the bacteria count on the therapist's palms increased during and after massage whereas the bacteria count on the client's skin decreased during and after massage. After handwashing with water for 20 seconds after each massage session, bacteria were still present on the therapist's palms.

Recent Fractures

Fracture is the break in the continuity of the bone. In initial stage, massage should not be given as it disturbs the healing process (Liston, 1995). The shearing movement of the massage may retard the organization of hematoma and callus formation. It may sever the delicate capillaries as well as the bridging tissues and may damage the flexible granulation tissues that bridge the fracture at an early stage. This may lead to nonunion or malunion. Further, it is very painful and uncomfortable to tolerate massage if administered in the vicinity of a recent fracture.

However, if the fracture is immobilized, massage may be administered to the area proximal to the fracture site. It gives comfort to patient by reducing swelling and relieving tension and pain in the area, but the fractured site must be avoided always.

Varicose Vein

This is a condition in which due to incompetency of valves, veins become dilated and tortuous. This results in the venous congestion and walls of vein become thin. In this condition, massage may provoke complications like hemorrhage and phlebitis.

Thin veins may not tolerate even minor trauma. It may rupture and due to high pressure in congested vessels, profuse bleeding may result. The vein may become extremely tender and firm. Overlying skin becomes red and edematous. So, in severe varicose vein, massage is an absolute contraindication (Liston, 1995).

Thrombosis and Arteriosclerosis

This condition is characterized by formation of fatty plaque in arterial lumen. This is known as thrombus. Massage should not be given in the presence of thrombus as emboli may break off from the wall due to mechanical squeezing of blood vessels. It may travel to some other parts of the body through bloodstream and block the circulation of vital organs, i.e., brain, heart and lungs giving rise to serious consequences (pulmonary embolism).

Myositis Ossificans

In this condition, there occurs callus formation in the soft tissues. The joint capsule and periosteum are stripped from the bone by violent displacement. Blood collects under the stripped soft tissue forming hematoma. The hematoma is invaded by osteoblasts and becomes ossified. This gives rise to limitation of movement and pain. The risk of formation of hematoma should be minimized by ensuring complete rest.

Strain and stretching of soft tissue might provoke further bleeding beneath the soft tissue and may exaggerate the condition. This condition is more common around the elbow joint. So, massage should not be given around elbow joint after any injury.

Malignancy

Metastasis (spread of tumor cells from one area to the other) is the essential feature of all malignant tumors. Tumor cells disseminate through lymphatic and hematogenous pathways. Therefore, anything which increases the lymphatic flow also, increases the chance of spread of tumor. In order to avoid the movement of abnormal cells to other areas, massage is contraindicated in malignant conditions (Liston, 1995; Knapp, 1990).

Weiger et al. (2002) commented that though no evidence indicates that massage promotes tumor metastasis, it is prudent to avoid massage directly over known tumors or even predictable metastasis and special cautions should be exercised in patients with bony metastases as they are prone to fracture.

Open Wound

Massage over open wounds, cuts, and bruises is not only painful, but may further damage the healing tissue. Mechanical movement to wound which massage will produce is an established causative factor for delayed healing of tissue. Therefore, over the damaged skin, massage is a contraindication (Knapp, 1990).

Poisonous Foci

Massage should not be administered in case of snake bite, stings, and insect bites (Liston, 1995). Massage increases the circulation and may facilitate the release of poison into the circulation, leading to serious systemic effects.

Other Conditions

Specialized massage techniques, such as connective tissue massage acupressure, trigger point massage, etc. can elicit adverse autonomic response in pregnancy, cardiorespiratory conditions, and psychological disorders, such as panic attack. Therefore, the specialized techniques of massage should not be administered in these conditions.

CHAPTER 5

Techniques

The nomenclature of basic techniques of the classical massage have remained unchanged for centuries, though a consensus on the exact way of performing these techniques is not available in the literature. Various authors have described the various techniques in different manner. This chapter presents a detailed discussion on each technique of classical massage which includes definition, description, physiological effects, therapeutic uses, specific contraindications, and commonly used variations. The aim is to present all the relevant information about a technique in one place.

The basic techniques of classical massage described in this chapter are:
- Stroking
- Pressure manipulation
- Tapotement
- Vibration

The special techniques of massage, such as connective tissue massage, etc. are not discussed in detail in this book, though an outline of these techniques is presented in a separate chapter.

STROKING GROUP OF MANIPULATION

This group includes two techniques—superficial stroking and deep stroking or effleurage. In both the techniques, one uninterrupted linear movement of hand or its part covers one aspect of a whole segment. The uninterrupted linear movement of hand along the whole length of a segment is called "stroke". The essential features of this group of techniques are even pressure, equal rhythm, and constant contact of therapist's hand with the patient's body. On the basis of amount of pressure applied and the direction of movement of hand, this group consists of two basic techniques:
1. Superficial stroking, and
2. Effleurage or deep stroking

These two techniques can be modified in a number of ways.

Superficial Stroking

It is the rhythmic movement of hand or parts thereof over the skin with the lightest amount of pressure in order to obtain sensory stimulation. The strokes can be applied from proximal to the distal part or *vice versa*. The rate of strokes per minute, i.e., speed can be slow or fast, but the rhythm must be maintained throughout. The variation in the direction and speed of this technique depends on the desired effect.

Technique

Superficial stroking is best performed with the palm of hand or with the pulp of fingers. However, the use of heel of hand, edge of hands, ball of thumb, and knuckles in stroking have also been mentioned by some authors (Kellong, 1919; Wood and Becker, 1981).

Therapist should position himself in a comfortable position. Since, usually the strokes cover the entire length of segment in one go, the walk standing or fall out standing is preferred. In these two positions, the most proximal parts of the segment can be reached with one outstretched and upper limb without putting undue strain on the back of the therapist. Direction of stroking can be centripetal or centrifugal. In the author's opinion, for best effects, it should be performed in centrifugal (i.e., from proximal to distal) direction. Therapist should keep his hand fully relaxed. The fingers should be kept slightly apart and flexible, so that they can be molded according to the contour of the body.

At the beginning of technique, the pulp of right hand of therapist should be placed on the most proximal end of the segment to be massaged; this can be achieved by flexion of right shoulder and extension of right elbow. The left hand should remain in air, it should be placed near to the most distal part of the segment. This can be achieved by flexion of left elbow and extension of left shoulder **(Fig. 5.1)**.

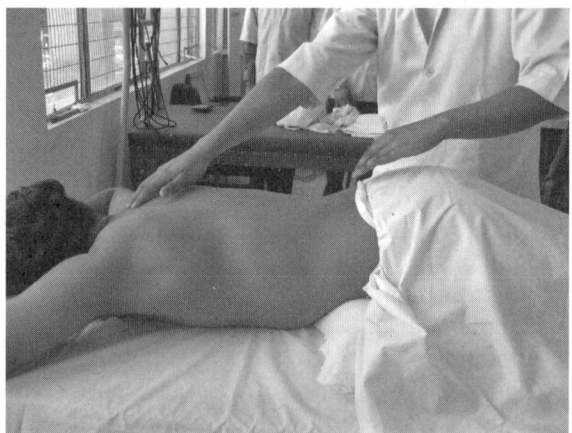

Fig. 5.1: Superficial stroking: Starting position.

The stroke is initiated by controlled extension of right shoulder, so that hand is gently lower down in order to make contact with skin. The contact should be gentle and essentially without any pressure. This "just touch no pressure" contact should be maintained throughout the stroke. Controlled and combined flexion of right elbow and extension of right shoulder ensure the passage of hand over the skin.

As the right hand moves toward the distal part, the left hand should also move in the proximal direction by a controlled and combined extension of left elbow and flexion of left shoulder **(Fig. 5.2)**. This is essential to ensure that at the end of stroke, the position of both the hands is reversed, i.e., left hand assumes the proximal position and right hand comes near the distal most part, so that when right hand breaks the contact with the most distal part, left hand immediately establishes the contact with proximal part and starts the stroke **(Fig. 5.3)**. The stroke should end with a smooth lift of hand. The movement of two upper extremities should be well-timed and controlled in order

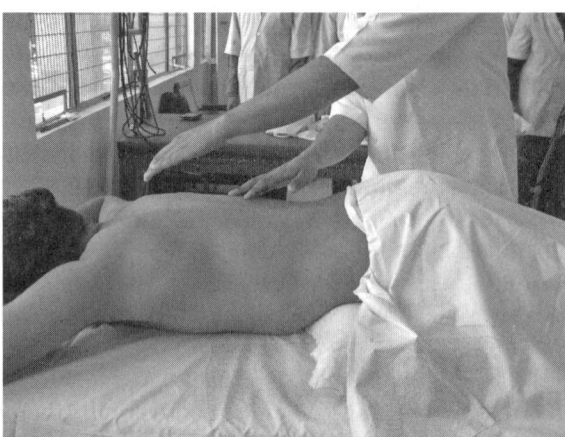

Fig. 5.2: Superficial stroking: While proximal hand goes down, the distal hand moves up but does not touch the skin.

to ensure that at no time, both the hands neither make nor break the contact with skin simultaneously. And at a time, only one hand slides over the patient's skin. Making and breaking of contact should be very gentle, so that patient does not perceive the change of hand.

This alternate movement of right and left hands over the skin must be performed with a constant rate or rhythm. Mennell's recommended a rate of 15 strokes/min for stroking from shoulder to hand, whereas Wood and Becker determined that movement of hand at the rate of seven inches per second produced the desired effects. However, depending upon the desired effects, the rate can be varied. The slower strokes (12–15 strokes/min) are more sedative while for stimulating effects, faster strokes (30–40 strokes/min) should be preferred.

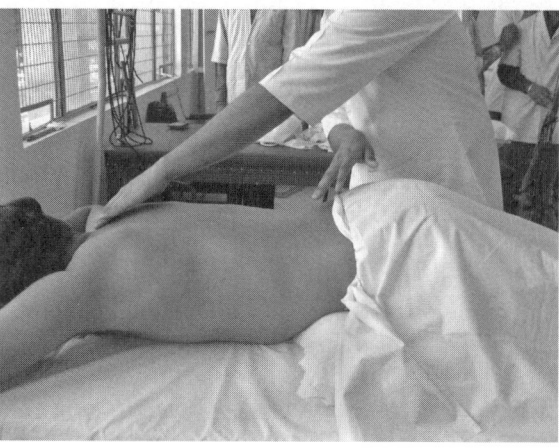

Fig. 5.3: Superficial stroking: Finish—note the complete reversal of the position of hands of therapist.

Variation

The stroking may be performed using:
- Entire palm—over the broad and highly muscular areas, i.e., back, thigh.
- Knuckles—seldom used in massage treatment except in stimulating massage of back. It can be used in sports massage set up.
- Ball of thumb—it can be used over confined area.

Techniques of Thousand Hands

In this technique, the entire length or segment is not covered in one stroke. Rather, the technique involves several small and overlapping strokes. Strokes are applied with both the hands wherein strokes of one hand overlap with the strokes of other hand and the strokes moved down to cover the entire length of part. It is used for relaxation (Hollis, 1987).

Physiological Effects

1. Superficial stroking stimulates the cutaneous touch receptors. It has a sedative effect on the body and if applied in a proper manner, it has soothing and reposing effects.
2. Superficial stroking also indirectly improves the circulation by activating the axon reflex.
3. It exerts a facilitatory effect on the motoneuron pool and facilitates the contraction of the muscles. Superficial stroking, if performed faster, can have a stimulating effect as against the relaxing effect, when it is done slowly.

Therapeutic Uses

a. In patient's assessment, information about contour, texture, tone, temperature, etc. can be obtained by superficial stroking which can be used both to identify the problem area and to determine the effect of treatment used.
b. It is used owing to its sedative effect.
   1. Prior to any massage procedure, to relax the muscles, and to accustom the patient to manual contact.
   2. In sleeplessness, gentle stroking of the forehead and the back offers great relief.

3. In anxiety, tension, and psychological stress, slow rhythmic stroking for a prolonged period can be very useful.
4. In hypersensitivity, stroking is used to decrease the hypersensitivity of part. In nerve injuries and after amputation, phantom limb, the patient is asked to do frequently stroking of the part. This accustoms the part to touch and desensitizes the hypersensitive areas.

c. Owing to its facilitatory stimulating effect, fast stroking is used in all facilitation techniques to elicit contraction in the hypotonic muscles.

Cautions

This technique is a light and stimulating maneuver. This may produce a ticklish sensation. So, it should not be applied in:
1. A hypersensitive person where this may produce unwanted and excessive tickling.
2. Severe spasticity where superficial stroking may elicit flexor withdrawal.

Effleurage or Deep Stroking

It is the movement of the palmar aspect of hand over the external surface of the body with constant moderate pressure in the direction of the venous and lymphatic drainage.

It is one of the main maneuvers of massage. In fact, every massage begins and ends with effleurage. It is a maneuver in which the relaxed hand of therapist slides over the patient's skin with firm pressure without attempting to move the deep muscle mass. The strokes are applied in the direction of the lymphatic and venous drainage. Each stroke begins from the distal end of the segment and is completed at the proximal end usually at the site of a group of lymph nodes. The direction of movement of hand in this technique is always from distal to proximal. Contact and continuity must be even throughout the stroke.

Technique

Depending upon the area being massaged, the effleurage can be performed with one or both hand(s). Usually, the palmar aspects of hand, fingers, or thumb are used.

The therapist should be positioned in a comfortable stance. Like superficial stroking, in this technique also, the entire length of segment is covered in one go. Therefore, the walk standing position is preferred. This not only ensures a better reach of the distal part, but also facilitates sufficient and controlled application of pressure without putting undue strain on the back of therapist.

The hand/hand(s) of therapist should be relaxly placed over the distal most part of the segment to be massaged. It should be molded to the contour of the part, so that all parts of hand maintain an even contact with the skin. Stroke is initiated with the combined and controlled flexion of shoulder and extension of elbow, to slide the hand forward over the skin in the distal to proximal direction. Pressure is applied by transfer of the body weight to the subject's skin through the upper extremity of therapist (**Fig. 5.4**). At no time, the therapist should use muscle force from upper extremity to apply pressure. This is tiresome and effleurage cannot be performed for a longer duration.

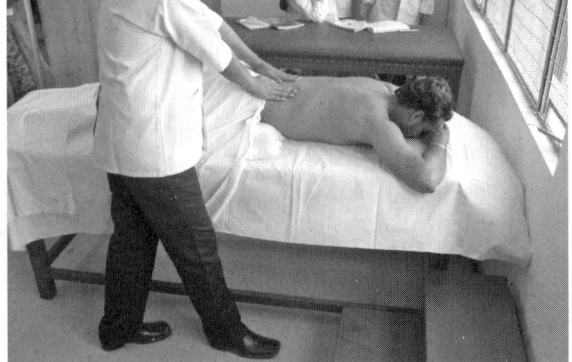

Fig. 5.4: Effleurage of back: Initial stance.

The hand of therapist should remain rather relaxed and as the strokes advance forward, its shape should be molded to maintain a perfect and even contact with the skin according to the variation of the shape of body part. As the hand moves forward, the body weight should also be shifted from rearfoot to the front foot in order to ensure an even application of pressure to the skin. This can be achieved by either controlled flexion of the knee of forefoot or by lifting the heel of rearfoot by plantar flexion. Toward the end of stroke, weight should be completely transferred to the front foot from the rearfoot **(Fig. 5.5)**. Stroke is terminated with a little overpressure near the lymph node. After this, the hand is brought back to its starting position with a returning stroke. Controlled extension of shoulder and flexion of elbow execute this returning stroke.

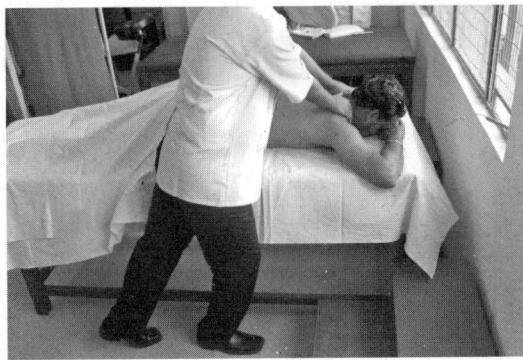

Fig. 5.5: Effleurage of back finish: Note that the rearfoot is plantar flexed to apply compression without bending the spine.

At the end of restoring stroke, the foreknee comes back in extended position and the rear heel touches the ground.

This returning stroke is essentially a superficial stroking where no pressure is applied to the skin. If pressure is applied during returning strokes, it will interfere with the venous and lymphatic refilling and will decrease the effect of effleurage. Few authorities also advocate that while returning back to its previous position, the hand should remain in air. While this ensures no pressure on skin, it can only be used when one hand is used for stroking. When both the hands are used in same direction, the lifting of hand while returning will break the continuity of contact.

The pressure applied during each effleurage stroke should be as deep as can be applied without causing discomfort to the patient. The rate of stroking should essentially be slow (10–12 strokes/min) in order to allow sufficient time for refilling of the venous and lymphatic channels.

As the direction of effleurage is similar to that of venous and lymphatic drainage, the therapist should be thorough with the anatomy of venous and lymphatic systems.

Variation

The basic technique of effleurage described above can be modified in the following ways depending on the area to be treated:

1. Both hands can be used on the opposite aspect of the segment, such as medial and lateral aspects of thigh.
2. One hand may follow the other with both the hands ending stroke within a short interval of time **(Fig. 5.6)**.
3. Only one hand can be used. The other hand is used to support or change the position of massaged segment. This variation is suitable for the upper limb **(Fig. 5.7)**.

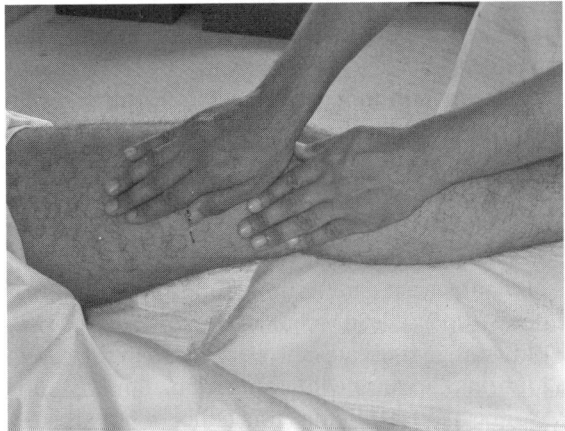

Fig. 5.6: Both hands effleurage: Right hand follows the left hand.

4. Limbs can be held in the first web space between the thumb and other fingers, so that the hand assumes the shape of letter "C" **(Fig. 5.8)**.
5. Indian effleurage: In this variation of effleurage, the direction of stroke is reversed, the extremity is grasped with C grasp, and pressure is applied from proximal to distal part. It is most commonly used over babies. It is claimed that this technique improves the flow of arterial blood to the massaged part. However, this variation of effleurage has no place in the classical therapeutic massage.
6. Cross-hand effleurage or effleurage of knee: For the drainage of areas surrounding knee joint, special positioning of hands is used. Both the hands are placed just above patella in such a way that they cross each other without overlapping **(Fig. 5.9A)**. During effleurage, both the hands are drawn backward **(Fig. 5.9B)** on each side till their heels come in contact with each other just below patella **(Fig. 5.9C)**. Thereafter, the fingers are moved forward and posteriorly to terminate the stroke in the popliteal fossa (behind the knee) **(Fig. 5.9D)**.

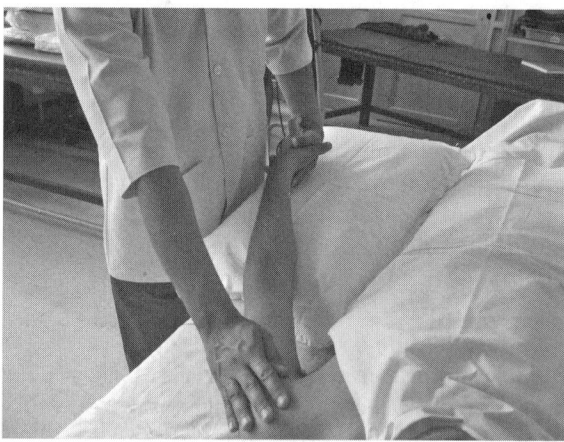

Fig. 5.7: Upper limb effleurage: One hand changes the position of patient's limb while the other executes stroke.

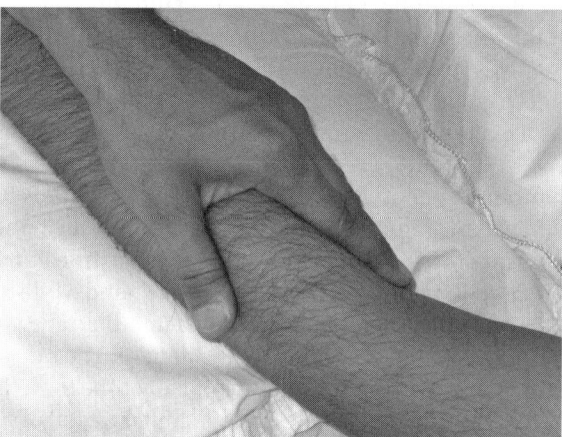

Fig. 5.8: C grasp for forearm effleurage.

Physiological Effects

The effects of effleurage are more pronounced on the circulation to the area and skin of the massaged area.
1. Effleurage produces squeezing of the veins and lymphatics and forces the venous and lymphatic fluids toward the heart. As a result of which:
   a. The chance of accumulation of waste is prevented/minimized
   b. Stagnation of blood and lymph is reduced
   c. Improves venous and lymphatic drainage
   d. Reduces edema
2. Effleurage has a mild stimulating effect on the vasomotor nerves supplying the blood vessels and skin and leads to elicitation of axon reflex.
3. Effleurage facilitates the circulation in the capillaries.
4. It brings about the liberation of histamine (substance) due to the stimulation of mast cells and causes erythema (this effect of effleurage varies from individual-to-individual and is maximum when the therapist's hands are tense; increasing friction between the hand of therapist and the skin of patient).

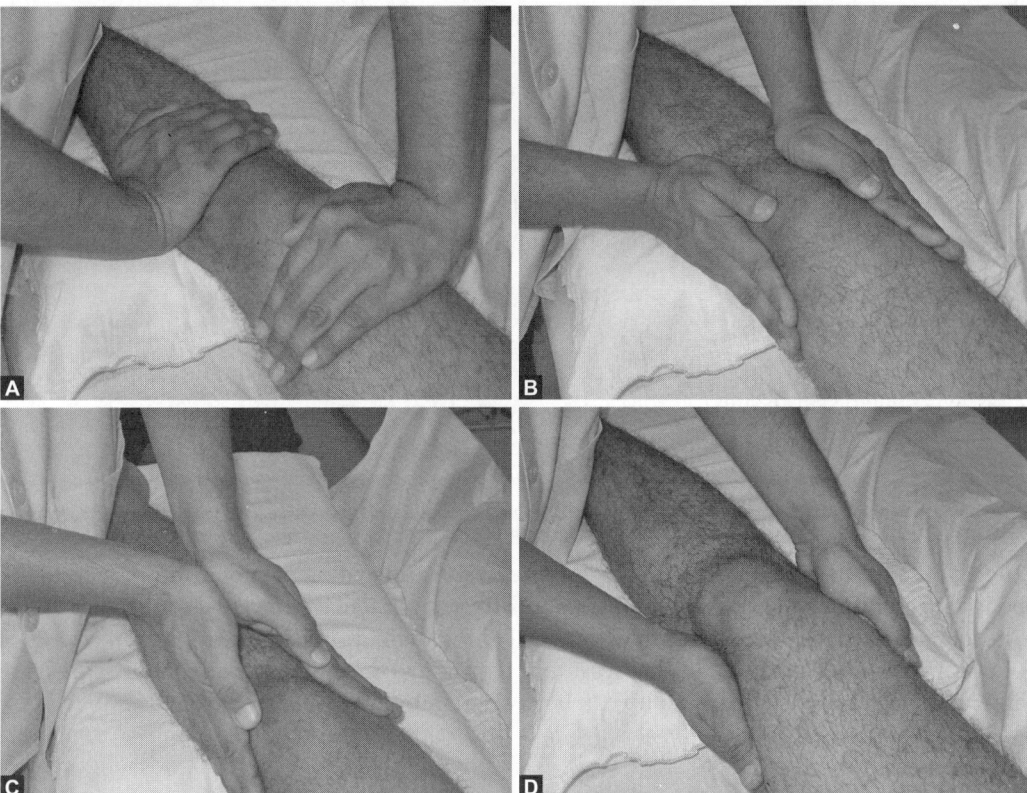

Figs. 5.9A to D: Effleurage to knee. (A) Initial position of hands; (B) Movement of hands toward patella; (C) Heels of both the hands almost come in contact with each other near the tibial tuberosity; and (D) End of the stroke directed at popliteal fossa.

5. Effects 2, 3, and 4 collectively improve arterial circulation which overall improves the nutrition of the part.
6. Improved lymphatic and venous drainage resulting from effleurage may increase the venous return and cardiac output to a slight extent.
7. By exerting a stretching effect on the subcutaneous tissue, effleurage improves the elasticity and the mobility of the skin.
8. Stimulation of touch and pressure receptors during effleurage brings about a sedative effect which serves to sooth, decrease pain, and lessen muscle tension.
9. It facilitates the removal of dead cells of skin and improves the activity of sweat and sebaceous glands.

Therapeutic Uses

1. To search for the area of muscle spasm, soreness, and trigger points that help determine the further management.
2. To reduce edema in:
   - Mild varicose ulcer
   - Gravitational edema and paralytic edema associated with paralysis and muscle weakness
   - Radical mastectomy, etc.

3. To assist the absorption and removal of metabolites and inflammatory products in:
   - Muscle fatigue following severe exercise
   - Subacute and chronic inflammation
   - Soft tissue injuries
4. To accustom the patient to the touch of the therapist and to evenly distribute the lubricant over skin if used.
5. To link up and join various manipulations during massage.
6. To lessen the negative effects of immobility and lethargy associated with psychological distress (Liston, 1995).

Specific Contraindications

In conditions where there is a danger of peeling off of the skin, effleurage should not be used, e.g.,
- Newly healed scar tissues
- Recent skin grafts
- Open wounds

PRESSURE MANIPULATIONS

The essential feature of this group of techniques is the application of deep compression to the body with constant touch. These techniques are directed particularly toward the muscular tissue. The maximum mechanical movement between different fibers is achieved in these techniques by the application of deep localized pressure. According to the nature and direction of pressure application, techniques of this group can be divided into three major subgroups:
  i. Kneading
 ii. Petrissage
iii. Friction

These techniques produce almost similar physiological effects on the soft tissue. Kneading and petrissage involve application of intermittent pressure, whereas in friction, the application of pressure is constant.

Kneading

In this technique, tissues are pressed down onto the underlying structures and pressure is applied in a circular way along the long axis of the underlying bone, so that the comparison is vertical. The pressure is increased and decreased in a gradual manner.

Relaxed hands are placed over the skin. The tissues are compressed against the bone and the hands are moved in a circular direction, so that the deeper tissues are compressed and moved in a circular way. The hands should be placed firmly on the skin, so that the movement can take place only in the deeper structure and not over the skin.

The whole maneuver consists of several small concentric circles performed parallel to the body surface and each circle overlaps the previous one. The pressure is gradually increased during one-half of the circle till it reaches to the maximum level at the top of the circle. Similarly, during the other half, pressure is decreased gradually till it reaches a minimum at the bottom of the circle. Thus, each circle has two phases:
1. Phase of compression
2. Phase of relaxation.

During the phase of relaxation, where the pressure reaches the minimum, the hand slides smoothly to the adjoining next area.

The body weight is used to apply the pressure. The therapist usually adopts a walk standing stance and applies the pressure by shifting the body weight alternately on both the legs.

Therapist may begin the kneading either from proximal or distal part of the segment, but the increasing pressure should always be applied in centripetal (i.e., proximal to distal) direction (Wood and Becker, 1981). For example, in treating an extremity, the kneading may be started from the proximal part and each succeeding movement proceeds over the adjacent distal area or vice versa. If kneading starts at proximal end, pressure should be applied in latter half when hand relaxes to proximal position. If the kneading starts from distal end, the pressure should be applied in the initial half when hand moves to the proximal position (**Fig. 5.10**).

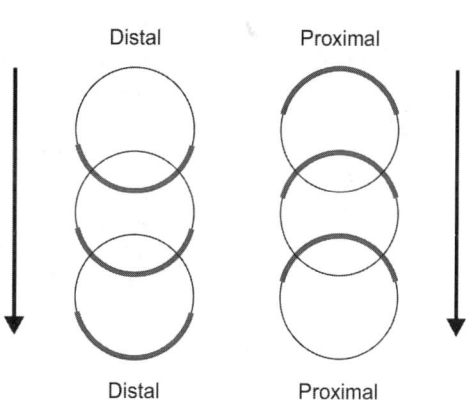

Fig. 5.10: Circular movement of kneading where pressure increase in one-half and decrease in other half. Direction of the pressure is always centripetal.

The small circular movement of kneading can be performed with part of fingers, thumb, or palm of one or both the hand(s). When using both hands, either both the hands can make the circle simultaneously or alternately. One hand may support the tissue while other hand makes the circles. Depending on the size of area to be massaged either whole finger, thumb, or a part thereof can be used to make circles.

According to part of hand used during maneuver, the kneading can be classified in the following three techniques:
1. Palmar kneading
2. Digital kneading
3. Reinforced kneading

Each technique can be varied in a number of ways.

Palmar Kneading

It is performed with either whole of palmar or with the heel of hand. It can be performed with one or both hands and usually used over the large areas, such as thigh, calf, arm, etc.

Technique

Therapist positions himself in a comfortable position. Walk standing is preferred. Both the palms are placed relaxly on the opposite aspect of limb segment (e.g., right hand on the medial and left hand on the lateral aspect of thigh). The fingers and thumb are not kept in contact with the skin (**Fig. 5.11**).

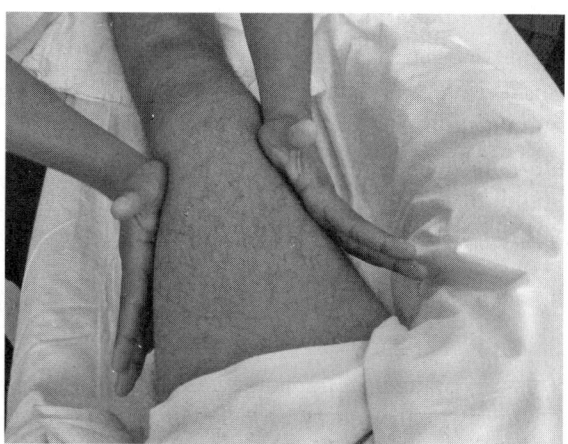

Fig. 5.11: Both hands palmar kneading: Fingers and thumb are off contact with thigh.

Manipulation is initiated by making a small circle first with one hand than with other hand without applying any pressure. This no pressure circle helps to coordinate the action of two hands and to assess the condition of part to be massaged.

Circular movement of palm over skin is produced by the coordinated flexion and extension of shoulder combined with elevation and depression of scapula. It is the shoulder girdle where therapist produces the actual movement. Position of hand over skin should not be changed and throughout the maneuver, the hand and skin should move as one.

After ensuring that both hands can perform coordinated circular movement, the therapist proceeds to perform actual kneading movement. Both the hands make circle in opposite direction (i.e., clockwise with right hand, anticlockwise with left hand). Pressure is applied to the circle by transferring the body weight in such a way that during one-half, the pressure builds up gradually out while in another half, it recedes gradually. When the pressure reaches to it minimum at the bottom of circle, therapist slides his hand over the skin by gentle flexion or extension of elbow in order to perform next circle over the adjoining area. He should ensure that next circle should also overlap at least half area of the previous circle.

This process is repeated and the hand is advanced to cover the entire length of the segment.

The rate of making circle and application of intermitted pressure should be kept constant. Slower rates allow better penetration to the deeper tissue.

Digital Kneading

In this group, the kneading movements are executed either with thumb or fingers and accordingly there are following two subcategories of this group:
a. Finger kneading
b. Thumb kneading

Finger Kneading

This technique utilizes the contact of palmar aspect of either whole finger or a part thereof to apply pressure. Only one finger may be utilized or two or three fingers can be used together to increase the contact area. Little finger is usually not used, considering its short length and inability to apply sufficient pressure. Depending on the part of finger which remains in contact with skin during kneading, this has following subgroups:

Whole Finger Kneading

Otherwise also called flat finger kneading, this technique is usually performed with palmar surface of 2, 3, and 4 digits which are held together to make a broad contact area. The thumb and palm remain off the contact with skin. This is usually applied over the less muscular or poorly padded area, i.e., mandibles **(Fig. 5.12)**.

Finger Pad Kneading

This technique uses the contact of pulp of finger which is otherwise called finger pad and more appropriately can be described as the palmar surface of distal phalanx. Depending upon the area to

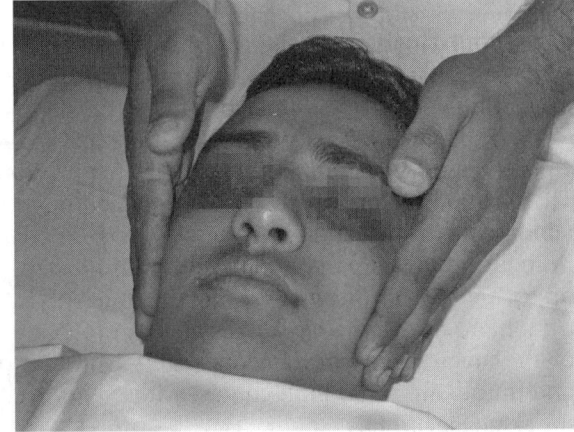

Fig. 5.12: Whole finger kneading over mandible: All the fingers are joined together to increase the contact area.

be massaged, either one finger can be used or two or three can be held together to cover the larger area. During this technique, the distal interphalangeal (DIP) and proximal interphalangeal (PIP) joints of the kneading finger should be kept little flexed in order to allow adequate contact of pulp with skin and to relieve strain of ligaments of interphalangeal (IP) joint **(Fig. 5.13)**.

It is used around the joint line, extensive scar, and along the line of ligaments.

Fingertip Kneading

In this technique, only tip of the pulp remains in contact with skin. Usually done with only one or two fingers, this technique is the technique of choice when kneading needs to be performed over a localized area, e.g., long and narrow interosseous space and over localized thickening fibrositis nodules **(Fig. 5.14)**.

Thumb Kneading

Depending upon the size of area to be treated, the pulp or the tip of one or both thumbs may be used to knead. Alternately, one thumb may be placed over the other to reinforce the moving in contact thumb, the other finger should either remain off the contact with skin or be placed on little away from the area to be massaged (preferably on the opposite side of extremities). Following are the two variations of this technique:

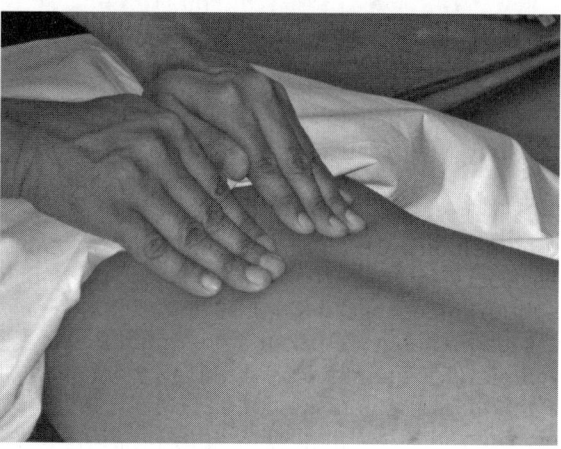

Fig. 5.13: Finger pad kneading over paraspinal area.

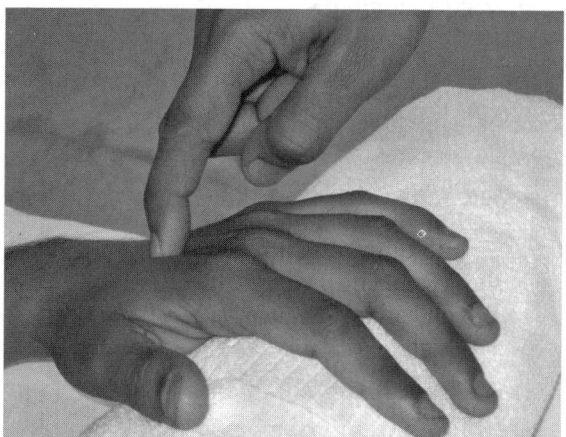

Fig. 5.14: Fingertip kneading over the interosseous space of dorsum of hand.

1. Thumb Pad Kneading

The whole pulp of thumb, i.e., palmar surface of proximal and distal phalanx of thumb is kept in contact with the skin. It is used over smaller and muscular area, such as thenar and hypothenar eminences **(Fig. 5.15A)**.

2. Thumb Tip Kneading

Usually performed with the side of thumb tip, it is used like fingertip kneading over the long and narrow areas, such as interosseous spaces **(Fig. 5.15B)**.

During these procedures, the therapist should keep his IP joint little flexed. This helps to protect the palmar ligaments which may be injured if kneading is performed with extended finger for a prolonged duration. Most commonly, these digital kneading techniques are used around the joints, localized areas, face, and the paravertebral area of spine. Digital kneading maneuvers are the technique of choice when a localized area is to be mobilized.

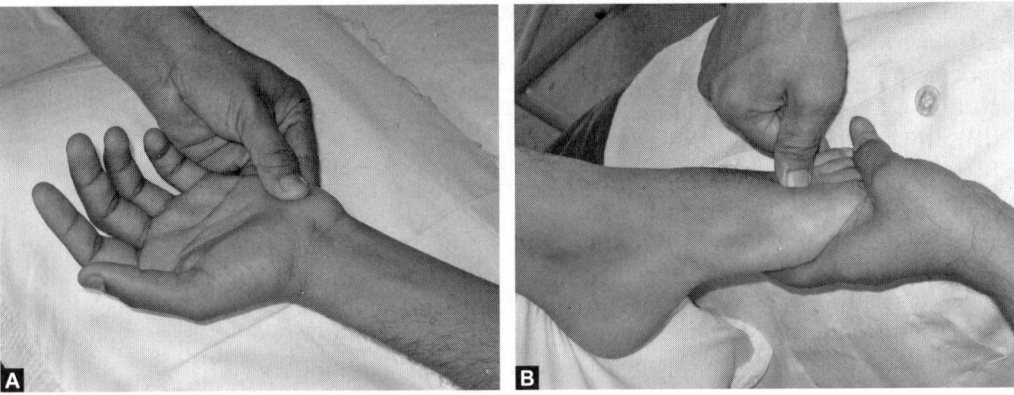

Figs. 5.15A and B: (A) Thumb pad kneading over hypothenar eminence; (B) Thumb tip kneading over interosseous space of foot.

Reinforced Kneading

This is also called ironing which utilizes both the hands while kneading. It transmits pressure to the very deep structures and used when greater depth is required. Most commonly, this technique is performed over the back.

Technique

Therapist adopts a walk standing stance. The hands are placed over each other and lower hand remains in contact with the skin. The hand should be placed that side of spine which is nearer to the therapist. Elbow of the therapist is kept in complete extension **(Fig. 5.16)**. Intermittent circular pressure in increasing and decreasing order is transmitted to the body through shoulder and elbow by controlled shifting of the body weight from one leg to the other. The extremity which remains in contact with skin, executes the circular

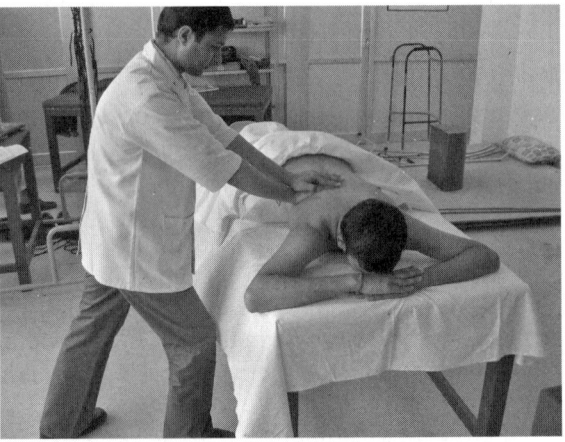

Fig. 5.16: Ironing/reinforced kneading of back.

movement while the other hand is used only to reinforce the contact hand. After one circle, the hand slides over to the next area of the near side of the back. This sliding movement of hand results from controlled flexion or extension of shoulder. At no time, the elbow should be allowed to flex as this will interfere with the effective transmission of pressure.

The area near side of back is worked in this stance. For other side of back, therapist should shift his position to the other side of couch without losing contact with the skin. This is important in order to apply equal pressure on both the sides.

Variation of Kneading Techniques

Palmar and Digital Kneading

i. Both the hands can be used simultaneously or alternately one after the other.
ii. One hand makes the circle while other hand only supports the body part.

iii. When both the hands are used simultaneously, the direction of their circle can be same or different, i.e., both the hands move in anticlockwise or clockwise direction or one hand moves in clockwise circle and the other moves in anticlockwise direction.

Reinforced Kneading

It can be performed in both the near and far side of back without changing the side. In this case, therapist adopts a walk standing stance across the back to the circles on the opposite side and a walk standing stance obliquely to the couch to treat the near side. However, in this way, the elbow cannot be maintained in extended position throughout the maneuvers and the effective transmission of pressure to all areas of back cannot be ensured.

The selection of any of these variations is purely based on the comfort of patient as well as ease and familiarity of the therapist with the technique.

Petrissage

According to the Chambers Dictionary (1983), the word petrissage is derived from the French word "Petrir" meaning "to knead". There is no agreement among various authors in the exact description of the petrissage and often just opposite views have been expressed regarding this technique. Few authors have described petrissage as a kneading technique (Lehn and Prentice, 1994) while others describing the picking up, skin rolling, and wringing which have omitted the use of word petrissage (Thompson et al., 1991). Some authors (Kuprian, 1981) have also used the term "working" for petrissage and kneading (Hollis 1987). Under the heading petrissage, it described all deep techniques, such as wringing, and picking up including kneading.

It is only the direction of application of pressure that differentiates petrissage from kneading. Mennell's states that while in kneading, the compression is vertical, petrissage involves a picking up movement of soft tissues with a lateral compression (as quoted in Wood and Becker, 1981). In kneading, the tissues are compressed down onto the underlying bone, whereas in skin rolling, picking up and wringing the tissues are lifted away from the underlying bone. Thus, these three techniques have one element in common, i.e., the direction of application of pressure which differentiates them from kneading maneuvers. Therefore, it is rational to group these techniques under petrissage.

Thus, in petrissage group of techniques, the tissues are lifted away from the underlying structures and intermittent pressure is applied at a right angle to the long axis of the bone. The different techniques of this group are:
- Picking up
- Skin rolling
- Wringing

Picking up

This technique involves lifting of the tissue up at right angle to the underlying bone, squeezing and releasing it. It is most commonly performed with one hand only. It is one of the most difficult techniques of massage to master.

Technique

Therapist adopts a walk standing stance. The hand is placed on that body part in such a way that the web space between thumb and index finger lies across the central line of the muscle bulk and skin to be lifted. The thumb and thenar eminences are placed on one side and index middle finger with hypothenar eminence is placed over the other side of the central line. Arm is kept in a position of slight abduction and elbow in the semiflexed position. The wrist should remain in slight extension.

Transfer of body weight to skin through upper extremity to apply compression initiates the technique. At the same time, the grasp of hand is tightened along with little extension of wrist. This produces the simultaneous lift and squeeze of the grasped tissue **(Fig. 5.17)**. Then, the grasp is loosened and transfer of body weight releases the compression again. With the release of compression, the relaxed hand slides over to the next adjacent area without loosing contact and conformation with the skin and the same maneuver is repeated. In this way, the sequence of lift, squeeze, and release is performed. During the picking up, the web space between the thumb and the index finger should always remain in contact with the skin. The therapist should avoid the contact between two bony prominences (i.e., anteromedial aspect of proximal phalanx of thumb and anterolateral aspect of second metacarpal head). The contact between the bony prominences transmits localized force to the skin and produces pain. During picking up, the pressure should be evenly distributed to all the lifted tissue.

If pain is felt during the maneuver, then either the pressure should be reduced or the amount of grasped tissue should be lessened.

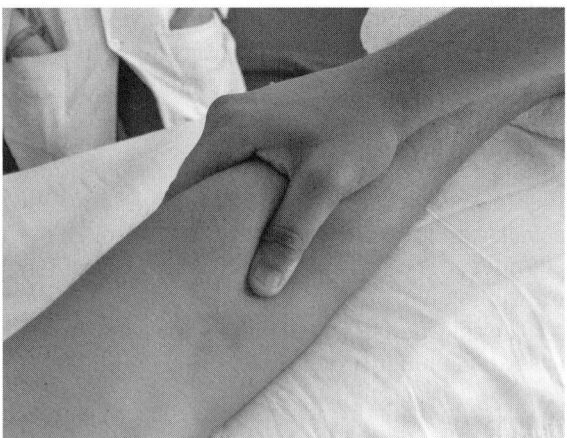

Fig. 5.17: Single-handed picking up to forearm: Note total web space is in the contact of skin.

Variation

On larger areas, such as thigh, hand may be joined together to produce a larger grasp. Thumb of left hand lies under the heel of right hand alongside the hypothenar eminence while the thumb of right hand lies alongside the index finger of left hand. This produces a larger grasp and tissues are lifted and squeezed between medial part of palm and medial three fingers of both the hands **(Figs. 5.18A to C)**.

Skin Rolling

This technique involves lifting and stretching of the skin between the thumb and the fingers as well as moving the skin over the subcutaneous tissue. The therapist lifts up and moves the skin and superficial fascia with both the hands keeping a roll of the skin raised continuously ahead of the moving thumb.

Technique

Both the hands are placed on the skin with thumb abducted in such a way that tip of thumb and index finger of both the hands touch each other maintaining a full palmar contact with the skin **(Fig. 5.19A)**.

The technique is initiated by pulling the finger backward with sufficient pressure, so that skin is pulled up. If done correctly, it lifts up of the skin. At the same time, the thumb is adducted and opposed with downward pressure over the underlying skin. The coordination of finger and thumb motion lifts off a roll of skin from the underlying structures **(Fig. 5.19B)**. Next, the palm is gradually lifted off the skin, so that the lifted roll of skin remains between the tip of fingers and thumb. Then, the thumbs are moved forward to roll the lifted skin against the fingers **(Fig. 5.19C)**.

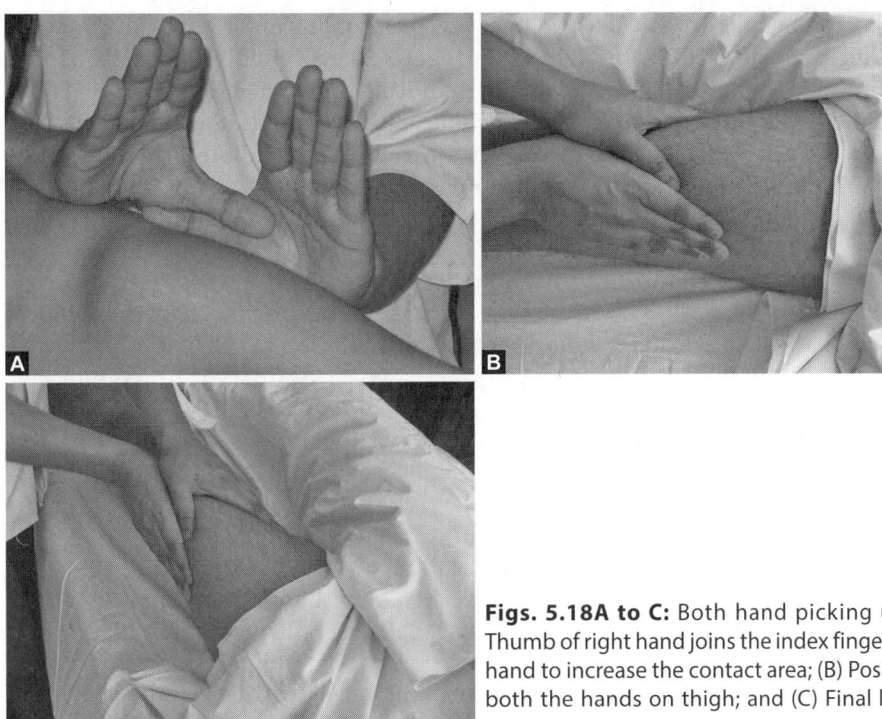

Figs. 5.18A to C: Both hand picking up. (A) Thumb of right hand joins the index finger of left hand to increase the contact area; (B) Position of both the hands on thigh; and (C) Final lift and squeeze.

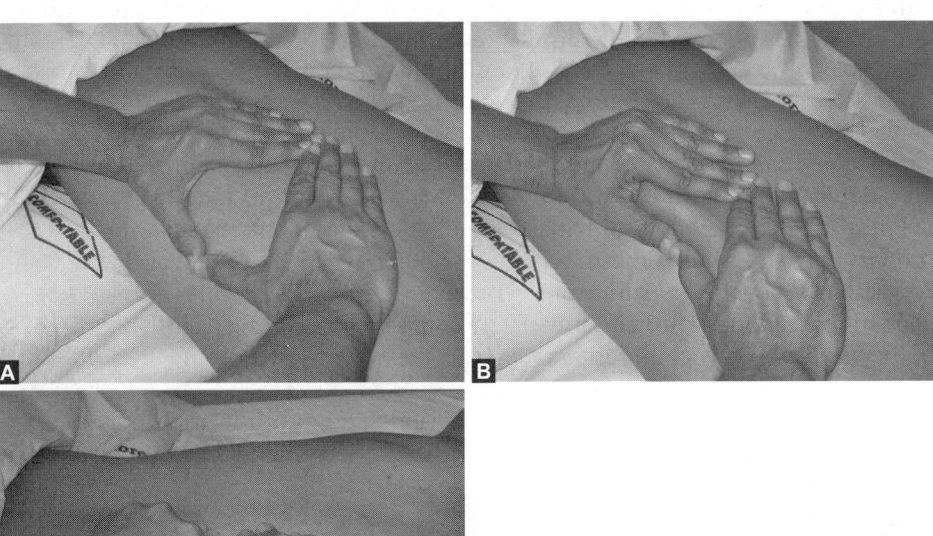

Figs. 5.19A to C: Skin rolling. (A) Initial complete contact of palm with skin; (B) Lifting a roll of skin with thumb and fingers; and (C) Rolling of skin: Note the center of palm does not come in contact with the skin.

More skin can be rolled in one grasp in persons with mobile skin, whereas in adherent skin, only little skin can be lifted up. In the areas where there is excessive subcutaneous fat deposition, such as lateral abdominal wall, the skin rolling is difficult and produces pain.

The main effect of this technique is to stretch the cutaneous and subcutaneous tissues and induce relaxation. It is most often performed over the back. It can also be used around superficial joints and on the thickened and shortened scar tissue in a modified form.

Variations

1. Skin rolling can be performed by single hand also over small area, such as foot and wrist.
2. Over arm and calf, thigh, instead of lifting the skin, the whole muscle can be lifted slightly up between tip of finger and thumb using the similar grasp. Then by alternately applying and releasing the pressure with thumb and fingers, the muscle fibers can be rolled from side-to-side. This variation is called muscle rolling (Hollis, 1987) **(Fig. 5.20)**.

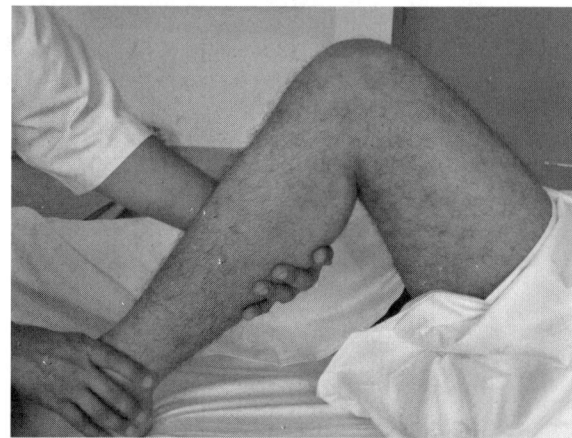

Fig. 5.20: Muscle rolling to calf.

Wringing

This technique resembles somewhat with the activity of twisting and squeezing a wet towel. Both the hands are placed on the opposite aspects of the limb and moved in opposite direction, i.e., one in forward and the other in the backward direction. This is done so that the tissues are lifted and twisted.

Technique

The grasp and placement of hand are similar to that of picking up with only difference that in this technique, both the hands are used. Hands are placed on the skin with abducted thumb in such a way that fingers and thumb of both the hands face each other but remain slightly apart. The therapist adopts a walk standing stance and uses the body weight to apply compression. Technique is initiated by pulling the fingers of right hand to pull and lift the skin from underlying structure. At the same time, left thumb pushes the skin in opposite direction **(Fig. 5.21)**. This produces the stretching of the lifted tissue. Thereafter, the finger of left hand pushes and right thumb pulls the tissues. The process is repeated several times before the hands move over to the next area. It is an extremely useful technique for mobilization of the adherent skin.

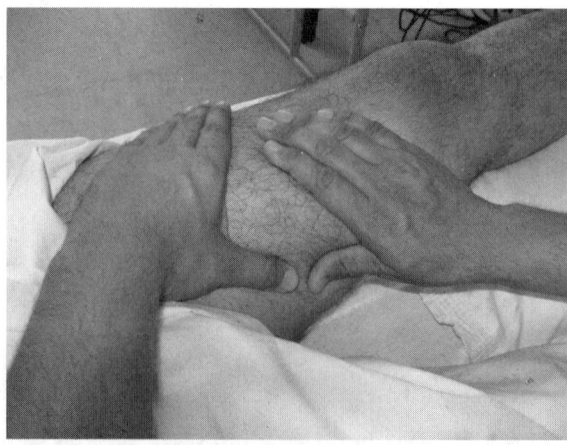

Fig. 5.21: Wringing to thigh.

Physiological Effects of Kneading and Petrissage

Effects of these techniques are more pronounced on the deeper tissues.
- Techniques of this group produce a local increase in the flow of blood due to the pumping action, liberation of H-substance, and elicitation of axon reflex. This also decreases the stagnation of fluid and edema as well as improves the nutrition of the area.
- It stretches the tight fascia and helps in restoration of mobility of skin and subcutaneous fascia.
- Various maneuvers of this group stretch the constituent fibers of muscle and other connective tissue in different directions which help in preventing the consolidation of edema fluid and thus adhesion.
- The fibrin formed during chronic edema gets stretched and softened. This helps in breaking the adhesion and increasing the mobility of adherent structures.
- The intermittent pressure may also stimulate tension-dependent mechanoreceptor, i.e., Golgi tendon organ, etc. and decrease the excitability of motoneuronal pool in neurologically healthy individuals. This helps in decreasing the tension of muscle.
- Improved mobility of soft tissue, decreased edema, and muscle tension as well as stimulation of touch and pressure receptors associated with these techniques collectively contribute to the reduction of pain.

Therapeutic Uses

i. To mobilize adhesion and soft tissue showing adoptive shortening, e.g., chronic inflammation, organized edema, and traumatic adhesion.
ii. To improve mobility of skin by loosening and softening the scar in:
   - Burns
   - Postoperative scar
   - Fibrosis following soft tissue injury and laceration.
iii. To improve circulation particularly in the muscle in:
   - Fatigue following intensive muscular activity
   - Disuse atrophy
iv. To reduce muscle tension in:
   - Spasm associated with pain
   - Tension headache

Caution

Deep pressure maneuvers should be used with caution over the areas afflicted with flaccid paralysis because the excessive stretch to flaccid muscle may prove to be counterproductive.

Friction

This technique consists of small range of oscillatory movement which is applied to the deeper structures with pressure by thumb or fingers. According to the direction of movement, there are two types of friction:
1. Circular friction
2. Transverse friction

Circular Friction

This was advocated by Wood in 1974. This resembles the digital kneading with the only difference that it has no phase of relaxation and a constant deep pressure is applied to the tissue during the whole procedure. The fingertips are placed over a localized area and along with the application of little pressure downward, the skin and the fingers are moved as one in a circular direction. The amount of pressure is gradually increased as the superficial structure becomes relaxed.

This technique is applied around localized area, i.e., joints, muscle attachments, over fibrositis nodules, and its vicinity, etc. It is most useful when a nerve trunk is imbedded in consolidated edema fluid. It is used to produce localized affect on muscle which is in a prolonged state of tension, e.g., paravertebral muscle (Thompson et al., 1991).

Transverse Friction

This technique was advocated and popularized by Dr Cyriax of England in the early half of this century. Here, the direction of the movement is transverse, i.e., across the long axis of the structure to be treated. It can be performed with:
- Tip of the thumb **(Fig. 5.22)**
- Index or middle finger which can be reinforced by placing one over the other **(Fig. 5.23)**
- Two or three fingers
- The opposed finger and thumb.

The other parts of the hand should not come in contact with the skin. The fingers are placed across the length of the structure. With pressure either forward or backward, movement is performed in small ranges, so that the patient's skin and the therapist's fingers are moved as one. The movement should take place only between the affected structures (muscle, tendon, and ligaments) and the underlying parts. It should never take place between finger and skin. The direction of the movement is the single most important factor which decides the efficacy of this maneuver. Before starting the friction, the anatomical structures to be moved are identified and according to the arrangement of the fibers present in that structure, the fingers are placed transversely along the long axis of the structure.

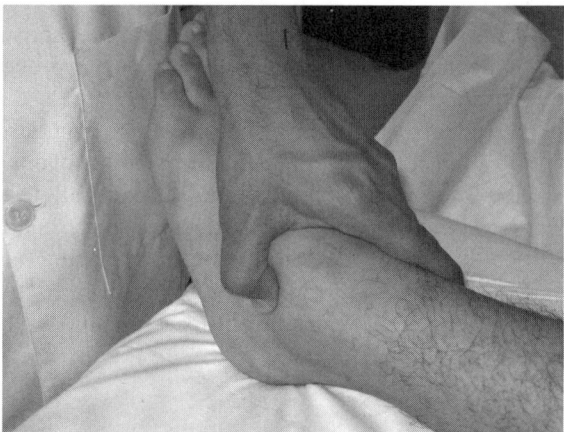

Fig. 5.22: Transverse friction at ankle with thumb: Note that PIP joint thumb is flexed.

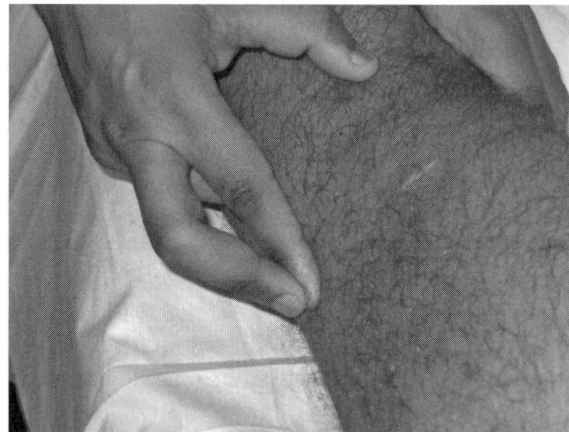

Fig. 5.23: Transverse friction of collateral ligaments of knee with two fingers reinforcing each other.

While applying friction to the soft tissue, the positioning of the patient should also be decided carefully to ensure perfect movement. The noncontractile structures, i.e., ligaments and the tendons are placed in fully taut position, whereas the contractile tissue, i.e., muscles should be fully relaxed. Explaining the importance of positioning, Cyriax (1998) commented that relaxation of target muscle is paramount. Otherwise, the forces of friction will not penetrate deeply and broadening out of individual fibers will not be achieved.

The fully stretched position of ligaments and tendons provides an immobile base against which the ligaments/tendons can be moved effectively. This is a painful procedure and the patient should be informed about it prior to the application of the maneuver.

Technique

In general, the digits, hand, and forearm should form a straight line, being kept in parallel to the movement imparted. The DIP joint being slightly flexed, much extension at wrist, or flexion at MP joint reduces the strength and friction and forces DIP joint into full extension, painfully straining it (Cyriax, 1998).

The forces of friction can be generated by alternate flexion and extension movement of finger/thumb or by wrist, elbow, shoulder, or trunk movement while keeping the finger/thumb firmly against the structure to be treated unduly strain the hand, muscle and cannot be performed for longer duration. Cyriax advocated the use of latter as in this method, more power is achieved with less effort.

Physiological Effects

1. It forcefully broadens out the structure.
2. It moves the individual collagen fibers over the underlying structure and keeps the structure free from adhesion.
3. It breaks the intrafibrillary adhesions. The to and fro motion helps to smoothen the rough gliding surfaces and ensures pain-free mobility of the individual collagen fiber.
4. Pain produced during this technique may facilitate the release of enkephalin/endorphin.
5. Deep friction results in increase in the local blood supply and induces hyperemia. The mild erythema may also be produced.

Uses

It is mostly used in the treatment of subacute and chronic lesions of muscles, tendons, ligaments, capsules, nodules, adhesions, etc. It is much useful in localized pain (trigger points).

Cyriax has strongly advocated the use of transverse friction in traumatic muscular lesion, tendonitis, tenosynovitis, and ligament sprain. He has listed as many as 22 soft tissue lesions where he claims that transverse friction is much more beneficial than other modalities including steroid infiltration. Some of these sites are musculotendinous junction of supraspinatus, biceps, psoas, anterior and posterior tibial muscles, peroneal muscles, muscle belly of brachialis, supinator, interossei of hand and foot, intercostal muscles, oblique abdominal muscles, subclavius, ligaments around carpal bones, coronary ligament of knee, posterior tibiotalar ligament, and anterior fascia of ankle joint.

Specific Contraindications

1. Traumatic arthritis at elbow
2. Calcification or ossification in soft tissue, e.g., calcification at supraspinatus tendon. Calcification at collateral ligament of elbow.
3. Rheumatoid arthritis—to the joint capsule
4. Inflammation due to bacterial infection
5. Bursitis
6. Pressure on nerve

Clinical presentation of these conditions mimics those soft tissues lesion where transverse friction is indicated. However, in the above first 3 conditions, it is harmful while in the rest 3, it is not effective.

Caution

1. Vigorous friction may give rise to blister formation.
2. Risk of blister formation is more when the friction is performed on a moist skin. In order to reduce moisture, the area should be made dry before application of friction using spirit or powder.

PERCUSSION OR TAPOTEMENT

These are French words which when translated in English mean—the striking of two objects against each other. Characteristic feature of this group of techniques is the application of intermittent touch and pressure to the body surface.

All techniques of this group utilize the controlled movement of wrist and forearm to strike the patient's body surface rhythmically. Mild blows are applied with various pressures and in different manner.

It must not be confused with the diagnostic percussion in which the fluid containing cavities of the body (the heart, lung, and abdomen) are tapped and the sound produced is used to diagnose the case.

The essence of these techniques is to use the different parts of the hand to strike the body. The names of these techniques are given according to the part of the hand used to strike the surface. Various techniques of this group are:
- Clapping
- Hacking
- Tapping
- Beating and pounding
- Tenting
- Contact heel percussion

Clapping

It is a very common and useful tapotement technique that finds an important place in the management of chronic respiratory disorders which often leads to sputum retention. In this technique, the slightly cupped hands strike the chest wall one after the other in a predetermined rate.

Technique

Therapist adopts stride standing stance. Arm is kept at 30° angle of abduction and elbow is kept flexed at 90° angle. The hands are cupped so as to trap air inside the hollow as it comes in contact with the skin. For this purpose, fingers and thumb are kept adducted and the metacarpophalangeal (MP) joint of index, middle, and ring fingers are kept slightly flexed. In this position, when hand rests over the body, the center of hand does not come in contact with the body surface and only border of hands, fingers, and heel of hand strike the body surface **(Fig. 5.24)**.

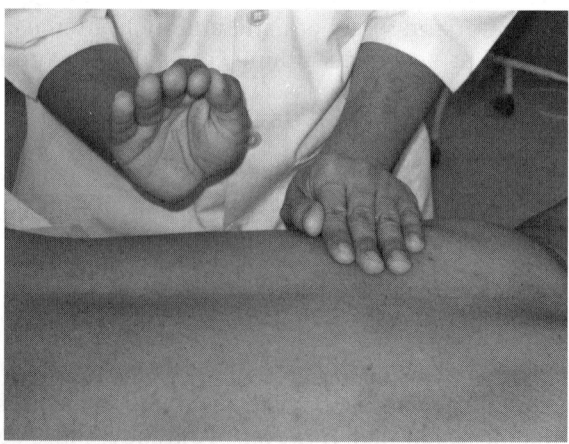

Fig. 5.24: Clapping: See when hand strikes, the center of hand does not come in contact with skin.

The technique is executed by the controlled and rapid flexion and extension of wrist. At no time, movement at elbow should be allowed. For an effective correct, a free fall of extended hand is required. This is achieved by actively extending the wrist and thereafter allowing it drop under the influence of gravity without attempting to produce active flexion of wrist. Hand should create an air cushion between the hand and the chest wall on impact. It is performed during both inspiration and expiration and should not apply undue pressure on the soft tissue of chest wall. Manual percussion is normally performed at a rate of 100–480 times/min and is reported to produce between 58 N and 65 N of force on the chest wall (Mackenzie, 1989). If applied in a proper way, it produces a characteristic sound which can easily be differentiated from that produced in slapping when the whole palmar aspect of hand comes in contact with the skin. Production of appropriate sound is important because it indicates that adequate negative pressure (suctioning) is achieved which produces the mechanical effect of loosening the secretion.

Clapping is performed over the chest wall. Preferably, it should be applied over the blanket or towel covering the chest. It helps to avoid sharp skin stimulation and pain. Clapping can be taught to the patients suffering from chronic respiratory disorders, so that they can self-percuss and loosen up the viscid secretion.

It should not produce pain to the patient and need not be forceful.

Variations

1. While cupping, some therapists fix the wrist in neutral position and use alternate flexion and extension of the elbow to perform the technique. However, if not properly controlled, clapping performed in this manner can transmit excessive force to the chest wall and may traumatize the tissue.
2. It can be performed over the bare chest wall.
3. In children or infants, percussion can also be applied using various cup-shaped objects, such as medicine pot padded with gauge, bell of a stethoscope, infant facial mask, etc.

Caution

Clapping should not be avoided over the anterior chest wall as it may induce cardiac arrhythmia. The sensitivity of skin is also more on the anterior aspect; therefore, caution must be taken.

Hacking

In this percussion technique, only the ulnar border of medial three fingers (little, ring, and middle) are used to strike the skin. The fingers are held loosely apart, so that the ulnar border of middle, ring, and little fingers come successively in contact with skin during each strike. This produces a peculiar sound.

Therapist adopts a stride standing stance. He keeps his shoulder at about 30° angle of abduction and fixes the elbow at 90° angle of flexion. Hand should be completely relaxed with fingers held loosely apart. Alternate supination and pronation of the forearm combined with ulnar and radial deviation of the wrist, respectively produce the hacking. Movement of elbow is not allowed at all **(Fig. 5.25)**.

As the hacking advances, the movement at shoulder moves the hands forward or backward or sideways.

This technique is very useful from relaxation point of view and is employed over larger areas, such as back, thigh, etc.

Tapping

This technique is useful when intermittent touch and pressure are to be applied over a small area. In this technique, only pulp of fingers strike the body part. Either one or both the hands may be used. Fingers are held loose and are relaxed.

Alternate flexion and extension of the MP joints produce the tapping. The wrist and elbow should be kept fixed and no movement is permitted in these joints.

Commonly, it is used over face, neck, and other smaller areas. It can be conveniently used on children.

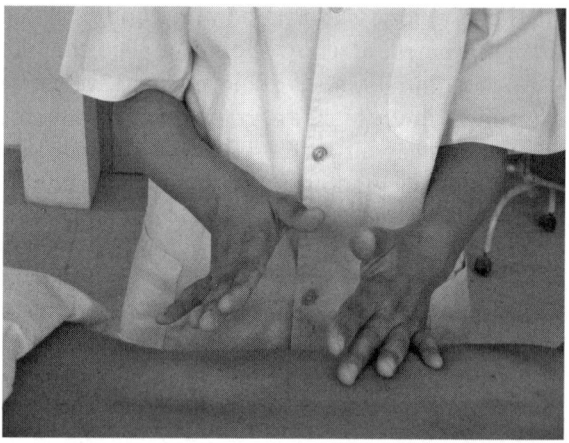

Fig. 5.25: Hacking.

Beating and Pounding

In these techniques, a loosely clenched fist is used to strike the body part. Either one or both the hands may be used. Depending on the part of clenched fist striking the body part, two techniques are named:
1. Beating—the anterior aspect of fist strikes the part
2. Pounding—the lateral aspect of fist strikes the part.

Beating

Therapist adopts stride standing stance. He keeps his shoulder in abduction of about 30° angle and the elbow is kept in 90° angle of flexion. In making a fist, the fingers are flexed at PIP and MP joint but the DIP joints are kept extended, so that a flat surface composed of dorsal aspect of two distal phalanxes is produced on the anterior aspect of fist. The beating is produced by the alternate flexion and extension of wrist as used in clapping. Movement at the elbow is not permitted as it may transmit excessive force (**Fig. 5.26**).

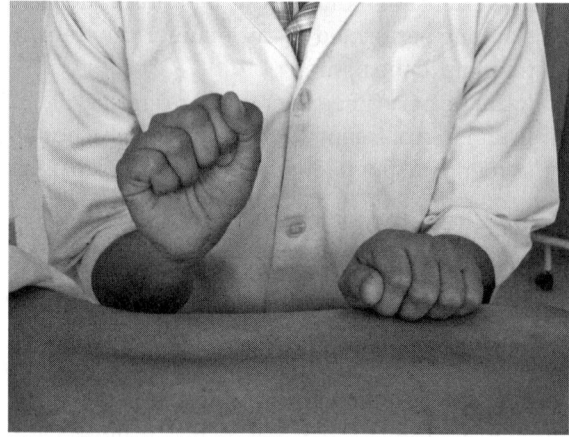

Fig. 5.26: Beating: Anterior part of clenched fist comes in contact with skin.

Pounding

Therapist adopts stride standing stance. The elbow and shoulder are kept at 90° angle of flexion and 30° angle of abduction, respectively. Here, in making the fist, all the finger joints, i.e., MP, PIP including DIP are flexed. Thumb rests over the ring finger.

Supination and pronation of forearm combined with ulnar and radial deviation of wrist, respectively produce the pounding. The action in pounding is similar to that used in hacking (**Fig. 5.27**).

These two techniques are commonly used over the back, thigh, and other fleshy and broad area of body to obtain relaxation.

Tenting

This technique is a modification of clapping. Here, the concavity is produced between the index and the ring finger with the middle finger is slightly elevated and placed over them **(Fig. 5.28)**. This technique is often used over the smaller chest of the newborn baby or a premature infant and it is very effective for loosening of viscid secretion.

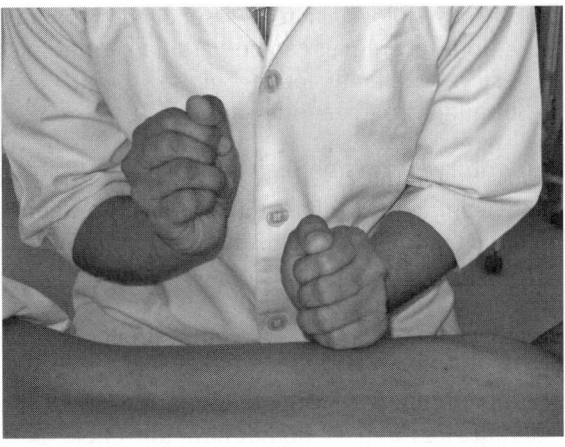

Fig. 5.27: Pounding: Lateral part of clenched fist strikes the skin.

Contact Heel Percussion

This is again a modification of the clapping technique. Here, the chest wall is struck with a concavity produced between thenar and hypothenar eminences.

Physiological Effects of Percussion Techniques

In general, percussion techniques bring about the following effects:

1. Tapotement (clapping) is thought to create a negative pressure into the lung through the chest wall. Like suction, it helps to loosen the viscid and tenacious sputum.

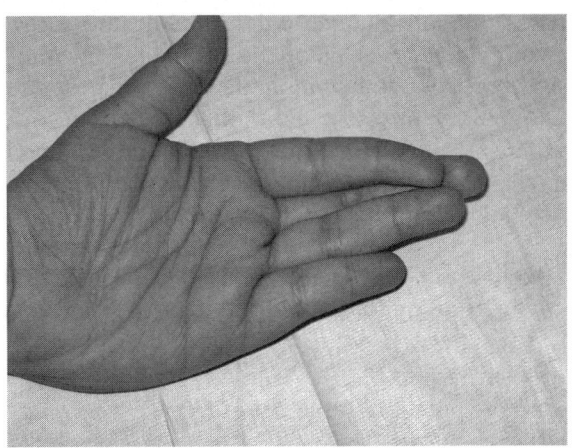

Fig. 5.28: Tenting: Position of fingers.

2. After removal of secretion, the gaseous exchange becomes efficient which improves ventilation and arterial oxygenation.
3. It results in intrathoracic pressure alteration in the range of 5–15 mm of H_2O (Imle, 1989).
4. In some patients of chronic lung disease, clapping may induce bronchospasm and a subsequent fall in FEV1.
5. The rhythmic intermittent touch associated with these techniques stimulates the low threshold mechanoreceptors which help to diminish the perception of chronic pain.
6. Cutaneous vasodilation is produced by elicitation of axon reflex and the release of H-substances. The latter effect is more pronounced when the techniques are not executed properly.
7. Percussion techniques may facilitate the contraction of muscle by decreasing the threshold of anterior horn cells.
8. Techniques of this group induce relaxation and calm the mental state of the patient. If applied properly, its rhythm and graduated pressure contribute a lot to induce sleep and relaxation.

If the physiological effects associated with individual percussion techniques are analyzed, the various techniques can be classified under following two subgroups:
1. Respiratory percussion technique
2. Stimulating percussion technique

Respiratory Percussion Technique

These techniques are directed toward lung and utilize the sound energy to dislodge the sputum from the bronchial tree. Only used over the chest wall, these techniques also have widespread effect on the hemodynamic system. Clapping, tenting, and contact heel percussion can be included in this group.

Stimulating Percussion Technique

Techniques of hacking, beating, tapping, and pounding can be included in this group. These techniques essentially do not have any effect on the respiratory system. Their main effect is to produce sensory stimulation and induce relaxation. From therapeutic point of view, these techniques do not offer much. Rather in 1967, the Education Committee of Chartered Society of Physiotherapists, London while investigating the value of different ways of giving massage had recommended to abandon the technique of beating, hacking, and pounding as the examination subjects of physiotherapy students (Cyriax, 1998).

However, in sports setup, these techniques can be utilized effectively to rejuvenate an exhausted athlete and to relieve his pre- and postcompetitive anxiety and tension. Even if mere placebo, the effect associated with these techniques can be of great help in tackling the psychological problems of the athletes.

Specific Contraindications of Respiratory Percussion Techniques

Specific contraindications of respiratory percussion techniques are the following:
- Hemoptysis
- Pleuritic pain
- Acute pulmonary tuberculosis
- Osteoporosis
- Rib fracture
- Over surgical incisions
- Metastatic deposition in ribs and spine.

Cautions

1. Indiscriminate use of clapping may provoke:
   a. Onset of cardiac arrhythmia with a subsequent fall in cardiac output and partial pressure of oxygen in arterial blood.
   b. Bronchospasm occurs following excessive and rapid clapping.
2. Hacking, beating, and pounding may induce flexor withdrawal and aggregate spasticity in the patients affected with spastic paralysis. Therefore, the application of these techniques in spasticity should be avoided.

VIBRATORY MANIPULATIONS

In this group of techniques, the vibration of the distal part of upper limb is used to transmit the mechanical energy to the body. Vibration is produced in hands and fingers using the generalized co-contraction of the upper limb muscles which are in constant contact with the subject's skin. However, it is the position of the forearm which differentiates its two techniques. The movement of hands during vibration is in upward and downward directions and forearm is kept in full pronation so that when complete palmar contact of hand establishes with the patient's skin, the wrist assumes the position of above 70–90° angle of dorsiflexion, whereas in shaking, the forearm is kept in midprone position so that the wrist assumes a position of 0–10° angle of dorsiflexion. As a result of which, when vibration is produced in the upper limb, the hand moves relatively in the mediolateral direction. This technique is mainly directed toward the lung and other hollow cavities.

Vibration

This technique involves constant touch of therapist hand or a part thereof with the patient's skin and the application of rapid intermittent pressure without changing the position of hand. Most commonly used over the chest wall where both the hands of therapist are used, the vibration can also be produced by one fingertip or palm, though the fingertip vibrations are rarely used in therapeutic massage.

Technique

For chest wall vibration, the therapist adopts a walk standing stance keeping his elbow completely extended and the shoulder fixed in little flexion. One hand is placed over the other which remains in contact with the chest wall of patient. To perform vibration, therapist transfers his body weight to the patient's chest through the extended and stabilized upper extremities and tenses up all the arm and shoulder muscles in a co-contraction. This produces oscillatory movement of his hand in upward and downward direction and transmits the mechanical energy to the patient's chest **(Fig. 5.29)**. Vibration is always performed during the expiratory phase of respiration. Patient is asked to inhale deeply and then blow out all the air through mouth. Vibration is initiated just before the expiratory phase and extended to the beginning of inspiration phase. Manual vibration operates at the frequency of 20 Hz (Imle, 1989).

Using co-contraction of upper limb muscle, vibration can also be produced in fingertips or single palm.

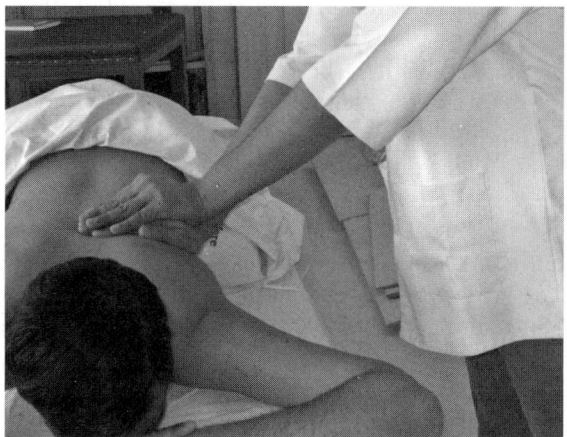

Fig. 5.29: Vibration to upper chest wall.

Physiological Effects
1. The transmission of vibration energy helps to dislodge the thick sputum from the bronchial wall.
2. It has finer action than shaking; therefore, it is used in some conditions where shaking or percussion is contraindications.
3. It may facilitate the movement of liquid and gases in the body cavities.

Therapeutic Uses
1. To mobilize the viscid secretion from lung
2. Postoperative sputum retention

3. Chronic obstructive pulmonary disorder
4. Cystic fibrosis
5. Neonatal respiratory distress associated with sputum retention.

In these conditions, vibration is commonly used along with clapping, postural drainage, shaking, and coughing techniques to clear the lungs.

Cautions

Chest wall vibration should be administered with caution in:
- Unstable thoracic spine injuries
- Rib and sternal fractures
- Persons receiving prolonged steroid therapy.

Shaking

This technique also transmits oscillatory mechanical energy to the chest wall like vibration. However, there are two basic features which distinguish this technique from vibration:
a. Oscillation produced in shaking is coarse as compared to that produced in vibration.
b. Unlike upward and downward movement of hand, in this technique, the direction of oscillation is sideways which may be produced by radial and ulnar deviations of wrist.

Technique

Therapist adopts either a walk standing or fall-out standing stance. Both the hands are placed over the chest wall over the affected lobe. Shoulder is adducted and elbow is kept slightly flexed. Placement of hand can be done in one of the following ways:
a. Patient is positioned in supine lying:
   1. Place both the hands on each side of anterior chest walls **(Fig. 5.30)**,
       or
   2. Place one hand on anterior and other on the posterior wall of same side.
b. Patient is positioned in side lying:
   1. Place both the hands on the upper lateral chest wall,
       or
   2. Place one hand on anterior and the other over posterior chest wall of upper side.

Shaking is done only during expiration phase. Therapist transfers body weight to patient's chest and tends to produce upward and downward movement of upper extremity. This shakes the chest wall vigorously.

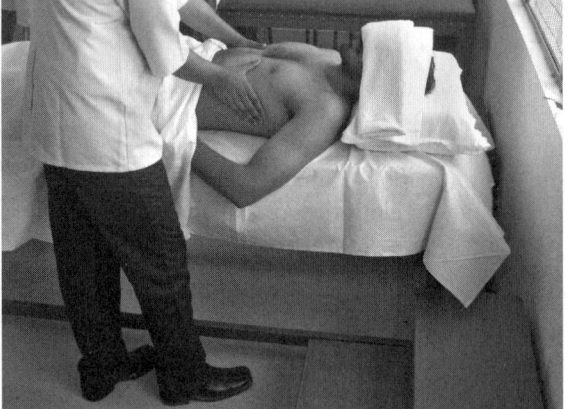

Fig. 5.30: Shaking on lateral chest wall of a supine patient.

Physiological Effects

1. Shaking produces coarse vibratory movement, and transfers mechanical energy to the lungs which help to dislodge the thick secretion from the bronchial tree.

2. It mechanically shifts the sputum from the smaller to the larger bronchioles which can then be cleared off by coughing.
3. Shaking over the sternum during respiration stimulates a cough.

Therapeutic Use

This technique is used in chest clearance programs along with all other respiratory techniques of physiotherapy.

Contraindications

Shaking should not be used in:
- Severe hemoptysis
- Acute pleuritic pain
- Active pulmonary tuberculosis
- Fractured rib
- Osteoporosis

CHAPTER 6

Practical Aspects of Massage

Success of a massage therapy depends upon several factors. Careful selection and correct application of various techniques no doubt are the most essential factors to elicit the desired effects. However, several practical points which are often ignorantly considered trivial also, influence the outcome of massage therapy. The position of patient, stance of therapist, proper support to body parts, congenial environment of treatment room, and attitude and appearance of therapist, etc. are not related to the various techniques of massage, yet play an important role in determining the efficacy of massage treatment. Position of patient and placement of pillows significantly influence the amount of muscular relaxation and the depth of tissue approached during therapy. A congenial atmosphere not only helps to win the confidence of patient, but also exerts a strong placebo effect. If the stance of therapist is not proper, he may be successful in relieving the symptoms of patient but he may himself become a victim of postural strain at the end of a prolonged session. Therefore, a thoughtful attention to these so, called trivial but practical points is essential for the intelligent and successful application of massage.

This chapter deals with some of those practical points which must be given due consideration during massage therapy session. The flowchart of massage treatment **(Flowchart 6.1)** and the sequence of different techniques often used in the general massage of upper limb, lower limb, back, and face are given at the end of the chapter. This aims at helping the beginner to learn the practice of massage.

POSITIONING OF THE PATIENT

Depending upon the age, sex, condition, and the part to be treated, patient should be placed in a suitable and comfortable position. The aim of this positioning is to ensure the following:
1. The part to be treated should be fully supported to ensure relaxation and to gain the confidence of patient.
2. The body part should be easily approachable to the therapist, so that he does not face any difficulty in proper administration of the techniques.
3. It should not hamper the continuity of massage.

Following are the different positions adopted for the therapeutic applications of massage:
- Prone lying: For back and posterior aspect of lower limb.
- Supine lying: For anterior aspect of lower limb, upper limb, and face.
- Half lying: For lower limb, upper limb, and chest.
- Side lying: For upper limb, chest, and lower limb.
- Sitting: For upper limb, upper back, and face.

Chapter 6: Practical Aspects of Massage

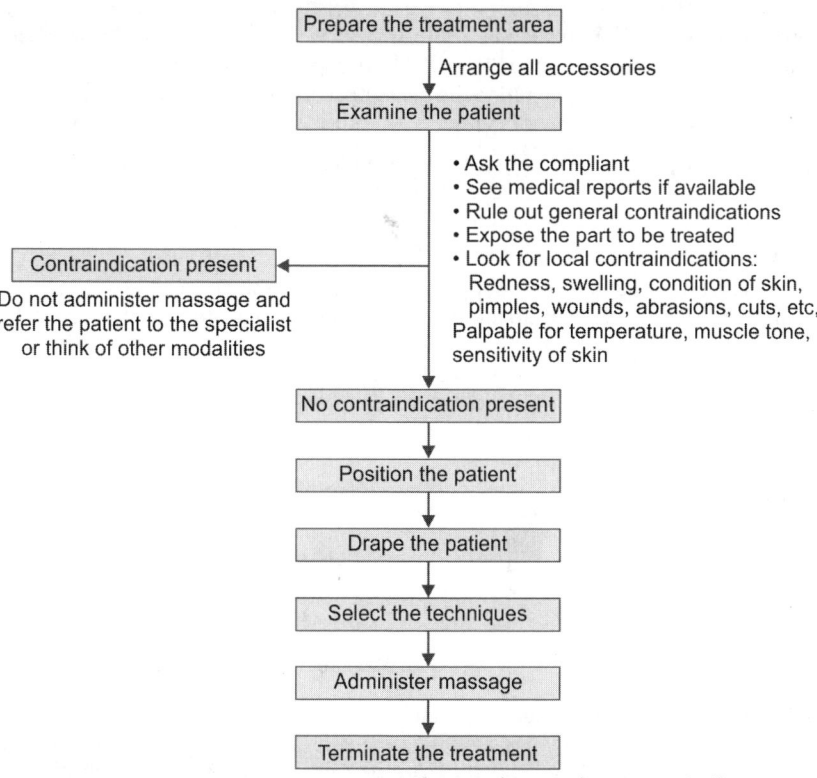

Flowchart 6.1: Steps of massage treatment.

Adequate number of pillows should be placed according to body contour to ensure proper support, complete relaxation, and gravity-assisted drainage.

Prone Lying (Fig. 6.1)

In this position, the patient is placed on a couch or bed with the face down. Most commonly used in the massage of back, it can also be used for the posterior aspect of lower limb (Table 6.1).

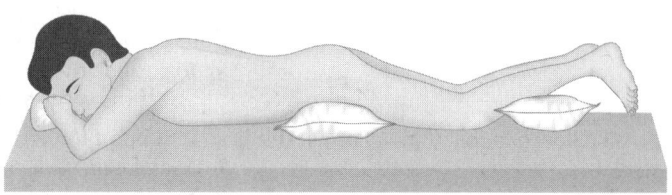

Fig. 6.1: Patient's positioning in prone lying.

Precautions

1. While placing pillows under the abdomen, care should be taken to avoid pressure over the:
   - Scrotum in male
   - Breast in female (pillows are kept little higher up to prevent pressure on breast).
2. This position should not be used for the people afflicted with heart or respiratory disorders because in this position, the abdomen and the chest are compressed by the body weight and inspiration is difficult.

Table 6.1: Rationale of pillow placement in prone lying.

Support	Purposes
One pillow under the abdomen	• To flatten the back and to obliterate the lumbar lordosis by tilting the pelvis posteriorly. This helps to relax extensor muscles of the spine
Pillows under lower legs	• To support the legs and to maintain knee in flexed position. It relieves the tension of hamstring muscle • To reduce pressure over the anterior aspect of ankle and to keep the toes free as well as to relieve tension of dorsiflexor muscles
Two pillows crossing one another at 90° angle under the forehead or Dorsal aspect crossed hands of patient under the forehead	• To support the neck in neutral position • To minimize the tension of posterior neck muscle • To ensure the easy access to the posterior neck • To facilitate easy breathing by not allowing compression of the nose

Supine Lying (Fig. 6.2)

This position is used for massage of the lower limb, upper limb, and face **(Table 6.2)**.

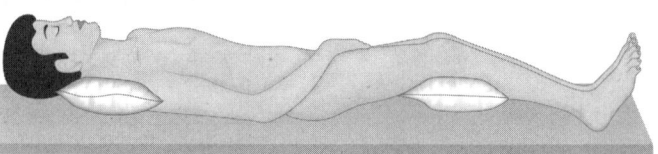

Fig. 6.2: Patient's positioning in supine lying.

Table 6.2: Rationale of pillow placement in supine lying.

Support	Purposes
Pillow under knees One long pillow across the couch under both the knees or Two small pillows along the couch under the knees	• To keep hip and the knee in slightly flexed position • To relieve the tension in the hamstrings, rectus femoris, and iliofemoral ligament • To tilt the pelvis posteriorly to avoid back hollowing and relax lumbar extensors • To position the thigh in elevation, so that the gravity assists the venous and lymphatic drainage
Small pillow or a rolled towel under the neck	• To support the cervical lordosis • To maintain neck in neutral position • To relax the muscles around the neck

Precautions

This position is not suitable for those patient's afflicted with respiratory and cardiac disorders as they may experience breathlessness (orthopnea).

Half Lying (Fig. 6.3)

This position is suitable for elderly, cardiac, and respiratory patients, as the breathing becomes easier in this position. It is most commonly used for arm and chest massage.

Patient is positioned in such a way that his trunk is about 45° angle in relation to lower limbs with pillow under both the knees. In this position, the back is completely supported and the

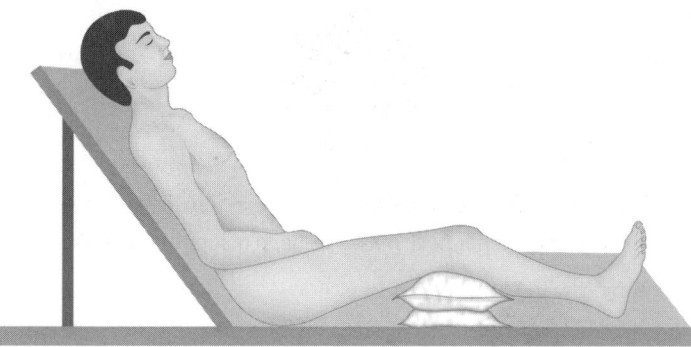

Fig. 6.3: Patient's positioning in half lying.

knee and hip are flexed. This helps to achieve relaxation of the abdominal muscles and makes the respiration easier.

Side Lying (Fig. 6.4)

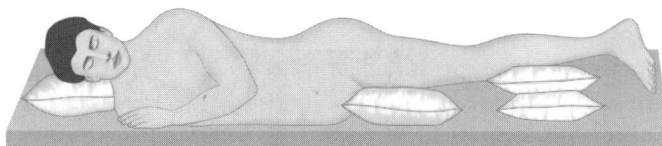

Fig. 6.4: Patient's positioning in side lying.

This position is used for the massage of the upper extremity, chest, and the posterior aspect of the lower limb **(Table 6.3)**.

Table 6.3: Rationale of pillow placement in side lying.

Support	Purposes
• Pillow under head	• To maintain alignment of neck in neutral position and to relax the neck muscle
• 2–3 pillows under the upper most, lower limb: One under thigh, two under legs	• To completely support the hip in line with the trunk

Sitting

This position is most commonly used for the massage of the upper extremity and the posterior neck massage.

a. When used for upper limb massage, the limb has to be placed on the plinth over prearranged pillows to maintain about 90° angle of flexion and abduction at shoulder joint, with elbow extended and wrist and fingers supported. This is the position of the ease which also elevates the arm, so that gravity assists the drainage **(Fig. 6.5)**.
b. When used for the posterior aspect of neck and the upper back, the patient should face the plinth and support is given to the forehead in one of the following way:
   i. Placing the forehead over the dorsum of both hands which are crossed and kept over the plinth **(Fig. 6.6)**

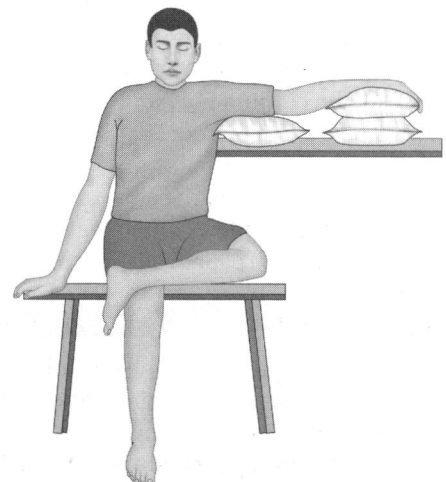

Fig. 6.5: Patient's positioning in sitting for massage of upper limb.

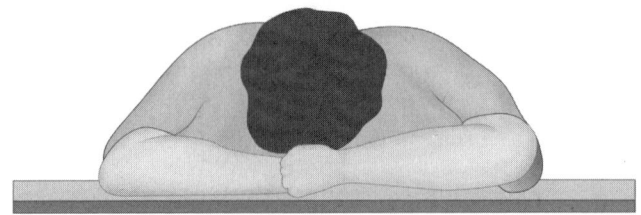

Fig. 6.6: Positioning for posterior neck massage, head is supported on the crossed hands.

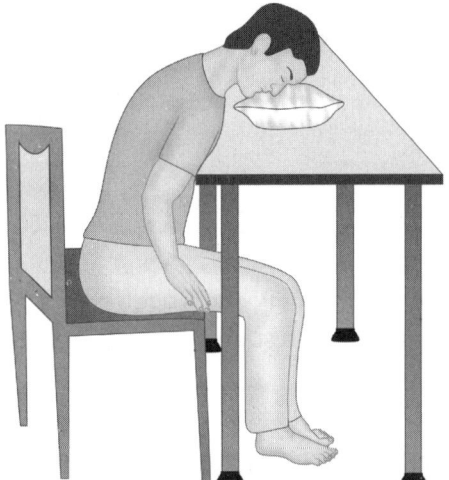

Fig. 6.7: Positioning for posterior neck massage, if the patient has shoulder stiffness.

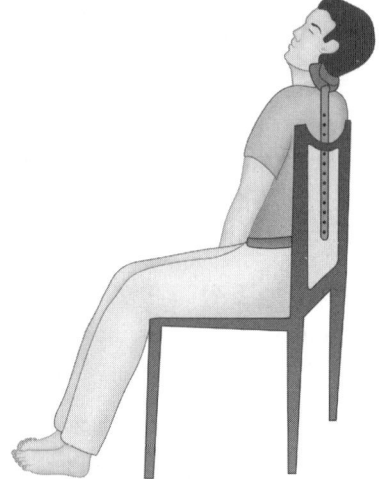

Fig. 6.8: Positioning for facial massage using headrests in sitting position.

    ii. Placing the forehead on pillows or (rolled towel) placed over the plinth (if the shoulder mobility is restricted) **(Fig. 6.7)**.
This serves to obliterate cervical lordosis to relax neck muscles and to give complete access of the posterior neck to the therapist.
  c. For facial massage, the posterior neck can be supported on the headrest **(Fig. 6.8)**. The face is, thus, exposed for the therapist to carry out the procedure.

Note: When elevation of part is required in treatment of edema, number of pillows in the distal part should be increased. For example, for lower limb massage in supine lying, the arrangement of pillow could be as follows:
- One pillow under knee
- Two or three pillows under leg and ankle.
Alternatively, if patient does not have any complications, the foot end of the bed may be raised.

DRAPING

The part to be massaged must be fully exposed, so that therapist can thoroughly look over the part and rule out the contraindications. Any adverse effects produced during manipulation can also be noticed immediately.

However, any undesired exposure of the body parts must be avoided. The other parts of body must be draped properly using appropriate draping material, such as bedsheets, towel, etc. This draping or covering up of the patient helps:

- To honor the modesty and privacy of the patient
- To keep the patient warm (in winter).

The draping of patient should not be done in a clumsy way; rather it should give an esthetic pleasure which helps to achieve proper relaxation and to create a congenial atmosphere **(Table 6.4)**.

STANCE OF THE THERAPIST

Economy of muscle work must be considered before starting manipulation, so that fatigue and discomfort for the therapist can be minimized during prolonged session of therapy. While performing massage, the therapist should adopt a position which can provide:

Table 6.4: Draping of various regions during massage therapy.

Parts to be massaged	Exposed parts	Draped parts
Back **(Fig. 6.9)**	From occiput to posterior superior iliac spine	Lower limbs up to gluteal region and upper limb up to shoulder joint
Lower limb **(Fig. 6.10)**	From toe to groin	Contralateral lower limb, trunk, and genitalia
Upper limb **(Fig. 6.11)**	Tip of finger to axilla and supraclavicular fossa	Contralateral upper limb, trunk below clavicle

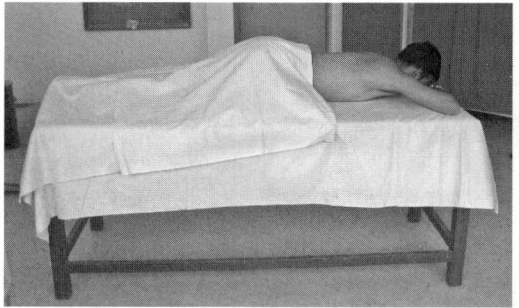

Fig. 6.9: Draping for back massage.

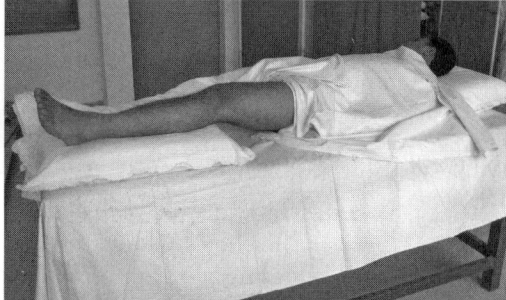

Fig. 6.10: Draping for lower limb massage.

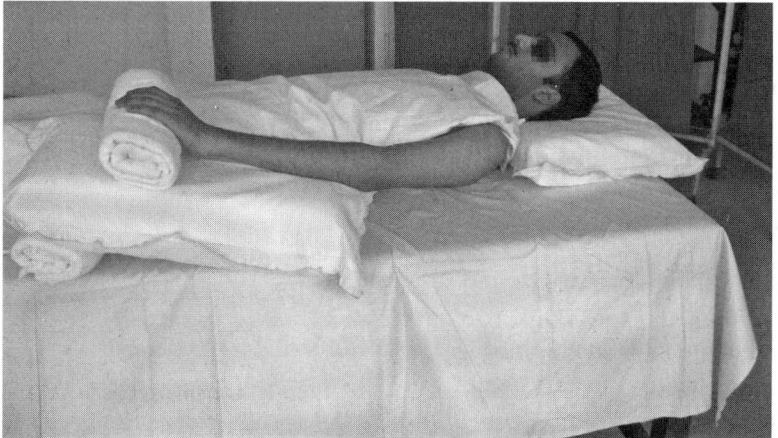

Fig. 6.11: Draping for upper limb massage.

- Wide base to ensure proper stability during manipulations
- Free body movement to have rhythm and maintain the continuity of massage
- Effective use of the body weight to minimize muscle work while applying pressure.

Flexion attitude of spine during massage strains the back muscles and adds to the discomfort of therapist. Therefore, it should be avoided as far as possible.

Generally, the therapists during the practice of massage adopt the following modification of standing:
- Stride standing
- Walk standing
- Fall-out standing

Stride Standing (Fig. 6.12)

The lower limbs are abducted at hip joint, so that feet are placed almost two feet wide apart.

In this stance, the base is widened laterally, so that the stability in the frontal plane is increased. Movement can be carried out effectively in mediolateral direction.

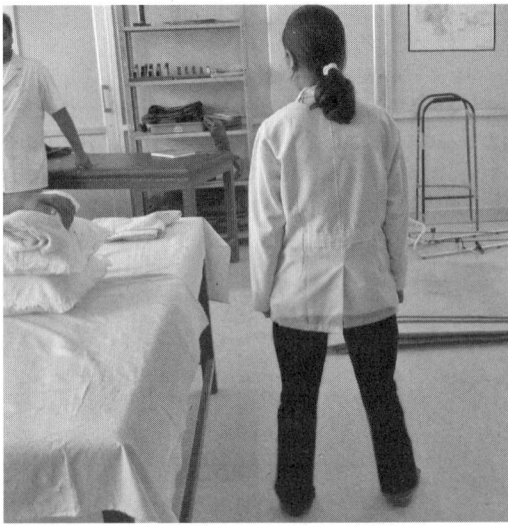

Fig. 6.12: Stride standing stance.

It is an effective stance to perform percussion maneuvers, skin rolling, and vibration. It is most commonly used for the massage of the back and the face.

Walk Standing (Fig. 6.13)

One leg is placed directly forward to the other leg in such a way that the heels of both the legs are placed in the same line and are almost two feet length apart.

In this stance, the base is increased in anteroposterior direction. Pelvis is stabilized so that the movement of spine can be effectively localized and rotation of spine and the movement in anteroposterior direction can be carried out efficiently. It is most suitable and commonly used position for the effleurage and stroking maneuvers where whole length of the segment is to be covered in one move.

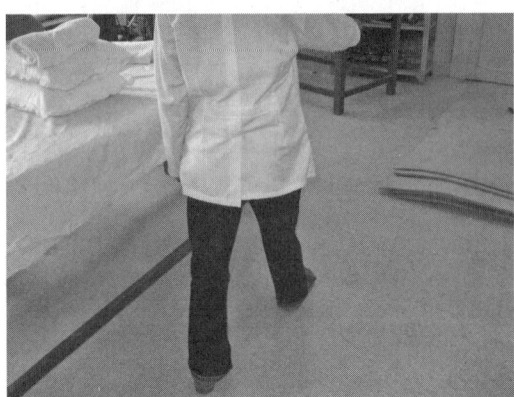

Fig. 6.13: Walk standing stance.

Fallout Standing (Fig. 6.14)

One lower limb is placed directly forward by the flexion of hip joint so that the feet are almost two feet length apart. Knee of the forward leg is slightly flexed while the other knee remains in extended position. The body is, thus, inclined forward.

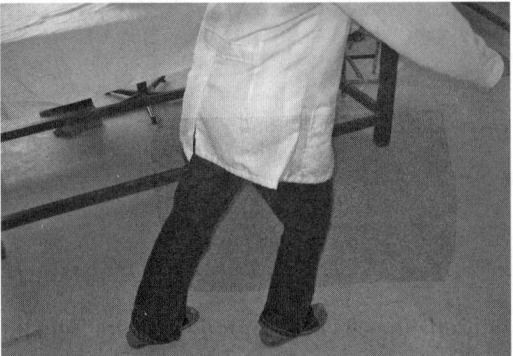

Fig. 6.14: Fallout standing stance.

If the arms and shoulders are properly supported, the body weight of the therapist can be effectively utilized in this position for applying the pressure.

ATTITUDE OF THE THERAPIST

- Therapist should be completely relaxed.
- His/her manners should be pleasant and courteous.
- He/she should be confident and give necessary instructions to the patient in an effective manner.
- His/her voice should be clear, low-pitched, and soothing.
- As far as possible, he/she should avoid conversations/discussions during the session.
- The instructions should be given in language which patient can understand.
- These instructions should be simple, short, and self-explanatory.

APPEARANCE OF THE THERAPIST

- Nails of therapist should be short and clean, as long nails may scratch the body and create discomfort during treatment.
- Therapist should also remove all the rings, bangles, watches, etc. for the similar reason.
- Hair of therapist should be preferably short or it should be properly arranged, so that it does not dangle over the patient's body and irritate him.
- For the same reason, ornament like necklace, long ear rings, etc. either should be removed or arranged properly.
- The sleeves of therapist's apron should be either half or folded up to arms in order to increase the efficient use of the hand.
- In order to avoid any chance of cross-infection, the hands should be washed and dried up before and after massage. If this is done before the patient, it helps to win the confidence.
- When the climate is cold, therapist's hands must be warm.
- Therapist should not touch the patient's skin with cold hands. He should make them warm by rubbing against each other. This is essential to avoid the unnecessary stimulation of cold receptors which may produce discomfort and increase the muscle tension of the patient.
- Therapist should avoid any sort of perfumes as they can have a nauseating effect on some patients due to allergy.

CONTACT AND CONTINUITY

"The fingers of a good rubber will descend upon an excited and painful nerve as gently as dew upon the gross, but upon a torpid callosities as heavily as the hoop of an elephant".
William Beveridge (1774–1839)

Massage at no time should cause pain or discomfort. Even during the friction, unbearable pain should not be elicited. The hands of the therapist should be relaxed and molded to the parts.

The amount of pressure applied during manipulations needs not be the same. It should be modified accordingly to the condition of the structures being treated. Initially the massage may start with less pressure and as the superficial tissues become relaxed, the pressure could be increased gradually in order to approach the deeper structures.

Massaging a patient is a continuous process. There should not be any break in the continuity of massage. The change of techniques should not be perceptible to the patient. Irrespective of the condition of body part, massage should always be practiced in a rhythmic manner. The speed of rhythm may vary according to the effects desired. For a stimulating effect, quicker and stronger strokes should be used while for a soothing effect, slower and light strokes are applied.

While the contact and continuity should be maintained throughout the session, there should be no aimless wandering of the hands over any area of patient body. It is unethical and can seriously endanger the reputation of the therapist.

SELECTION OF A TECHNIQUE

Before starting the treatment, the technique which is to be used during a session has to be carefully selected. The technique should be directed toward the condition in order to achieve only the desired physiological effect. For this purpose, patient should be examined thoroughly. Contraindications should be ruled out and the aims of treatment should be defined. The technique used during massage session should then be selected considering all these factors. **Table 6.5** illustrates the reasoning involved in selection of techniques in some of the conditions.

Table 6.5: Rationale behind the use of techniques in different conditions.

Conditions	Desired effects	Techniques to be used
1. Paralytic or gravitational edema	To increase drainage, to prevent the consolidation of edema fluid	Effleurage and kneading
2. Adhesion/contracture	To mobilize the individual fibers of adherent structure and breakdown the adhesion	Kneading, friction, and wringing
3. Bronchiectasis	To mobilize the viscid secretion from the lung	Clapping, vibration, and shaking
4. Decreased arousal of athlete	To induce peripheral vasodilatation, and induce psychological stimulation	Hacking, tapping, and fast speed superficial stroking

LUBRICANT

It is a common believe in medical and nonmedical circle that massage with different oil has some curative value and the effect of massage can be enhanced with the use of specific medicinal oils. Massage with various oils is a common prescription in various Indian medicinal systems where it is recommended in several systemic diseases including stroke.

Massaging babies with various types of oils is a common practice in several communities in the Southeast Asia. The reason for this practice is the presumptions that oil massage helps prevent hypothermia, increase growth pattern, improve sleep, and in general affect the health of the baby in a positive manner. In the recent years, these practices and claims about the baby oil massage have been investigated scientifically which lay some credence to this age old practice as far as the baby massage is concerned. In an interesting study, Agrawal et al. (2000) investigated on a sample of 125 full-term infants of 6 weeks of age, whether massage with oils commonly used in the community for massage in infancy is beneficial. Four groups of infants were massaged for 4 weeks with herbal oil, sesame oil, mustard oil, and mineral oil whereas the fifth group did not receive massage and served as control. The investigators observed that massage improved the weight, length, and mid-arm and mid-leg circumferences as compared to infants without massage. The femoral artery blood velocity, diameter, and flow were improved significantly in the group with sesame oil massage as compared to the control group. The postmassage sleep of infants was also improved. The study concluded that massage with oil in infancy improves growth and postmassage sleep.

Soriano et al. (2000) in a trial of 60 preterm neonates reported significantly higher weight gain over a 30 days period in the oil massage group as compared to those who received routine care (703 + 129 g vs. 576 + 140 g; $p < 0.05$). They also demonstrated a significant increment in length, triceps skinfold thickness, and mid-arm circumference after 30 days of oil massage in preterm neonates. Field (1980) in a review of supplemental stimulation of preterm neonates has identified two controlled trials that had used only tactile stimulation as an intervention. Each of these studies enrolled 48 subjects. Both had reported greater weight gain in infants receiving stimulation as compared to controls after a 10-day intervention period.

A nonsignificant increase in the body weight of premature infants following massage with oil as compared to massage without oil was reported by Arora et al. (2005) who concluded that oil application may have a potential to improve weight gain among preterm very low birth weight neonates. Solanki et al. (2005) in a controlled clinical trial of the effect of two kind of oil showed that topically applied oil can be absorbed in neonates and is probably available for nutritional purposes. The fatty acid constituents of the oil can influence the changes in the fatty acid profiles of the massaged babies. In a sample of 120 babies, they observed significant rise in essential fatty acids (linolenic acid and arachidonic acid) in the blood of babies massaged with sunflower oil and of saturated fats in babies massaged with coconut oil group. This study provides some evidence to believe that the composition of oil has a role to play in bringing about the cutaneous as well as systemic effects.

In the study of Satyanarayanan et al. (2005), coconut oil massage resulted in significantly greater weight gain velocity in the preterm as well as in the term babies as compared to mineral oil and placebo (powder). Coconut oil massage group also showed a greater length gain velocity as compared to placebo group. Improved weight gain following oil massage in preterm babies was also reported in other studies (Arora et al., 2005; Vaivre-Douret et al., 2009; Kumar et al., 2013).

In addition to the advantage of weight gain, it is also assumed that oil massage may have the potential to prevent nosocomial infection in premature babies by improving skin barrier. Darmstadt et al. (2005) reported that infants treated with sunflower seed oil were 41% less likely to develop nosocomial infections than controls. These studies while hinting at the possible benefit of the use of oil during massage also demand cross-validation on a larger sample and further investigations into the role of oil in massage as far as the treatment of various disorders are concerned.

The purpose of using the lubricating contact media during massage is mainly to:
- Make skin soft and smooth
- Reduce friction between therapist's hand and patient's skin
- Gain placebo effect.

The indications for the use of lubricants in massage are the following:
- Presence of excessive sweating either with the patient or with the therapist
- Poor condition of the skin. For example, dry, rough, scaly, and fragile skin. The commonly used lubricants in the practice of massage are: Powder, oils, and creams.

Powder

Preferably, it should be a nonperfumed one, as many people are allergic to the fragrance. French chalk or talcum powders are commonly used in the presence of profused sweating as it very readily absorbs the moisture.

Oils

The oil is helpful when the skin is dry and scaly. For example, after removal of the plaster cast. Most commonly used oils are edible oils (mustard and coconut oil, olive oil, etc.), mineral oil (liquid paraffin), and some medicinal oils. All these oils exert a drag effect on the skin and provide smooth gliding. For this effect, oils can also be used in the presence of a very hairy skin.

The use of edible oil in therapy is avoided because they have a peculiar smell which may be allergic to some people. They may also attract insects which may produce injuries in persons with anesthetic skin, such as paraplegic, leprosy patients, etc. Therefore, in these conditions, massage with edible oils should not be considered at all.

Cream

Lanolin or lanolin-based creams are suitable for the mobilization of scars due to burns and surgical trauma.

ACCESSORIES

Following accessories are essential in the practice of massage (**Fig. 6.15**).

Low Stool or Without Arm Support Chair

It is used in positioning of patient in sitting during the massage of the face and upper limb and the upper neck.

Couch

It should be well-padded. The top of couch should be covered with washable plastic or rexine to facilitate cleaning and disinfection. Height of the couch should

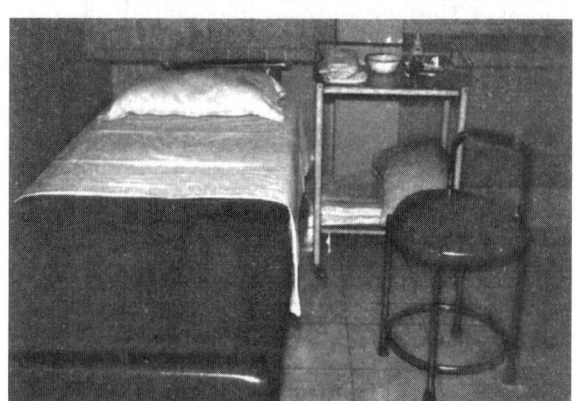

Fig. 6.15: Treatment area and accessories.

be adequate, so that the therapist need not stoop (when the couch is too low) or reach up (when the couch is too high) to perform the maneuvers. It should be wide enough to allow the patient to turn sides. A couch of 6.5 feet long, 2.5 feet wide, and 2.5–3 feet height is adequate for the most therapists of average height. Wider couch will have a disadvantage that each time patient turns the therapist which has to bring him closer toward the edge. Ideally, the couch should have shelves incorporated into it where linen, pillows, lubricants, etc. can be stored. Alternatively, a movable trolley can be used to keep the accessories near the couch.

Bedsheet

Six to seven, easily washable large bedsheets are required to drape the patient. One bedsheet should be placed over the plastic surface of couch to facilitate patient's comfort. This also absorbs the perspiration. In winter, the use of one or two large light blanket over the couch will add to the comfort of the patient.

Towel

Three to four, large size, and 3–4 small size towels are required to drape and provide support to the patient. The small towels can be used to remove the extra lubricants from the patient's skin.

Pillows

Seven to eight soft pillows with washable covers are essential for positioning of the patient.

Small Kidney Tray or Bowl

It is used to keep lubricants.

Soap

A nonperfumed soap should be used to wash the hands of therapist before and after massage.

Water Tap

Therapist should have access to a running water tap to wash the hands. Alternatively, water can be kept in a small plastic container.

SEQUENCE OF THE MASSAGE

Upper Limb (Fig. 6.16)

- *Superficial stroking:* From shoulder to fingers 4–5 strokes covering all aspects of the upper limb.
- *Effleurage:* Performed with only one hand, the other hand holds the patient's hand and changes the position of patient's forearm. It consists of 4–5 strokes each ends at axilla. Strokes are performed in following order:

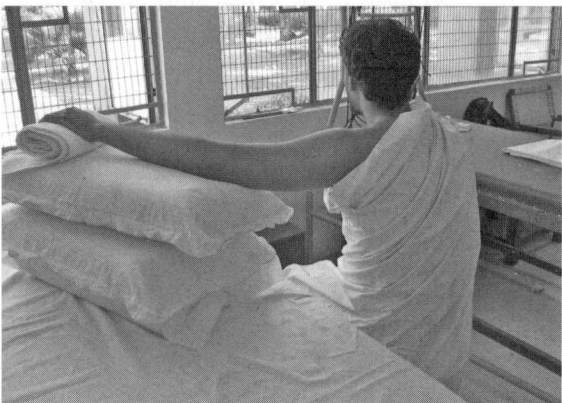

Fig. 6.16: Preparation of patient for upper limb massage.

Forearm Pronated

I. Starts from posterolateral border of hand → ulnar border of forearm → medial surface of arm → axilla
II. Dorsum of hand → posterior surface of forearm → posterior aspect of arm → axilla.

Forearm Midpronated

Lateral border of hand including thumb → radial border of forearm → lateral surface of arm → axilla.

Forearm Supinated

I. Palm of hand → anterior surface of forearm → anterior aspect of arm → axilla
II. Anteromedial border of hand → anteromedial aspect of forearm → medial surface of arm → axilla.

- Kneading:
  a. Double-handed finger kneading—around shoulder joint
  b. Single-handed finger kneading over deltoid
  c. Alternated handed palmar kneading over—biceps and triceps
  d. Palmar kneading—to upper part of forearm
  e. Fingertip kneading—on the interosseous space
  f. Thumb kneading—over thenar and hypothenar eminences.
- Picking up: To deltoid—triceps—biceps brachii—flexors of forearm and brachioradialis.
- Hacking: It is performed first on one aspect of the upper limb then the position of forearm is altered and other aspect is approached.
  i. Forearm pronated: Starts from posterior wall of axilla → posterior deltoid → triceps → forearm extensors.

ii. Forearm supinated: Starts from anterior wall of axilla → anterior deltoid → biceps—forearm flexors—palm (all bony prominences should be avoided) during hacking.
- Effleurage to whole upper limb again (distal to proximal ending at axilla).

Lower Limb (Fig. 6.17)
- *Superficial stroking:* From the thigh to toe 3–6 strokes covering all the aspects of the lower limb.
- *Effleurage:* Performed with both the hands alternatively or simultaneously, consists of 3–6 strokes each starting from toe and ending at the inguinal lymph nodes (femoral triangle).

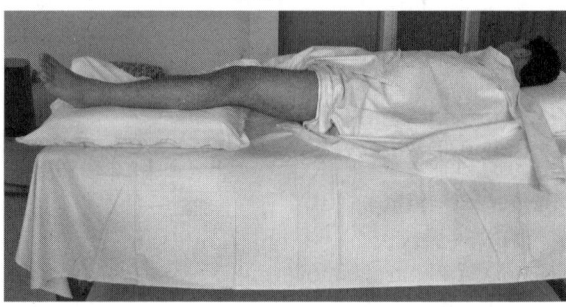

Fig. 6.17: Preparation of patient for lower limb massage.

Over Thigh
- *Effleurage:* It consists of 3–6 strokes covering all aspects of thigh. Stroke ends at inguinal lymph nodes.
- *Kneading:* Double-handed palmar kneading to:
  i. Anteroposterior aspect together
  ii. Mediolateral aspect together
- *Picking up:* On quadriceps, adductors, and hamstrings
- Hacking
- Beating
- Effleurage

Over Knee
- *Effleurage:* Performed by crossing both the hands above patella, stroke ends at the popliteal fossa.
- *Thumb kneading:* Around margin of patella.
- *Finger kneading:* Around medial and lateral collateral ligaments of knee joint.
- Effleurage

Over Leg
Effleurage: Starts from toe or ankle; stroke ends at popliteal fossa. Rotate the limb into lateral rotation to approach the posteromedial aspect of leg.

Over Calf Muscles
- Palmar kneading on the upper calf/thumb or finger kneading on the lower calf.
- Picking up
- Hacking

Rotate the leg into medial rotation to approach the posterolateral aspect of leg.

Over Tibial and Peroneal Muscles
- Palmar kneading on the upper half/thumb or finger kneading on the lower half.
- Picking up
- Hacking
- Effleurage

Over Foot
- *Effleurage:* Stroke ends at ankle
- *Fingertip kneading:* On the interosseous space and over extensor digitorum brevis
- Effleurage to whole lower limb.

Back
The back can be divided into 3 areas—thoracolumbar, gluteal region, and the neck. Massage may be performed in the following sequences in the respective areas:

Thoracolumbar Region
1. *Superficial stroking:* From proximal to distal.
2. *Effleurage:* Performed with both the hands working together, it consists of 3 strokes executed in the following order **(Fig. 6.18)**:
   i. Starts from the most lateral lumbar region—goes up to axilla.
   ii. Central lumbar region—up to axilla.
   iii. From posterosuperior iliac spine → midline of back → neck → supraclavicular nodes.
- *Ironing:* Over the entire back, therapist should change his side while approaching the opposite side.
- *Finger kneading:* Over paravertebral area, both the hands are used simultaneously preferably starting from lower back and proceeding gradually toward upper back.
- *Hacking:* Entire back leaving the spinous processes and scapulae.
- Beating or pounding.
- Skin rolling:
   a. From side to midline or *vice versa*
   b. In midline from distal to proximal.

For beginner, respiratory massage techniques, i.e., clapping, vibration, and shaking can be included in massage of upper thoracic region for the sake of mastering the techniques.

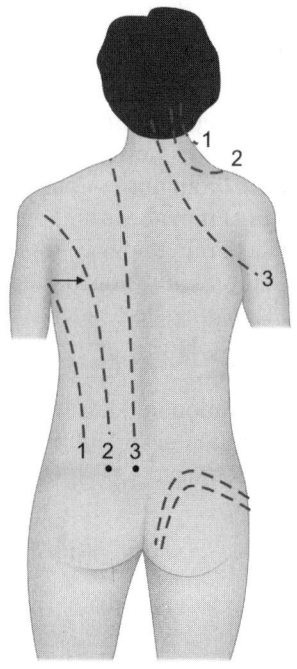

Fig. 6.18: Direction of effleurage strokes in the region of back.

Gluteal Region
- *Effleurage:* It consists of 3 curved strokes performed with one hand, each stroke ends at the groin. Direction of strokes is from PSIS to iliac crest upward and from iliac crest to groin obliquely downward in order to terminate at inguinal lymph nodes **(Fig. 6.16)**.
- *Palmar kneading:* Over gluteal muscles
- Ironing
- *Finger kneading:* Over the margin of iliac crest
- Picking up
- Wringing
- Hacking
- Effleurage

Neck

- *Effleurage:* Performed with palmar aspect of adducted fingers. It consists of 3 strokes in the following order. The direction of stroke is from upper to lower neck **(Fig. 6.16)**:
    i. Side of neck → supraclavicular area
    ii. Back of neck → supraclavicular area
    iii. Midline → side of neck → scapular muscle → axilla.
- Finger pulp kneading to—occiput, upper trapezius—midscapular muscles
- Picking up—to upper fiber of trapezius
- Hacking
- Effleurage

Face

- *Effleurage:* It consists of 4 strokes directed from midline of face to the submandibular lymph nodes performed in following order:
    i. Starts from midline of forehead → downward → below the ear
    ii. From nose → cheeks → submandibular nodes
    iii. From above and below mouth → submandibular gland
    iv. From under chin → submandibular gland.
- *Finger kneading:* In the same line of the stroke of effleurage
- *Wringing:* Performed with pulp of index finger and thumb over the entire face
- Skin rolling
- Tapping
- Vibration and kneading with one finger over the exit of trigeminal nerve, i.e., supraorbital submental and infraorbital foramina and facial nerve, i.e., stylomastoid foramina
- Effleurage

CHAPTER 7

Therapeutic Applications of Massage

This chapter deals with the application of massage in pathological conditions. The different techniques of massage as applied in various conditions are described. The emphasis is given on the patient's positioning, techniques to be used, and their sequences as well as on the aims of treatment. This arrangement is intended to serve as a guideline to all those who have learned the basic techniques of massage and now want to apply their knowledge in the treatment of some disorders.

However, one should remember that the techniques mentioned or the massage itself constitutes only an adjunct to the total therapy plans in many conditions. For example, in the treatment of venous ulcer, massage can be effective only if supplemented with elevation, elastic bandage, dressing, and medication.

Therefore, while administering massage, this fact should always be kept in mind and massage should always be supplemented/combined with other physical modalities as and when required.

The methods of application of massage for the following conditions are described in this chapter:

- Edema
- Radical mastectomy
- Venous ulcer
- Lower motor neuron lesion
- Bell's palsy
- Sprain
- Tenosynovitis
- Tendinitis
- Muscle injury
- Traumatic periostitis
- Fibrositis
- Painful neuroma
- Engorged breast
- Flatulence
- Relaxation
- Pulmonary conditions

EDEMA

When massage is used to reduce edema, it is often combined with elevation, active exercises, passive movements, and elastic compression to have the lasting effect.

Prior to application of massage, all the restrictive clothing, such as tight garments, underwears, etc. should be removed in order to provide a resistance-free drainage pathway.

The edematous part should be kept in elevated position by pillows placement, elevating bed ends, or by the suspension slings, latter is useful for the heavy limbs. This position should be maintained for 15–30 minutes before the massage is administered, so that the gravity will assist the drainage.

The patient is instructed to perform deep breathing exercises throughout the treatment. Deep inspiration decreases the negative pressure of the mediastinum. This facilitates the flow of lymph and venous blood from the adjacent parts toward the center which is at higher pressure.

The massage is administered in the form of deep effleurage, kneading, picking up, and friction. For soft edema, the effleurage is used frequently along with light kneading, while for indurated edema, the emphasis is given to deep kneading and friction interspersed with effleurage.

The proximal area should be drained first, and then the distal area is approached. To end with, the whole area should be drained once again.

These principles can be utilized in various conditions where reduction of edema is the main goal, e.g., arm edema following radical mastectomy, venous ulcer, gravitational and paralytic edema, etc.

RADICAL MASTECTOMY

It is the en bloc resection of breast tissue along with its lymphatic glands. This surgical procedure is used in the treatment of malignant breast tumors.

The removal of axillary glands destroys the lymphatic channels through which the lymph returns from the upper extremity. This results in intensive lymphatic congestion and massive swelling of the arm. The edema persists until the new lymphatic channels are formed through axilla to the thoracic duct or the lymphatic duct.

Aims of Treatment

To facilitate the lymphatic drainage and relieve congestion in the upper limb.

To raise the pressure in the lymphatic vessels in order to assist in the formation of new drainage pathways.

Position

Patient lies supine or in-side lying with arm in elevation and supported by pillows or suspension sling. Tight undergarments, brassieres, and banians should be removed.

Techniques

- Effleurage—slow and deep
- Kneading—slow and deep
- Friction around the joints.

Sequence

Effleurage is given to the whole upper limb followed by effleurage to the arm to empty the proximal vessels into the axilla.

At the end of each stroke, the patient is asked to take deep breath. This sequence should be repeated until the whole length of arm is treated. After 2–3 strokes of effleurage, slow and deep kneading and picking up are given to squeeze out the edematous fluid and to make the tissues soft and pliable.

Friction around the shoulder, elbow wrist, and the small joints of hand can be used for the similar purposes.

If the swelling is present over the chest, back, and the side, similar manipulations may also be used. In these areas, effleurage must accurately follow the direction of lymphatic drainage of the part.

Care should be taken not to stretch or damage the surgical incision. Medical advice should always be taken before attempting the massage in the immediate neighborhood of scar.

VENOUS ULCER

In this condition, the chronic venous congestion persists due to incompetency of the valve and failure of calf muscle pump which slows down the blood flow and diminishes the nutrition of the part. As a result of which, cells necrose; skin breaks down and ulcer is produced. Later on, microorganisms also invade which irritate the normal tissue and facilitate the spread of ulcer.

The treatment for gravitational venous ulcer by deep massage was first put forward by *Bisgaard* of Denmark in 1923.

Aims of Treatment
- To reduce edema and relieve congestion
- To improve circulation of the lower limbs
- To mobilize the soft tissue
- To mobilize the indurated ulcer.

Procedure
Position: All bandages and dressings are removed. The wound should be cleaned scrupulously with an antiseptic solution. It should be covered with sterile gauge before the application of massage.

The lower limb should be well-supported and elevated from the hip by pillows, suspension sling, or by simply raising the foot end of the bed.

Techniques
- Effleurage—slow and deep
- Kneading—slow and deep
- Picking up
- Wringing
- Friction

Sequence
General massage is given first to the whole lower limb in the following order to enhance the circulation:
- Effleurage to whole lower limbs
- Effleurage to thigh
- Effleurage to knee and legs.

Effleurage to thigh, knee, and leg draining into deep inguinal lymph nodes and slow kneading followed by picking up and wringing.

Special attention should be paid to the dorsum of foot, region of tendocalcaneus, and behind malleoli.

Then the region of ulcer is treated.

Finger and thumb kneading is given from the periphery to the edge of the ulcer. The fingers and thumb of the therapist should be placed on the either side of ulcer and ulcer is moved from side-to-side.

These manipulations soften the induration and increase the local circulation.

Cautions
- Care should be taken if the skin is unhealthy and fragile
- Support the ulcer from one side if kneading is painful

- If the ulcer is infected, manipulations in the region of ulcer should be avoided as it may spread the infection to the other part of the lower limb.

LOWER MOTOR NEURON LESION

In the case of flaccid paralysis due to lower motor neuron lesion, massage is indicated with the aim of hastening the absorption of tissue fluid as a substitute for the pumping action of muscle keeping the muscle/soft tissue supple and adhesion free and improving nutrition of the part.

Massage should be combined with passive movements of joints and passive stretching of the tight structures as and when required.

Procedure

Position: The paralyzed part should be well-supported. Care should be taken while positioning to avoid the stretch on the paralyzed muscles. For example, in flail lower limbs, the foot must not be left hanging at the edge of bed. As in this position, gravity stretches the anterior tibial muscles. Rather, in this case, the ankle and foot should be kept in neutral position by proper support with sandbag or footboard.

Techniques

Kneading, petrissage, mild percussion interspersed with effleurage, and superficial stroking.

Sequence

Superficial stroking should be given from proximal to distal area followed by light effleurage. Direction of effleurage should always be from distal to proximal in the direction of lymphatic drainage of the part.

Kneading, picking up, wringing, and skin rolling should be given thereafter. Care must be taken not to stretch the atonic muscle and throughout these maneuvers, the use of deep pressure can be avoided.

Tapotement in form of hacking is given after the pressure maneuvers. Massage session ends with general effleurage of the affected segment.

Cautions

- Sensitive areas like elbow, quadriceps muscle, and adductor region of thigh should be treated with extra caution as the chances of myositis ossificans are more in these area.
- Excess pressure and stretch during manipulation must always be avoided.

BELL'S PALSY

It is a condition in which facial nerve is affected and the muscle supplied by it, i.e., the muscles of facial expression are paralyzed. Due to the nonspecific inflammation, the facial nerve becomes swollen within the limited space of facial canal which prevents conduction of the impulses and results in the paralysis of facial muscles.

Aims of Treatment

- To maintain suppleness and elasticity of the skin and muscles
- To improve the circulation
- To reduce the swelling due to inflammatory deposit at the stylomastoid foramen.

Position
Patient sitting on a chair or preferably supine lying with head supported over the pillows.

Techniques
Stroking/effleurage, gentle kneading, tapotement, circular friction, and petrissage.

Sequence
Stroking is given in the following order:
- From chin upward to the temple, and
- From middle of the forehead downward to the cheek. It should be gentle but firm and stimulating.

Effleurage is given considering the lymphatic drainage of different parts of face. Small circular kneading is given all over the affected side of face but deep pressure is always avoided.

Tapotement may be administered in the form of quick and light finger tapping. Over the area of face where only a very thin layer of skin covers the bone, i.e., forehead and supraciliary ridge, tapotement should be very gentle. Circular friction and kneading are given at the point where the nerve enters the face (stylomastoid foramen) in order to soften any inflammatory deposit present over there, followed by effleurage to drain them. Gentle picking up and skin rolling can also be practiced.

Normal side of the face should be supported with one hand covered with a layer of cotton. The use of vibration performed with tips of one or two fingers over the nerve trunk has also been advocated (Wale, 1968).

Caution
Care should be taken while working in the vicinity of eyes as little neglect or inattentiveness of therapist may produce serious damage to eyes.

SPRAIN

It is an injury to a ligament produced by the violent stretching in which some of ligamentous fibers are ruptured within the outer sheath of the ligament. The posttraumatic adhesion is formed, and if allowed to consolidate, glue the fibers together. The mobility of ligament is reduced and there occurs chronic pain whenever ligament is put under stretch.

Aims of Treatment
- To disperse the inflammatory exudate and reduce edema
- To mobilize the ligament

Techniques
Effleurage, kneading, and transverse friction

Position
Affected ligament should be placed in a slightly stretched position.

Procedure
Subacute stage: Effleurage and kneading are given gently along with the other modalities to disperse the inflammatory exudate. Gentle friction to the injured ligament can also be given to maintain the mobility of the ligament.

Chronic stage: Transverse friction is the treatment of choice. Chronic sprain results from scars holding the ligament, abnormally adherent to underlying bone (Cyriax, 1998). Transverse friction is aimed at rupturing the adhesion. Adequate attention should be given to localize the site of adhesion by careful examination. Direction of friction should always be at the right angle to the long fibers of the ligament to be treated.
Duration: 10–15 minutes on alternate days.

Caution

In acute and subacute stages, massage should be used with extreme caution and if at any time the pain or swelling is found increased, it should be stopped.

In acute and subacute stages, massage should be used along with other modalities, such as ice, etc.

In chronic sprain, massage is painful so the patient must be warned before hand. Ice application over the sore area can be used if the pain is unbearable.

TENOSYNOVITIS

It is the nonspecific inflammation of synovial sheath of a tendon. There occurs roughening of gliding surface which produces eruption when the tendon is moved within its sheath. It is the movement between the close fitting tendon sheath and the tendon that causes the pain.

Aims of Treatment
- To restore pain-free mobility of tendon within its sheath
- To smooth off the two sliding surface, i.e., inner surface of sheath and outer surfaces of tendon by breaking down the inflammatory deposition.

Technique
Transverse friction

Position
Tendon should be held in a stretched position. When taught, the tendon provides an immobile base against which the tendon sheath can be moved.

Procedure
Deep transverse friction is applied across the affected tendon. This moves the sheath repeatedly across the tendon and smoothens the roughness.

Caution
Taught: Position of the tendon should be maintained throughout. Otherwise, sheath and tendon may be rolled as a one against the underlying surface and no benefit will occur as the movement will take place at wrong site.

TENDONITIS

It is the inflammation of the tendons which do not have sheath. It is produced due to trauma, sudden stretch of contracting muscle, or the degenerative changes. Some of the tendon fibers are torn and a low-grade inflammatory change takes place resulting in adhesion formation and scarring. Painful scar often forms in the substance of tendon or at the tenoperiosteal junction

(Cyriax, 1998) which binds the tendon to the surrounding structure and every active movement involving that tendon produces sharp pain.

The tendons that are commonly affected by this condition are supraspinatus, infraspinatus, common flexor origin, common extensor origin, biceps femoris, tibialis anterior and posterior, and peroneal muscles.

Aims of Treatment

- To regain mobility of the affected tendon by breaking the adherent scar.
- To relieve pain

Techniques

Kneading, effleurage, and friction

Procedure

Position: The affected tendon should be held in a stretched position with the part to be treated in a comfortable position.

Gentle circular kneading and effleurage are given in the vicinity of the area to mobilize the soft tissue and to clear edema.

Transverse friction at tenoperiosteal junction or over the tendon in the region of scar adhesion and scarring is administered vigorously.

Caution

Friction must be given to the right spot only otherwise it will cause unnecessary discomfort without any result.

Pressure of friction must be deep enough to reach the structure.

MUSCLE INJURY/STRAIN

Scar results following healing process due to muscle strain. The intrafibrillary adhesions are formed in the muscle which restrict the movement and cause pain whenever the muscle contracts or puts into the stretched position.

Aims of Treatment

- To prevent adherence of the granulation tissue
- To mobilize the adherent scar tissue
- To relieve pain

Techniques

Friction and kneading

Position

Patient should be put in a position where the affected muscle remains in fully relaxed position; otherwise, the force of friction will not penetrate deeply.

Procedure

Kneading and effleurage are given to disperse the edema, if any. Transverse friction is given perpendicular to the long axis of the adherent muscle fibers. The muscle fibers must be made to move within themself. Each fiber should be drawn away from its neighboring fiber at the site of painful area.

The muscle groups commonly affected and treated by this method are supraspinatus belly, brachialis belly, supinator, intercostal muscles, psoas muscles, oblique muscles of the abdomen, and gastrocsoleus.

Caution

In all soft tissue injuries, massage treatment is useful only in subacute and chronic states. Soon after the injury, massage in any form should be avoided, as it may exaggerate the inflammatory process. Before the application of transverse friction, the site of injury must be localized by proper assessment of the patient. Friction is often a painful treatment and it should be combined with the other pain relieving modalities.

TRAUMATIC PERIOSTITIS

A direct blow to the bone results in painful thickening of the periosteum. This condition is most often seen with tibia.

Aim of Treatment

To hasten the recovery by dispersing the localized edema/hematoma of the periosteal membrane.

Techniques

Effleurage, kneading, and circular friction

Sequence

Deep effleurage is given around the periphery of the lesion and gradually the center of lesion is approached.

Caution

In acute stage, massage should not be attempted. The process is painful, so patient should be warned beforehand and ice may be used after the massage maneuvers in order to reduce the postmassage soreness.

FIBROSITIS

Fibrositis is an ambiguous term. It is also known as nonarticular rheumatism or acute/chronic muscular rheumatism (Wale, 1968). Firm and localized tender nodules are present in the muscle mass. Causes for this condition include any trauma, exposure to cold, overuse of muscle, poor posture, etc. It is also suggested that these nodules are produced by local muscle spasm of reflex origin due to injury of intervertebral disk or spinal nerve root. Nodules are quite tender and sometimes also known as trigger points. Though this condition commonly presents in trapezius muscle, it can affect any muscle of the body.

Aims of Treatment

1. To break the nodules and mobilize the muscle fibers
2. To reduce muscle spasm and associated pain
3. To increase circulation of the part.

Techniques
Stroking, effleurage, kneading, and friction

Position
The position of the patient varies according to the muscle affected. Ideally, the position of patient should be such that muscle affected remains completely relaxed during the treatment.
    For trapezius, prone position with pillow support to neck and head is ideal.

Sequence
- First massage is given to the area above and below the affected area in the form of very light rhythmic stroking, gentle kneading, and effleurage. This preliminary massage helps to increase circulation, gain relaxation, and to prepare the patient for more specific friction massage.
- Tender area is approached gradually with care. First light stroking and gentle kneading are practiced over the painful site. Friction is added as soon as the patient is able to tolerate it. The depth of friction should be increased gradually.
- Treatment is concluded with a repetition of kneading and effleurage in order to sooth any soreness produced during the manipulation.

PAINFUL NEUROMA
It is a bulbous swelling at the severed end of a nerve. It often gives rise to tender amputation stump and painful phantom limb. It has been shown that repeated percussion in the form of tapping over the neuroma abolishes the symptom permanently.

ADHERENT SKIN
Any injury to the skin may lead to extensive scarring and subsequent induration. Scar formed during the healing of skin wound has a tendency to contract. An exaggeration of this wound contraction process often results in the formation of contracture which restricts the mobility of skin. This situation is commonly encountered in microsurgical procedure of hand, burns, skin grafting, and tendon repairs. The adherent skin not only restricts the mobility of adjacent joint, but may also binds the superficial tendons and leads to the insufficient transmission of the muscle force to its insertion point resulting in mechanical weaknesses of muscle. The massage techniques in later stage of these conditions are very helpful to prevent formation of adherent scar by reducing the stagnation of edematous fluid and to soften and mobilize the adherent tissue.

Techniques
Effleurage, kneading, and skin rolling

Burns
Procedure: Massage should not be given until the tissue can withstand it. Recently healed skin appears red. It is thin and very delicate which can be easily sloughed off if shearing forces are applied to it. Therefore, massage procedure should only be started when healing skin gains considerable strength.
    A lubricant is used in early stage to have a smooth sliding of the fingers of therapist over affected skin. The scar area is mobilized very gently with finger kneading, first at the periphery then at the center. There should not be any drag on the injured part.

As the skin becomes harder, the depth of kneading is increased to treat scar tissue vigorously.

Skin Grafting

Procedure: The aim of treatment is to soften and mobilize the grafted tissue and to improve nutrition.

Massage should not be attempted until graft is established, i.e., till 10–14 days after surgery. Otherwise, the shearing movements of massage will destroy the newly formed capillaries in the graft and lead to graft failure. Lubricant is applied at the edge of the graft. Finger kneading around the edge is used to mobilize the tissue, effleurage and rolling of grafted structure are also interspersed in between.

Small range of movement is used and pressure is kept superficial, in order to avoid the sliding of the fingers over the skin while applying pressure as it may cause blistering. In these cases, the overzealous and too early massage should be avoided as it may encourage the formation of the hypertrophic scars.

ENGORGED BREAST

After the childbirth, once the function of lactation is established, the milk may stagnate inside the breasts. This may be due to presence of some obstructions to the lactiferous duct, or sometimes the suckling of the child is inadequate enough to empty the breast properly. This produces considerable pain. In this condition, massage combined with hot bath may sometime offer considerable relief (Wale, 1978).

Aims of the Treatment
- To decrease congestion and reduce pain
- To increase the circulation.

Techniques
Kneading, picking up, stroking, and friction

Position
The patient lies on her side warmly covered up. Only the part to be treated should be exposed. The garment and bed cloth are to be carefully protected by macintosh and towel. A receiver or kidney tray is placed beneath the breast.

Sequence
Prior to the massage, hot water bath is given to the breast for about 10 minutes.
Lubricant is used in the form of oils.
- Stroking, kneading, and picking up maneuvers are applied from the circumference of the breast toward the nipple for 3–4 times.
- After this, friction may be given carefully over any hardened nodules located during previous maneuvers.
- Treatment finishes with the repetition of kneading, picking up, and stroking movements.

Lubricants are removed. Hot bathing sometime may also be repeated after the massage to enhance the circulatory effects.

This procedure can also be applied to increase the flow of milk. But in this condition, instead of hot bath, alternate cold and hot bathing are given in order to stimulate circulation of gland and massage technique are applied more vigorously.

FLATULENCE

Massages can be used in the treatment of flatulence which can cause severe discomfort in postoperative abdominal, gynecological, and urological patients where the distended abdomen puts strain on scar and produces pain (Hollis, 1987).

Aim of Treatment
To facilitate movement of gases in the abdomen.

Technique
Vibration

Position
Patient is positioned in crook lying to relax the abdominal musculature.
Sequence: Hand is placed on the side of abdomen and gentle vibration is given with single hand. Gradually, the hand is moved over the central part of the abdomen.
The depth of the vibration can be increased if the wind is voided or pain decreases.

Gentle vibration over the back interspersed with circular kneading with little upward pressure over the middle back can offer relief in babies with postfeeding wind (Hollis, 1987).

RELAXATION

Massage is most commonly used in the day-to-day life for the purpose of relaxation. There are various ways in which the technique of massage can be administered for this purpose. It is the choice of the therapist and preference of the patient which determines the selection of a particular sequence. The essential principles of massage in this area of application are as follows:
- The basic technique for relaxation, i.e., comfort, support, and restful atmosphere should always be utilized during treatment session.
- Patient should always be placed in a position of ease.
- Massage technique should be continuously applied without any interruption or change in the rhythm.
- Each technique should be repeated several times.

Following are the description of some sequence of administration of massage for the purpose of relaxation:
1. Patient is positioned in either prone or side lying. He is covered from neck to toe with blanket (in cold weather or bedsheet in warm weather). Stroking is given to each part of the body so that the body is stroked in following order:
   a. One hand each side at the center of back
   b. One hand each side over the scapula
   c. One hand each side in the midaxillary line
   d. One hand each side down the arm and outer side of leg
   e. Both the hands should work together and movements should be smooth and of the same depth
   f. Strokes may also be given with single hand alternately, i.e., one stroke to the right side and then to the left.
2. Patient positioned in the similar way described above. The length of the stroke is decreased and each hand performs a short stroke. Each hand overlaps the previously performed stroke. Strokes are repeated quite speedily for a long duration.

3. General massage of the face, lower limb, upper limb, and the back (as mentioned in Chapter 6) can relax a person considerably.
4. In very tensed persons, very slow facial massage (as described in Chapter 6) with emphasis on the slow and deep kneading over temporal region may be helpful in inducing relaxation.

REMOVAL OF SECRETION

For this purpose, the respiratory technique of massage is used in cardiothoracic units of hospitals and in chronic lung diseases, such as chronic obstructive pulmonary diseases, cystic fibrosis, etc.

Procedure

- The patient should be examined properly and the affected lobe should be localized by the auscultation and percussion.
- Patient should be positioned in postural drainage position, so that gravity will also assist the drainage of secretion.
- Contraindications should be ruled out and techniques are selected accordingly.
- Techniques used for this purpose are vibration, shaking, clapping, tenting, and contact heel percussion. The latter two techniques are much helpful over the chest of babies.
- Shaking and vibration should be given during the phase of expiration while, percussion is applied throughout the expiration and inspiration.
- These techniques are supplemented with the huffing and coughing techniques, breathing exercises, and humidifications.

Detailed discussion on the application of these principles in each chest condition is beyond the scope of this book. The interested readers may refer any book on chest physiotherapy for this purpose.

CHAPTER 8

History of Massage

The French colonists in India first used the term "massage" during 1761–1773, and included it for the first time in 1812 in a French-German dictionary. This accounts for the widespread use of French words in massage terminology. However, its uses were known from very ancient times. In Unani medicine, massage is referred as *Dalak*, whereas in Siddha system of medicine, it known as *Thokkanam*.

Initially, there was a dispute regarding the origin of this word. Few authors claimed it derived from the Arab word—Mass (to touch), others said it was from the Greek word—Massein (to knead). The Hebrew word—Mashesh (to touch, to feel, and to grasp), and the Sanskrit word—Makesh (to strike, to press) were also said to have been the original from which the word massage came.

The Arabic and Greek origin proposed by Savery in 1785 and Piory in 1819, respectively has been considered more authentic due to widespread use of massage in East and ancient Rome. This word according to the Oxford dictionary entered in the English literature in 1879.

The practice of massage has been mentioned in all the recorded ancient civilizations. In Babylon and Assyria, it was used principally to expel the evil spirit from the body of the patient, while in China it was used in a more scientific way. The oldest medical work of Chinese "Nei-Ching", written around 1,000 BC, mentions the use of massage in paralysis and in cessation of circulation. In about 619–907 BC, during Tang Dynasty, massage was recognized as a part of medical practice. The official repertory of the New Tang Dynasty describes that during those days, the department of massage had one professor and four masseurs. Degree was conferred after 3 years of study and a stiff examination. These professionals treated the cases of fracture, injury, wound, etc. and gave lectures on physical exercises.

However, after Sung Dynasty (AD 960–1279), practice of massage in China declined, and became the stronghold of the barbers. First in China, then in Japan, it was delegated to the blinds who went about the street soliciting patronage by shouting Amma-Amma (shampooing or massage).

In India, the uses of massage were well-known long before its modern name came into being. In Sanskrit literature, it is known as *Champan* or *Mardan* as well as *Abhyanga*. Its mention is found in *Ayurveda*—the medical part of *Atharvaveda*, supposed to have been written around 2nd millennium BC. Megasthenes and Alexander's description of India and the Buddhist literature and sculptures also depict its widely used status in India. Its use with different medicinal oils in the treatment of various disorder is still the mainstay in the practice of *Ayurveda*, naturopathy, and other traditional forms of Indian medicine system.

The Greeks and Romans were more interested in physical beauty and physical education than their contemporaries. Massage was very popular among them and desired by all classes. It was practiced by medical practitioners, priests, slaves, and anointers, whose main duty was to anoint the wrestlers before and after their exercises. Herodias made exercise and massage as a part of medicine while his pupil Hippocrates (460–375 BC), the father of modern medicine, was the first person who discussed the qualities and contraindications of massage. He recognized massage as a therapeutic agent.

Another Greek Physician Asclepius, who was great advocate of massage and physical therapy, had recommended this technique as the third most important treatment. It was he, who discovered that sleep might be induced by gentle "stroking". Galen (AD 125–195), the renounced Greek Physician after Hippocrates, wrote about 16 books related to exercise and massage. In these books, he discussed about the massage at length. He also classified this technique into three qualities and by different combinations, he found nine forms of massage, each of which had its own indications.

Greeks and Romans left behind a lot of literature in which they mentioned the use of massage in conditions like paralysis, cold extremity, muscle sprain, etc. which hold good even today. However, they also recommended it in condition like intestinal obstruction where now the use of massage is considered inappropriate. In these literatures, various nonmedical persons also spoke in favor of massage. This shows the popularity of massage in those days. Cicero (Greek King) considered his anointer equal to his physician. He even commented that he owed his good health as much to his anointer as his physicians. Julius Caesar had reported to receive daily massage by a specially trained slave in order to relieve his neuralgic pain. It is well-known that Julius Caesar was a patient of epilepsy.

After the fall of Roman Empire, massage and medical gymnastics went back to the level of folk medicine. There is no mention of massage in medical literature till fourteenth century. This period during which the progress in almost all branches of science came to a halt is referred in history books as the Dark Age. Toward the fifteenth century, people again started writing about massage. Antonius, Gazius, Hieronymus, Mercurius, and Ambroise Paré collected the teachings of Hippocrates and Galen, and started using massage in the various conditions. Ambroise Paré (1510-1590), who was a great surgeon, started the application of massage to surgical patients. In sixteenth century, Fabricius ab Acquapendente, who was the tutor of William Harvey (the discoverer of the blood circulation), wrote a book on massage in which he warmly recommended the use of massage as a rational therapy for joint affection. It was he who used the term "kneading" for the first time.

Francis Glisson (1597-1677) one of the founders of Royal Society, mentioned the use of massage and exercise in the treatment of rickets. Thomas Sydenham (1624-1689) also known as English Hippocrates was a strong supporter of physical therapy. During his time, several books were published where massage was mentioned in the care of almost all the diseases including syphilis.

Friedrich Hoffmann first said that human body is a machine which is subjected to mechanical laws. Nicolas Andry in his *L'orthopedie* published in 1741 described the effects of massage on the circulation and the skin color. He used these effects to soften the tendons and muscles.

In 1780, Joseph Clément Tissot published a book on exercise where he spoke of "Alternate Pressure and Relaxation" on external part which should cause a movement of the solids and liquids of the body and thus increase the circulation.

In nineteenth century, the person who contributed a lot in this field was Per Henrik Ling (1776-1839). He was a teacher in Physical Education. He started the Central Institute of Gymnastics in Stockholm in 1813 where he developed massage as a part of medical gymnastics and due to his efforts massage gained the attention of an increasing number of physicians. He classified the techniques of conventional massage and incorporated the French words, such as percussion, tapotement, effleurage, etc. in his Swedish system of massage. His pupils spread his teachings in the other European countries. His immediate pupils Augustus George published Ling's system in French under the term "Kinesitherapy". By the end of nineteenth century, Swedish massage had received international acclaim.

However, Ling did little to distinguish between exercise and massage and his system though generally known as a massage system that also included passive and active movements. It was left to Dr James B Mennell of England to distinguish between the massage, movement, and exercise during the years 1917 and 1940.

After 1850, the number of books, articles, and journals on gymnastics and massage increased remarkably. During this time, two important doctoral thesis on massage by Estraderf (in 1863) and Mezger (in 1868) were published, where massage was discussed in a more appropriate manner in the disorders of locomotor system. Mezger was a Dutch physician and probably it was due to his influence that the oldest association of *Masseur's* was formed in Holland in 1889. The oldest periodical of this profession was published in 1891.

In the last quarter of the 19th century, massage was studied in various research projects. Following is the list of work done by some researchers:
- Effect of massage on lymphatic flow—Lassar (1887)
- Circulatory effect of vibrations—Hassebrock
- Histological effect of massage on tissue trauma—Caster
- Physiological effects of massage—Piorry.

Toward the end of nineteenth century, massage was prescribed in combination with heat, exercises, and electricity. In this century, some workers attempted to establish a solid scientific basis of massage, but unfortunately a few misused and abused it. Several publications appeared in Germany, France, Italy, Denmark, England, and US reporting on the abuses connected with massage which ranges from quackery to prostitution.

History of massage in twentieth century was dominated by the development of new techniques and new systems namely:

- Sports massage
- Reflex massage
- Periosteal massage
- Connective tissue massage
- Acupressure
- External cardiac massage

Massage was taught in the schools of physiotherapy, medical gymnastics, and the schools of massage. In this century, the well-known figures in the field of massage were Rosenthal, Cyriax, Graham, and Mennell. Rosenthal gave scientific ground to massage and manipulation and is accredited for reintroduction of massage into mainline medical practice. Cyriax advocated the use of deep friction in periarticular lesions. Terrier combined massage and manipulative therapy more intimately and termed it as manipulative massage.

While the diversity of technique increased manifold, its uses in therapy were diminished throughout the world in the first half of the twentieth century. In fact, the history of massage has been dominated by a love-hate relationship between medical establishment and other groups who practice these techniques. Throughout the world, the so-called fitness centers, health clubs, and massage parlors have been mushrooming up where untrained people unethically practice some of the technique of massage as a mode of luxurious comfort. These centers have given a very bad publicity to this ancient mode of treatment. It is due to this, that in the late 1960s and 1970s, the soft tissue manipulation has been entered in the vocabulary of some physiotherapists in lieu of the term massage.

Nevertheless, in the late twentieth century, massage again received the attention of scientific investigators and a number of scientific papers have appeared in the literature. In most of these works, the effects of massage established till date by subjective and observational methods have been subjected to rigorous objective evaluation. With the advent of sophisticated instruments, it became possible to measure the physiological parameters associated with the effects of massage. Plethysmography, radioactive isotope clearance rate, Doppler ultrasound, etc. are now used to examine the effect of massage on the blood flow, whereas the effects of massage on neuromuscular system are evaluated by electromyographic techniques. The discovery of pain gate theory by Melzack and Wall gave a new credence to the role of massage in pain management. Studies have been conducted to see the cellular level changes in fibrous tissue after massage maneuvers using electron microscope. Several investigators have also attempted to evaluate and standardize the exact pressure applied during different maneuvers of massage using sophisticated pressure monitoring devices. Twenty first century is witnessing an explosion in the research related to massage. Animal models, genetic expression, immunological markers, histopathological technique, etc. are being used to explore the science behind massage.

These studies have been successful in their attempt to re-establish the scientific value of massage. However, the result of these sporadic studies is conflicting. Some of them have also challenged the basic circulatory effects of massage. It is essential that these reports are interpreted with caution in view of small sample size, nonstandardization of massage technique used in these studies, and more importantly the lack of cross-validation. There is an urgent need to conduct multidisciplinary studies aimed at exploring the various aspects of this ancient mode of treatment with the help of all available advanced technology.

Massage therapy has been subjected to alternating period of advocacy and denigration and current phase is one that of denigration. The development of pharmacological industries, intervention of new adjuncts in physical therapy, i.e. SWD, US, traction, IFT, etc. and moreover, the dehumanization of the patient and therapist relationship can be enumerated as few factors responsible for this state.

However, in the present era when the technological and pharmacological advances are fast approaching toward zenith, their limitations and drawbacks have also become the cause of concern for medical and nonmedical world. An increasing number of people throughout the world are now moving toward the drugless approaches of treatment. The trend of disease pattern is also witnessing a rapid change. Today man is subjected to far greater stress and strain than at any time in the history. Technological and economic advancement has created a pace and lifestyle which an individual often finds difficult to synchronize with. The incidence of stress, anxiety, and psychosomatic diseases is increasing at alarming rates. In this changing scenario, the role of human touch, in combating the dehumanization of modernity, is fast receiving attention. The physiological and psychological effects of massage can offer a solution to majority of these problems, if combined appropriately with other approaches.

Despite fluctuations in the support of massage, the utility of a few of its techniques in the management of certain type of soft tissue lesions has always been acknowledged. In these conditions, their effectiveness has been proved beyond doubts.

CHAPTER 9

New Systems of Massage

Classical massage techniques were advocated and standardized by PH Ling, otherwise called Swedish massage has witnessed a dramatic change in the twentieth century. Many new techniques have been evolved and are continuing to evolve which though use the basic principles of classical massage are essentially different from it. Although these methods are not very popular, they are widely used in some parts of the world and form an integral parts of the soft tissue mobilization. These have proved effective in certain conditions where classical massage is usually not used. Many of these techniques elicit vicerocutaneous reflexes and have been proved effective not only in disorders of locomotion system, but also in the dysfunction of internal organs. This chapter deals with few of those techniques of massage which do not fall under the classical massage. The essentials of these techniques are outlined briefly. For further details, the interested reader is advised to refer to the literature mentioned in Bibliography.

CONNECTIVE TISSUE MASSAGE

It is a specialized form of massage which utilize vicerocutaneous reflex for diagnosis and treatment. It was discovered in the 1930s by a German physiotherapist Miss Elizabeth Dicke. The main effect of this technique is to enhance the blood circulation of a target area by mobilizing the deeper layer of dermis which is said to have balancing effect on sympathetic and parasympathetic components of autonomic nervous system (Thompson et al., 1991).

Human embryo is composed of serially arranged several homogeneous primitive segments called metameres. This arrangement is concerned with the mesoderm and tissue region derived from it, that is, sclerotome, myotome, dermatome, angiotome, and nephrotome. The ectoderm participates in segmentation since in each of the metamere one spinal nerve enters. The skin over the segment is also innervated and in this way the segmentation is projected to the skin. This embryonic connection between metameres and the spinal nerves (dermatome) develops early and remains unchanged postembryonically. The internal organs that develop from endoderm correspond to certain spinal cord segments. The relationship between the functions of internal organs, vessels, and nerves as well as the tissue of the locomotor apparatus which descends from the same metamere is the scientific foundation of connective tissue massage (Chaitow, 1996).

The proponents of this system emphasize that the surface of body provides evidence of internal derangements and it is possible to influence the internal organ reflexly by the application of powerful stimuli to the surface of body. Practitioners of connective tissue massage have divided the external surface of body into several reflex connective tissue zones. It is claimed that disturbed organ function gives rise to altered connective tissue zone. These changes in connective tissue zone are palpable and may take any of the following forms (Chaitow, 1996):

- Drawn in bands of tissue
- Flattened area of tissue
- Elevated area giving impression of localized swelling
- Muscle atrophy or hypertrophy
- Osseous deformity of spinal column.

The practice of connective tissue massage involves the identification of the changes in the connective tissue zone related to a specific visceral organ and treatment of connective tissue zone by special kind of stroking in order to improve the function of that organ.

Evaluation is the most important part of an effective connective tissue massage program. Before the treatment is executed, the patient is examined thoroughly to find out:
- The affected dermatome
- The mobility of various layers of connective tissue
- The amount of tension present in muscular layers.

Lifting of skinfold, stretching of superficial tissue, and skin distraction are the three diagnostic techniques used in connective tissue massage.

The technique of massage consists of a special type of gliding and cutting strokes (Hollis, 1987), executed mainly with tips or pads of middle and ring finger of either hand which are placed at an angle of 30–40° from the body surface. Stroke applies a tangential pull on the skin and subcutaneous fascia in order to mobilize the superficial connective tissue (skin and subcutaneous tissue) over the deep connective tissue (fascia). The strokes are applied in a specific manner. They start from sacrum and buttock and may progress further upward up to the neck and upper limbs or downward toward the legs. Over the back, the strokes are applied along the dermatome whereas over the peripheral area, they are applied along the muscle fibers. Connective tissue massage stroking elicits a sharp pain and patient feels a scratching and cutting sensation.

Treatment is carried out two to three times per week and there should be a rest period of at least 1 month after fifteen sessions of connective tissue massage.

During and after connective tissue massage, a number of reflex reactions occur which include vasodilatation, diffuse or localized swelling, elevation of skin temperature, pleasant fatigue, decrement of edema, increased bowel movement, diuresis, etc.

Vasodilatation and increase in skin temperature often occur in the area distal to the massaged site. For example, when pelvis is treated with connective tissue massage, there occurs dilatation of blood vessels of upper extremities. Temperature of skin has been observed to increase half an hour after the termination of connective tissue massage, which persists almost for an hour.

It is observed that the vasodilatory effect of connective tissue massage is as permanent as that of lumbar sympathectomy. It is found very useful in conditions like varicose veins, thrombophlebitis, thromboangiitis obliterans, Raynaud's disease, and frostbite. Myocardial dysfunction, pulmonary dysfunctions, intestinal disorders, hepatitis, inflammation of ovary and uterus, and menstrual disturbances like amenorrhea and dysmenorrhea are the other indications for connective tissue massage where it is utilized owing to its autonomic effects.

It is a useful technique in dealing with the consequences of psychiatric disturbances, anxiety and agitation. Its effectiveness has been claimed in the problems involving sleep disturbances, chronic fatigue, and fibromyalgia of psychosomatic origin.

Since this massage technique provokes widespread autonomic effects, it must be learned under the direct supervision of an experienced expert.

This revolutionary technique of manual therapy was discovered in a dramatic way. The therapist, who discovered this technique, was herself suffering from endarteritis obliterans—a severe circulatory disorder of left leg. She was awaiting the amputation of her leg, which had the appearance of gangrene.

She was also experiencing severe low back pain after 5 months of recumbency. When in order to relieve her pain, she palpated her back, she found densely infiltrated tissue and an increased tension of skin and subcutaneous tissues over ileum and sacrum. She casually applied some pulling strokes over these hyperesthetic areas. Surprisingly, those strokes could not only disperse the dense infiltrated mass and relieve her backache, but also brought remarkable change in the condition of her leg. After some trial of these strokes, her affected ice cold leg felt warm and superficial venous circulation was reestablished. After three months, the severe manifestation of her disease dramatically subsided and amputation was avoided. After a year, she could resume her full-time duty as physiotherapist.

The work of Elizabeth Dick was investigated further by Dr Leube and Dr Kohlrausch, who gave scientific basis to the technique. In 1948, the first book on Connective Tissue Massage coauthored by Dick and Dr Leube was published. In English literature, the technique was fully described by Miss M Ebner in 1955 in her book "Connective Tissue Manipulations".

TREAD MASSAGE

In this type of massage, the soft tissues are manipulated not by the hand but by the feet of therapist. It is commonly applied to the back of patient. It can also be used for lower limbs. The therapist regulates the pressure by utilizing his/her body weight. For the application of maximum pressure, he/she may have to stand on the patient's back in order to use the total body weight. It is an ancient technique of massage most commonly practiced in the Eastern countries.

PERIOSTEAL MASSAGE

It is a type of reflex-zone massage described by Vogler in 1930s. It is a rhythmic massage technique applied to the bony prominence of the body by the tip of finger or thumb. The main effect of this technique, as claimed by Vogler, is to activate the local and vasomotor reflex by the stimulation of periosteum. The technique resembles very much with the kneading techniques.

The fingers, thumb, or knuckles are used to apply pressure over the periosteum near painful areas. Pressure is applied in small circles of 4–5 mm diameters. In half of the cycle, pressure increases and in other half it decreases. Massage progresses from the periphery toward the center of periosteal tenderness. The pain relief obtained by this technique is presumed to be due to the vasomotor reflex changes and the counterirritant effects.

STRIPPING MASSAGE

This specific form of massage is employed in the treatment of trigger points. It consists of specific type of stroking manipulations.

The fingers and thumb apply the slow and deep strokes along the length of muscle. The muscle to be treated is placed in a comfortably relaxed position but under moderate stretch. The fingers and thumb of both hands are placed over the well-lubricated skin at the distal end of the muscle and allowed to slide slowly toward the tender point. This is done in order to squeeze out the fluid content of the muscle.

Initially, the pressure is light which increases with the successive strokes. With the increase of pressure, the stroking fingers of therapists encounter a nodular obstruction at tender spot which may be due to stagnation of blood and other tissue fluids. Repeated strokes of this stripping massage are said to decrease the nodule and inactivate the trigger point.

HOFFA MASSAGE

Hoffa massage is the classical massage technique using a variety of superficial strokes including effleurage, petrissage, tapotement, and vibration (Lehn and Prentice, 1994). Albert Hoffa's text published in 1900 provides the basis for various massage techniques that have developed over the years.

The primary purpose of this massage is to increase circulation and decrease the muscle tone. The way of performing effleurage and petrissage of Hoffa massage has been described by different authors as follows:

Effleurage (by Hoffa)

The hand is applied as closely as possible to the part and glides on it from distal to proximal. The balls of thumb and little finger are used to stroke the muscle mass and at the same time slide along the edge of muscle. While the fingertips take care of the larger muscles, the stroke is applied upwardly.

Petrissage (by Tappan)

Apply both hands obliquely to the direction of the muscle fibers. The thumbs are opposed to the rest of fingers. This manipulation starts peripherally and proceeds centripetally, following the direction of muscle fibers. The hand goes first and tries to pick up the muscle from bone, moving back and forth in a zigzag path.

ROLFING

It is a system devised by Ida Rolf. Rolfing or structural integration is a system used to correct inefficient posture or to integrate structures. The basic principle of treatment is that if balanced movement is essential at a particular joint yet nearby tissue is restrained, both the tissue and the joint will relocate to a position that accomplishes a more appropriate equilibrium (Lehn and Prentice, 1994).

The technique involves manual manipulation of myofascia with the goal of balancing the body in the gravitational field. Rolfing is a standardized nonsymptomatic approach to soft tissue manipulation, with a set number of treatment sessions in basic and advanced sequences. The basic sequence usually involves 10 sessions, each focusing upon different aspect of postural integration. The advance sequence that is usually of 2–3 sessions followed by tone up sessions as and when required.

The 10 basic sessions include the following:
1. Respiration
2. Balance under the body (legs and feet)
3. Sagittal plane balance—lateral line from front to back
4. Balance left and right—base to body to midline
5. Pelvic balance—rectus abdominis and psoas
6. Weight transfer from head to feet—sacrum
7. Relationship of head to the rest of body—occiput and atlas
8. and 9. Upper half of body to lower half of the body relationship
10. Balance throughout the system.

Once these 10 treatments are completed, advanced session may be performed in addition to the periodic tone up sessions.

Structural integration of the body's fascia through deep tissue mobilization is used to reduce abnormal stress from postural deviation and restore vertical alignment. Rolfing is believed to be able to normalize the directional pull of the fibers within connective tissue and improve muscle tone extensibility and contractility. Rolfing pressure along the spine of scapula is utilized to realign the shoulder girdle.

MECHANICAL DEVICES OF MASSAGE

Usually massage is performed with hands, which consume time and energy. Moreover, the therapist cannot attend many numbers of patients in a day. Since ancient times, people have constructed many apparatus which can bring about the same effect, as massage, mechanically and save time and energy for the therapist. Modern mechanical devices of massage can be grouped under the following two types according to the effect produced:
1. Vibration devices
2. Compression devices.

Vibration Devices

These devices provide the oscillation of varying frequency and amplitude to the body. The effect produced by these devices can be compared with that of vibration and percussion.

These devices are either electrical or cell-operated. These can be handheld devices, which can be used and moved by the therapist, or they can be stationary devices against which the patient's body part is held or moved. Basically, a vibrating machine consists of a small motor, an applicator, and a control knob. Motor provides vibrations, the frequency of which can be regulated by the control knob. In handheld devices, there are several interchangeable applicators of different size, which are selected according to the need and contour of various parts of body.

The frequency and amplitude of vibration produced by these devices varies from machine-to-machine. Some devices provide oscillation of 100–200 Hz, while others can only produce oscillation of 10–20 Hz. The devices oscillating at lower frequency produce the effect of percussion manipulation and known as "percussor". By altering the frequency and amplitude, one changes into the other. Some devices incorporate a heating element also, which provides a low degree of heat along with massage.

Vibration devices find their use in many places. In motor dysfunction of various different neurological conditions, the vibrators producing fine oscillation have been used in order to stimulate the voluntary functions of paretic muscles. These vibrators are also used to induce reflex ejaculation in paraplegic and to assist in bladder emptying in neurological bladder, etc.

Percussor producing coarse vibratory movements are used to dislodge thick secretions from lungs in pulmonary conditions. For this purpose, vibrating pads are strapped over the dorsum of hand and therapist places his palm in contact with patient's skin. Some vibrating pads can be directly kept over the patient's chest. The mechanical oscillation provided by machine is smoothly transmitted to lungs through the chest wall without exposing the therapist to fatigue.

Vibrators are also used for obtaining general relaxation and relieving pain and fatigue in upper or lower back. It is for this purpose that these machines are commonly used nowadays in home and beauty parlors **(Fig. 9.1)**.

Compression Devices

Characteristics of these types of devices are to produce massage of pressure and release. These machines apply a rhythmic compression to the body segment. The effect produced by these machines can be compared with that of effleurage.

Basically, a compression device has a sealed doubled wall sleeve or hollow tube which encircles the patient's limb. The sleeve is attached to a pump, which regulates the entry of water (in hydraulic devices) or air (in pneumatic devices) into the sleeve.

When water or air enters inside, the sleeve inflates and compresses the encircled segment. This is followed by a phase of deflation in which water/air comes out of the sleeve. This way, the segment is alternatively compressed and released. The devices have a series of controls which regulates the time ratio of inflation/deflation (i.e. on/off ratio), the amount of pressure applied, sequence of compression (or rhythm), and the total duration of treatment.

According to the nature of applied compression, these devices can be grouped under following two types:
a. Intermittent compression devices
b. Sequential compression devices.

Intermittent compression devices: These devices are otherwise known as single cell compression devices. Here, the encircling sleeve has only one continuous compartment. The sleeve inflates and compresses the limb at chosen pressure and then deflates. A uniformly distributed pressure is applied to the whole limb at a time.

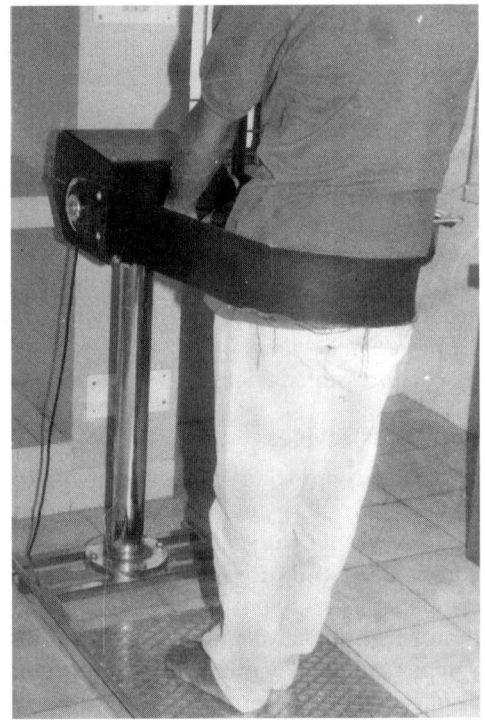

Fig. 9.1: Vibratory massage.

Sequential compression devices: Unlike the intermittent devices where the whole limb is compressed at a time, these devices provide a progressive pressure wave to the body, the encircling sleeve consists of a number of compartments, which can be inflated and deflated in sequence. As one compartment inflates, other deflates; a ripple or a pressure wave sets up. It compresses the encircled segment rhythmically. The overlapping cuffs are inflated sequentially in a centripetal direction. This helps to enhance the flow of body fluid toward the heart without allowing their backflow. The sequential devices can produce the milking effect of effleurage, which cannot be obtained in the intermittent compression devices.

The on/off timings, pressure duration, etc. can be adjusted according to the diagnosis, the extent of involvement, condition of tissue, and to the patient's comfort. Some machines provide an electronic control for these purposes while in some other the rhythm of pressure wave is synchronized with the ECG wave of the patient.

Originally designed in USA for the treatment of lymphedema following mastectomy, these devices are employed universally in the treatment of those conditions, where intermittent pressure helps to alleviate the symptoms. Some of these conditions are edema, chronic lymphatic obstruction, arteriosclerosis (pressure wave is applied from proximal to distal part), venous pooling, etc. It can be used for prevention of bedsore, phlebothrombosis, and pulmonary embolism. It is also used for shrinking of the amputation stump.

DIGITAL ISCHEMIC PRESSURE

This technique aims at evoking temporary ischemic reaction within the muscular tissue by application of a direct pressure. Fingertips are used to apply perpendicular pressure to the skin toward the center of a muscle for few seconds. The goal of this technique is to deactivate the sympathetic trigger points. The direct pressure over the localized painful area stimulates the tension monitoring receptors within muscle and leads to reduction of muscle tension. The ischemia also produces pain and facilitates the release of pain modulating substance. This may give a temporary analgesia (Brunker and Khan, 1993).

Primarily used for the management of trigger points, this technique can also be used to reduce muscle tone and to facilitate proprioception.

VACUUM CUPPING

In this technique, a vacuum pump is utilized to create a negative pressure over the skin. The different sizes of pads connected to the pump are placed over the patient's skin. When the negative pressure (suction) is applied over the body, the skin and subcutaneous tissues are lifted upward. This technique is used to release fascial cross-linkage and increases the mobility of the soft tissue restricted due to fascial tethering.

Initial application should be limited to one to five seconds at a very low negative pressure during which patient should not perceive a stretch in the tissue. This initial application serves to assess the tissue response to stretch. In subsequent application, the amount of negative pressure and duration of suction are increased gradually. The duration of suction can be increased up to 90 seconds while the magnitude of negative pressure can be increased up to a level where patient can perceive a comfortable tissue stretch.

Vacuum cupping is used in the conditions where fascial lengthening is required. Examples include anterior compartment syndrome of leg, muscle tightness at iliotibial band, etc. (Brunker and Khan, 1993). Correct placement of cups and selection of appropriate suction pressure are paramount as this technique can cause significant capillary rupture and damage to periosteum if used with excessive vacuum or with incorrect placement of cups.

STYLUS MASSAGE

Unlike all other systems of massage, this method uses a 12-cm long smooth surfaced, hardwood stick which is similar to a miniature Indian club, in order to intensify the local mechanical effect of therapist's finger. The wooden club called stylus has two ends, narrow and thicker ends. Narrow end has a spherical bulge that supports the tip of therapist's finger during massage. Narrow end is used to apply deep localized pressure whereas thicker end is used for mild and gentle treatment.

It is recommended only on particularly hardened area along with other maneuvers of classical massage with the aim of breaking the adhesions between skin, fascia, and capsules. It is claimed that this technique has the advantage of reaching the areas that would otherwise remain inaccessible to finger, such as under the shoulder blade, and of accurately estimating the location point and size of even smallest hardening and tissue disorder. It seems that this method relies heavily on the effects and uses of transverse friction because the only purpose of using a wooden stick is to apply more localized pressure without tiring the fingers.

However, this technique is full of hazards. Hematoma can result more easily, and an injury can aggravate. Inflammatory irritation, myositis ossificans, and Sudeck's atrophy are the other conditions which may also result after stylus massage. Therefore, majority of therapists and other professional groups outrightly reject stylus massage. The main contraindications of this technique include application over bone spur, spinous process, lymph nodes, veins, and breast.

The description of this method is found in the books of German authors. According to Kuprian (1981), E Densor, who was the masseur for many years to German national soccer team, first made the stylus massage known through his publication. Densor himself adopted the method from H Schult, an active masseur in 1936 Berlin Olympic who learned this technique from Japanese (Kuprian, 1981).

ACUPRESSURE MASSAGE

Acupressure massage can be considered as a type of reflex zone massage. Its principle is very much similar to that of the trigger point. It states that the dysfunction of internal or external organ is reflected as the alteration in the texture of skin, which may develop painful nodes. These nodules usually arise at a place distant from the site of original dysfunction and can be used successfully to alleviate the symptom.

This massage technique is based on the principles of acupuncture—an ancient Chinese method that believes that an essential life force exists in everyone, which control all aspects of life. This life force, called Chi in Chinese, can be considered as an equivalent of the Indian spiritual terminology *Prana*, which also describes the similar concepts. Chinese believes that Chi is governed by two opposing forces, Yang and Yin. Yang is the positive force whereas Yin denotes the negative force. These two forces flow through the 26 body lines called meridians. There are 12 paired and 2 unpaired meridians, which are associated with different parts of the body. An imbalance between these two forces is believed to be the causative factor for pain and disease.

Whenever such imbalance occurs, certain points along specific meridians become tender which disappear when the symptoms of disease subside. These points are called acupressure/acupuncture points. Several acupuncture points have been mapped out over the surface of body and each has been assigned a name and special identity in reference to a particular organ. It is claimed that stimulation of a specific acupuncture point either through needle or deep pressure can dramatically reduce pain and dysfunction in a distal area of body known to be associated with that particular point.

In acupressure massage, according to the symptom of patient, specific acupuncture points are selected. After locating the correct point by palpation or by electrical resistance testing, massage begins. Heavy pressures are applied using index middle finger, thumb, or even elbow in a circular direction over the point. Applied pressure must be intense and painful to the patient. It is often stated that if patient can tolerate more pressure, the treatment would be more effective.

Usually, a single point is massaged for about 1–5 minutes in one session.

In the recent years, this method has gained immense popularity throughout the world in both medical and nonmedical circles. The effects of this technique can be explained on the basis of pain gate theory, production of exogenous opioids, reflex, autonomic response, and placebo. Attempts have also been made to establish a correlation between trigger point and acupressure points.

EXTERNAL CARDIAC MASSAGE

Otherwise also known as closed chest cardiac massage, this technique is an essential component of cardiopulmonary resuscitation program. It is combined with mouth-to-mouth ventilation and they together form lifesaving techniques, which are simple, effective, and can be successfully administered even by a layman with little training.

It is indicated in sudden and unexpected cessation of effective cardiopulmonary performance, which is a medical emergency and is often encountered in drowning, cardiac patient, heatstroke,

diabetes, severe road traffic accidents, etc. Any person can be a candidate for cardiopulmonary resuscitation (CPR) if he/she suddenly develops the following signs:
- Loss of consciousness
- Loss of carotid and pulmonary pulses
- Loss of respiration
- Loss of heart beat
- Loss of blood pressure.

Unless immediate recognized and properly managed, these conditions can seriously jeopardize the life by restricted blood flow to brain and other vital organs.

The technique of external cardiac massage aims at forcing the blood out of both the ventricle by compressing the heart between the sternum and the vertebral column.

Procedure

Patient position

To effectively compress the heart, the patient should be placed supine, lying on a firm surface either on the floor or over a hardboard placed beneath the mattress. One hand of the operator should be placed under the neck and other on the forehead in order to tilt the head backward. This position lifts the tongue from back of throat and clears the airway. Any foreign body, froth, etc. should be cleared from the nose and mouth.

Technique

After proper positioning, mouth-to-mouth ventilation and external cardiac massage should begin simultaneously.

The best way of doing external cardiac massage is to place the heel of left hand over the sternum just above the xiphoid. Palm of right hand should be placed over the left hand. Elbow should remain straight. Rhythmic compression should be applied to the chest wall using the body weight. During compression, sternum should be pushed to a distance of about 1.5–2.5 inches. An effective compression will produce a palpable carotid and femoral pulses. Between compressions, the hand should just leave the chest wall.

Mouth-to-Mouth Breathing

Meanwhile, the mouth-to-mouth breathing should also start immediately. For this purpose, it is ideal to have two persons. Alternatively, one operator can also manage to administer both the procedures. The mouth of the operator should be placed over the mouth of patient, completely sealing the patient's mouth so that there occurs no leakage of air. Nostrils of patient should be closed by the fingers of operator. After this, operator should exhale a larger than normal breath into the patient's mouth. If the procedure is correct, a rise in the chest wall will be noticed.

In reference to external cardiac massage and CPR, the American Heart Association has issued the following guidelines for efficient results:
- About 80–100 external compressions should be applied per minute.
- About 50% of each compression-relaxation cycle should be compression.
- If two trained rescuers are performing CPR, then for every 5 compressions, one ventilation should be used.
- If CPR is performed by two lay rescuers or by one trained person, for every 15th chest compression two slow (1–1.5 seconds) ventilating breath should be given.

For every half minute, the procedure should be stopped temporarily in order to ascertain whether spontaneous beating has occurred or not. If there is evidence that efforts have been successful, one may stop and observe the patient for several seconds. On the other hand, if there is no change in the patient's status, CPR should continue till further advanced medical aid arrives. In any circumstances, CPR should not be halted for longer than 5 seconds.

Before starting CPR, it is worth trying the following two procedures which may restore the stopped heartbeat:
1. Elevation of legs for 30 seconds—it increases the venous return and if arrest is due to ineffectual myocardial contraction, it may sufficiently restore the weak beats and circulation.
2. Forceful thumping of the chest wall—a forceful direct blow delivered to the sternum by the heel of hand may revert the ventricular fibrillation, ventricular tachycardia, and asystole to the normal sinus rhythm. It may be repeated only once or twice if there is no response.

Most Common Errors

The most common errors while carrying out external cardiac massage are the following:
1. Failure to ensure that airway is closed
2. Not occluding the nose during mouth-to-mouth breathing
3. Failure to compress the heart sufficiently
4. Not allowing adequate cardiac filling by using a compression rate which is too fast
5. By not fully releasing the pressure on the sternum between each compression.

Complication of External Cardiac Massage

Complication, which may arise due to external cardiac massage, includes fractured ribs, hemothorax, pneumothorax, laceration of heart leading to hemoperitoneum, marrow embolism, and laceration of liver and other visceral organs. Many of these complications are trivial when compared with the seriousness of the emergency, which if allowed continuing for more than 3 minutes may result in death, or convert a healthy person to a neurologically vegetable throughout the life.

The practice of external cardiac massage has revolutionized the primary management of cardiac arrest. Before 30 years, the cardiac resuscitation was performed primarily by thoracotomy and open chest cardiac massage. Now, this kind of massage can successfully save a life even in the hand of a nonmedical layman. This important lifesaving technique must be learned not only by the medical and paramedical persons but also by all the educated persons of a civilized society.

UNDERWATER MASSAGE

Mode of application of pressure in this technique is the pressurized water stream, which is directed to the body parts submerged in a tub of warm water. This technique utilizes the relaxing effects of warm water combined with the mechanical compression of high pressure jet of water.

Equipment for this massage consists of a large tub, a pressure pump, a hose, and a set of different diameter nozzles (**Fig. 9.2A**). Tub has the capacity of 400–600 L and enough space to allow a subject to lie down comfortably. Pressure

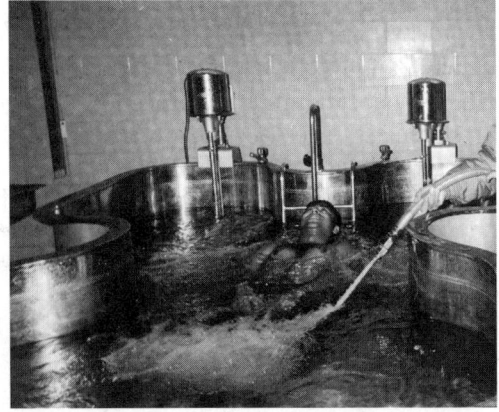

Fig. 9.2A: Underwater massage equipment.

pump is recirculating in nature. It draws the water in from the tub and returns it back under high pressure through a movable hose. The variable nozzles can be attached to the hose according to the amount of pressure required. The narrower nozzle increases the pressure of water stream and is used to obtain a localized penetrating and deep effect. The nozzles with medium to large diameter exert relatively less pressure and cover a wide area. The pressure of water stream may range from 0.5 to 7 bar. A manometer is incorporated in the pump in order to measure and regulate the amount of pressure.

Along with these essential components, few underwater equipment also has a heating element which keeps the water of the tub warm. Ideally, the temperature of tub water should be kept between 35°C and 38°C, i.e., a little above the temperature of body. The temperature of pressurized water jet can also be regulated and depending on the requirement it can be kept at either higher or lower temperatures with respect to the tub water.

Various natural or mineral extracts are usually added to the water with the intention of promoting relaxation, drainage, and rejuvenation.

Technique

Patient is asked to sit inside the water tub for 5 minutes before the actual underwater massage to accustom himself to the surrounding. Minimal clothing is allowed. Massage is administered in half-lying, supine-lying, and side-lying position. Prone position is not used because it interferes with the breathing. Besides, the buoyancy of water also places the spine in a hyperextended position and increases the lordosis in prone position. Half and supine lying are used to treat the front aspect of body, whereas for back and side of body side lying position is used.

Depending upon the type of treatment, the nozzle size and the pressure of water jet are adjusted. The movable hose is brought near to the body part to direct the pressured jet toward the target area. The distance between hose and patient skin should be 12–15 cm **(Fig. 9.2B)**. Adjusting the angle of water stream can vary the applied pressure. Stream striking the body at 90° angle applies more pressure than that striking at acute angles.

Considering these basic principles, practically effects of all techniques of classical massage can be produced during underwater massage. For the

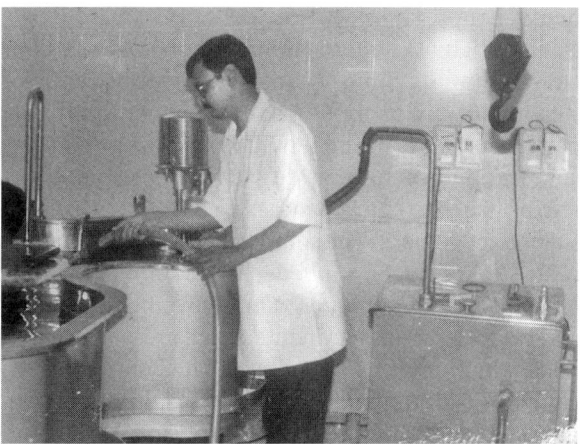

Fig. 9.2B: Underwater massage.

purpose of enhancing the lymphatic and venous drainage, the stream should be moved from the distal to the proximal area. It should constantly strike the skin at 50–75° angle. Stream can be moved in a circular direction with angle of strike, increasing in one-half and decreasing in other half circle. This produces the effects similar to that of kneading maneuvers. A high pressure stream striking the skin at 90° angle can be moved to-and-fro in small range, to have the effect of transverse friction.

Water jet should never be directed toward sensitive areas, such as female breast, genitals, anus, popliteal fossa, spinous processes, etc. in order to avoid injury.

The advantage of this technique includes preservation of energy of the therapist, enjoyable atmosphere, and facilitation of relaxation.

Routinely recommended to the athletes as an aid to recovery following intense physical activities, this technique can also be utilized in all other conditions where manual massage is indicated.

Apart from local and general contraindication of massage, adequate caution should be exercised to exclude the contraindication of hydrotherapy, such as cardiac disease, etc. because position in underwater strains the cardiovascular system. Athletes are not allowed to participate in intense physical activities for one to two days after underwater massage.

MANUAL LYMPHATIC DRAINAGE

The term manual lymphatic drainage (MLD) was first used by Dr Emil Vodder and his wife Estrid when they presented their work to a Paris Symposium in 1936 (Wittlinger et al., 2011; Korosec, 2004). This technique of massage uses light, gentle strokes in order to encourage natural drainage of lymph.

This technique of massage applies very little pressure on the skin. Compared to traditional massage, the pressure applied with manual lymph drainage is much lower in intensity and heavy pressure is discouraged (Kasseroller, 1998). The goal of these techniques is to manipulate the lymphatic structures located in the subcutaneous tissues. Practitioners of this system use their hands to move skin in the direction of lymphatic flow, either by pushing or stretching the skin. It is claimed that very light pressure involves only the skin surface not the subcutaneous muscles. In fact, so little pressure is used that when teaching this technique the practitioner of this system describes the touch on the skin: "...as light as a fly... a wasp would be too heavy" (Hansen, 2015) as higher pressures may compress the lymphatic vessels and thereby possibly hinder lymph transport.

The original Vodder Manual Lymph Drainage consists of four stroke techniques—stationary circle, pump technique, scoop technique, and rotary technique (Wittlinger et al., 2011). "Stationary circle" applies an oval-shaped stretching of the skin, using the entire hand or the palmar surface of the fingers. This stroke is primarily applied to the neck and the face. The scoop and the pump technique are used on the extremities. Pump stroke moves distally to proximally and utilizes the entire palm as well as the proximal phalanges whereas the scoop is a spiral-shaped movement. The rotary technique is used on flat body surfaces, such as the back. These basic strokes can be applied in any combination during treatment.

In all these techniques, hand movements are used to stretch the skin in specific directions and promote variations in interstitial pressures, usually without the use of oils (Williams, 2010). The techniques intend to manipulate lymph vessels located in the subcutaneous tissues. The common denominator of all strokes is the resting and working phase. In the working phase of the stroke, lymphatic structures located in subcutaneous tissues are stretched. The pressure in the working phase should be sufficient enough to stretch the subcutaneous tissues against the fascia but not large enough to manipulate the underlying muscle tissue. The amount of pressure needed in MLD is sometimes described as the pressure applied stroking a newborn's head. After the pressure phase, the therapist begins a relaxation phase. During this phase, the therapist maintains manual contact with the skin but does not apply any pressure (Hansen, 2015).

Apart from original Vodder techniques, different schools of MLD have been established. These include Földi, Casley-Smith, Leduc, and Fluoroscopy-guided manual lymphatic drainage (FG-MLD). The underlying features and principles of the MLD technique remain same in all these schools. Fluoroscopy-guided manual lymphatic drainage (FG-MLD) performs mapping of lymphatics before actual massage by injecting intradermally a fluorescent dye and then scan the area with a special infrared camera. This helps the specialist to visualize the superficial lymph channels.

The aim of MLD is to move fluid from the swollen area into a place where the lymphatic system is working normally. Therefore, before approaching the swollen area, the therapists work on the chest and neck and other proximal area in order to clear the lymphatic pathways.

The mechanisms through which MLD has its effect are not fully established (William, 2010). It is claimed that MLD produces stretching effect on lymph collectors and local smooth muscle and increases the frequency of contraction of lymphangions/lymph vessels and increased lymphatic transport capacity. Variations in interstitial pressures led to enhanced filling and emptying of initial lymphatic and accessory routes within the lymph drainage system that appeared to be "stimulated". Besides, it is claimed that MLD decreases sympathetic nervous system responses while increasing parasympathetic nervous tone (Korosec, 2004) which may produced a calming effect.

The main application of MLD is in the treatment of extensive lymphedema of the limbs that usually encountered after breast surgery although traumatic injuries, such as hematomas, distortions, muscle fiber tears, hyperkeratotic scars, cases involving subacute inflammatory conditions, fibromyalgia, and scleroderma are also said to benefit from this kind of massage. Manual lymphatic drainage is recommended for edema from different sources such as: Orthopedic, abdominoplasty PO, fleboedema, premenstrual edema, reflex sympathetic dystrophy, and fibromyalgia (Masson et al., 2014). In lymphedema treatment, MLD is often combined with compression bandaging, skin care, and exercise. The contraindication of this technique includes acute infections, thromboembolism, and edema caused by cardiac ailments and malignant tumors (Kasseroller, 1998).

CRANIOSACRAL THERAPY

Craniosacral therapy (CST) is an osteopathic approach to evaluating and treating dysfunction occurring within the articulations of the skull (Flynn et al., 2006). Practitioners of this system apply a gentle manual force to address somatic dysfunctions of the head and the remainder of the body (Jäkel and Hauenschild, 2012). It is based, in part, on the idea that physical manipulation of the meninges through the cranial vault sutures with low levels of force (< 5 g) can alter the rhythmic fluctuation of cerebrospinal fluid and intracranial pressure (ICP) (Downey et al., 2006).

Technique involves light holding of the skull and sacrum with almost imperceptible movements and gentle pushing and massaging of the skull, spine, and other parts of the body. CS therapists use "release" and "pumping" manipulation to produce motion in that particular body area (Zane, 2011). The practitioner of this system is said to use a soft touch which is generally no > 5 g and claim to release restrictions in the soft tissues that surround the central nervous system (Downey, 2004).

Craniosacral techniques can be indirect or direct. An indirect technique is one that releases a restriction by facilitating motion in the direction of ease. The practitioner "follows" the restriction into the direction of ease and gently holds it there. Craniosacral therapists believe that the inherent motion of the structure will attempt to return to neutral against the hold. Eventually, a release or "tissue softening" occurs. The opposite occurs with a direct technique in which the restricted structure is assisted to pass through the abnormal barrier in the direction of the restriction and then return to a neutral position. Some of the techniques utilized in this system are frontal lift, parietal lift, sphenoid compression, sphenoid decompression, temporal wobble and ear pull, and cephalad and caudal mandibular traction, still point induction, CV-4 technique, etc. (Downey, 2004).

The technique was developed by John E Upledger—an osteopath—in 1970 and it aims to enhance the body's own healing capabilities. Practitioners believe that the tiny manipulations of CST affect the pressure and circulation of cerebrospinal fluid. According to Upledger, CST works with natural and unique rhythms of various body systems to pinpoint and correct source problems. According to Zane (2011), CST is based upon following six assumptions:

1. The human brain pulsates unrelated to breathing or heart rate at about 10–14 cycles/min.
2. A person can feel such pulsations with one's fingertips in particular locations on the body.
3. The craniosacral system (cranium, joints, sutures, and spine) can move and can be moved by touching and massaging.
4. Restrictions of the natural movements of the cranial system restrict or prevent the flow of cerebrospinal fluid.
5. These presumed difficulties result in numerous problems such as learning disabilities, autistic symptomology (behavioral problems, poor social relationships, communication difficulties, and poor abstract thought), and other physical, social, and intellectual abnormalities.
6. With the pressure of about 5 g, therapists can remove restrictions and generate movement of the cranial system that results in improved functioning and the curing of disease.

Proponents of this system define the craniosacral system as a functioning physiological system that includes the meninges and cerebrospinal fluid surrounding the spinal cord and brain, the bones to which these membranes attach and connective tissue related to these membranes. This system is characterized by rhythmic, mobile activity, distinctively different from the physiological motions related to breathing and cardiovascular activity. An important component of craniosacral mobility is referred to as the primary respiratory mechanism (PRM), which manifests as palpable motion of the cranial bones, sacrum, dural membranes, central nervous system, and cerebrospinal fluid (CSF).

Proponents of this system believe that intrinsic rhythmic movements of the brain cause rhythmic fluctuations of cerebrospinal fluid and specific relational changes among dural membranes, cranial bones, and the sacrum (Hartman, 2006). Practitioners of CST claim that they can identify alterations in the movement patterns of the sacrum and cranial sutures through manual palpation (Flynn et al., 2006). Proponents assert that mobility restrictions or misalignments along the cranial sutures will disturb rhythmic flows of the cerebrospinal fluid, having in turn an adverse effect on health. Manual intervention, it is argued, has the ability to restore normal function within this system.

Craniosacral therapy is used to treat conditions ranging from headache pain and temporomandibular dysfunction to developmental disabilities. The conditions claimed to have benefited from this system include headache, visual disturbances, sinusitis, hay fever, asthma, cardiac and digestive problems, carpal tunnel syndrome, developmental disabilities, traumatic brain injury, dysmenorrhea, stress urinary incontinence, ankle sprain, torticollis, temporomandibular dysfunction, dyslexia, chronic back pain, depression, anxiety, colic, ear infections, irritability, vomiting, hypertonicity, hyperactive peristalsis, etc.

General contraindications to craniosacral therapy include patients with acute, unstable neurological signs, increased intracranial pressure, intracranial bleeding, and nonhealed fractures of the cranial vault or base. Seizure disorder is considered as a precaution (Downey, 2004).

Craniosacral therapy has received widespread criticism for its ostensible rationales and clinical claims (Green et al., 1999; Hartman, 2006; Flynn et al., 2006) which many called pseudoscientific (Earnest, 2012) due to absence of any scientific proof with regards to its basics tenet of cranial motion and palpation of craniosacral rhythm and ability to gentle touch to produce movement and sutures and influence the flow of CSF. On the other hand, proponents of this system held that CST can never be validly tested in a scientific way because the therapy technique will vary per patient therefore a controlled study of the CST methodology is unattainable (Jane, 2011).

INSTRUMENT-ASSISTED SOFT TISSUE MOBILIZATION

Instrument-assisted soft tissue mobilization (IASTM) has received much attention in the recent years. The concept of using equipment to deliver mechanical forces to the body is not new. The current practice of IASTM is in part based on the Cyriax theory of transverse friction where a mechanical force applied to deeper tissue through thumb fingers or elbow is used to break the adhesion and improves mobility of the soft tissue. IASTM is applied using especially designed instruments allowing deeper penetration and reducing imposed stress on the operator's hands (Cheatham, 2016).

There are various IASTM tools and companies, such as Graston, Técnica Gavilán, HawkGrips, Functional and Kinetic Treatment and Rehab (FAKTR), Adhesion Breakers, and Fascial Abrasion Technique augmented soft tissue mobilization (ASTYM), etc. (Kim et al., 2017). Each company has its own approach to treatment and instrument design in terms of shape and material of instruments. Most of these instruments are made of stainless steel and most of these techniques are trademarked and thus necessitates license from the parent organizations.

Graston technique uses six different stainless steel instruments (Stow, 2011) that have either a convex or a concave shape. It is claimed that the concave shape allows for the pressure applied by the clinician to be dispersed over a large area, whereas the convex shape concentrates pressure over a smaller surface area. The instruments have either a single-beveled edge or double-beveled edge.

The main use of IASTM is mobilization of scar tissue and promotion of soft tissue healing. It is postulated that heavy localized forces applied through instrument produce localized inflammation in the soft tissue that helps to restart the healing and produces better alignment of collagen. The IASTM treatment is thought to stimulate connective tissue remodeling through resorption of excessive fibrosis, along with inducing repair and regeneration of collagen secondary to fibroblast recruitment (Cheatham, 2016). Some studies conducted on rat model (Davidson et al., 1997; Gehlsen et al., 1999; Loghmani and Warden) supports this hypothesis where increased fibroblast proliferation and collagen repair have been observed in cases of enzyme-induced tendinitis following instrument-assisted soft tissue mobilization.

Bruising and soreness are the obvious side effects of IASTM. The contraindications of these techniques are no different from that of classical massage. Cancer, kidney dysfunction, pregnancy, rheumatoid arthritis, varicose veins, osteoporosis, lymphedema, fracture, and chronic regional pain syndrome are the relative contraindications whereas the absolute contraindications include the presence of an open wound, unhealed suture sites, thrombophlebitis, uncontrolled hypertension, skin infection, hematoma, myositis ossificans, and unstable fractures (Kim et al., 2017).

Relative contraindications include cancer, kidney dysfunction, pregnancy, rheumatoid arthritis, varicose veins, osteoporosis, lymphedema, fracture, chronic regional pain syndrome, and use of certain medications (e.g. anticoagulants, steroids, or nonsteroidal anti-inflammatory drugs). Absolute contraindications include the presence of an open wound, unhealed suture sites, thrombophlebitis, uncontrolled hypertension, skin infection, hematoma, myositis ossificans, and unstable fractures (Kim et al., 2017).

These techniques are now increasingly being used in management of sports-related soft tissue injury where the use of instrument-assisted soft tissue mobilization is integrated with strengthening, stretching, and cryotherapy. When IASTM is applied in sports rehabilitation, it generally goes through the following six different steps: Examination, warm up, IASTM, stretching, strengthening exercises, and cryotherapy. After identification of the correct lesion and ruling out contraindications, the patients are asked to warm up the area either actively (jogging or stationary bicycle) or passively through hot packs or ultrasound, the practitioner then rubs a cream on the patients' skin and applies the instrument at a pressure that the patient can withstand. Each lesion is treated for 30–60 seconds. After the completion of IASTM, stretching and muscle strengthening exercises targeting the treated area must be performed. Finally, cryotherapy is applied for 10–20 minutes (Kim et al., 2017).

ROLLER MASSAGE

According to Cheatham (2018), "roller massage is a type of self or assisted massage that uses a device to manipulate the skin, myofascia, muscles, and tendons by direct compression". In the recent years, roller massage has emerged as a popular technique for managing pain and aches of the musculoskeletal origin. According to the annual survey of worldwide fitness trends conducted by editors of ACSMs Health and Fitness Journal® (Thompson, 2017), roller massage has been one of the top 20 fitness trend in world over since last three years, i.e. 2016, 2017, and 2018. According to the Oxford Dictionary, roller is a cylinder that rotates about a central axis and is used in various machines and devices to move, flatten, or spread something.

The technique of roller massage involves rolling of a cylinder over a person's body. A cylinder of soft consistency is the device for this massage which is known as roller. These rollers are typically made of foam—thus the name foam roller—though the cylinders made out of rubber, plastic, and wood are also used over which a layer of foam or rubber is wrapped. Shape, and size of cylinder and the thickness, densities, and texture of covering wrap material vary considerable according to body part and purpose of use. Rollers have been designed for the low back, hips, and for larger muscle groups such as the hamstrings and the gluteal muscles (Thompson, 2017). There are three ways by which roller massage can be performed:

1. *Self-roller massage with bodyweight:* The clients may lay or position a body part on a roller and apply pressure with their bodyweight and counterbalance the body and the weight with their hands and feet.
2. *Self-roller massage with the hand:* The client rolls the handheld roller over specific body parts, such as thigh, shoulder, etc.
3. *Assisted roller massage:* Another person apply the roller device over the client's body.

Rolling over the cylinder produces compression and release of pressure over the body part and gives a massage-like feeling. It is postulated that during the rolling, direct and sweeping pressure and friction are exerted on the soft tissue that stretches the soft tissue, breaks the soft tissue adhesion, and restores the soft tissue extensibility. Depending on the pressure applied, both superficial and deep massage can be performed.

The reported effects of roller massage are similar to that obtained after a classic massage. It is postulated that roller massage increases the blood flow of the area, enhances the mobility of soft tissue, and stimulates the mechanoreceptor. Roller massage (RM) is often also referred to as self-myofascial release. Cheatham (2018) and the proponents of myofascial release postulated that roller massage may change the viscoelastic properties of the local myofascia by mechanisms such as thixotropy (reduced viscosity), reducing myofascial restriction, fluid changes, and cellular responses. The pressure on the fascia from rolling may allow fascia to become soft and lengthen, permitting for a larger stretch of the muscle and increased range of motion. It is claimed that rolling reduces local arterial stiffness, increases arterial tissue perfusion, and improves vascular endothelial function (Cheatham, 2015). The stimulation of cutaneous receptors by roller massage may also modulate pain and induce relaxation.

The roller massage is assumed to relieve muscle tightness, alleviate muscle spasms, improve circulation, ease muscular discomfort, and assist in the return to normal activity. Therefore, in sports setting, it is used during warm up and postexercise recovery. It is also used for improving the flexibility and increasing the range of motion. Certain clinical conditions such as fibromyalgia and myofascial pain syndromes (Cheatham, 2018) have also shown to be benefited from this technique of massage. The contraindications of this technique are similar to that of classical massage. Unlike instrument-assisted soft tissue manipulation, this technique does not produce soreness or bruising of the skin.

MYOFASCIAL RELEASE

Myofascial release (MFR) is a collection of approaches and techniques that focuses on the connective tissue, or fascia. Based on the concepts of osteopathic medicine where the term *fascia* is used almost synonymously with *connective tissue,* this approach views fascia as the unifying element of the body and postulates that all the peripheral and visceral structures are connected to each other by fascia (Schwind, 2006).

Fascia is a type of connective tissue that is divided into 3 layers: The superficial layer, a layer of potential space, and a deep layer (McKenney et al., 2013). The deep muscular fasciae are seen as coordinating elements for motor units (grouped together in myofascial units), uniting elements between unidirectional myofascial units (myofascial sequences), and connecting elements between body joints through myofascial expansions and retinacula (myofascial spirals) (Stecco and Day, 2010). Fascia modifies its consistency when under stress (plasticity) and is capable of regaining its elasticity when subjected to manipulation (Stanborough, 2004). Muscular stress, repeated inflammation, or psychoemotional tension alters the consistency of fascia (called densification) in which the ground substances of fascia lose its suppleness and collagen fibers are arranged haphazardly (Schwind, 2006). This densification of fascia produces restrictions in the smooth gliding movement of fascia.

Any obstruction to gliding between endofascial fibers and interfascial planes could cause anomalous tension within given fascial chain giving rise to altered proprioceptive signals resulting in nonphysiologic movements at joints. Such movements could cause inflammation within the joint of a malfunctioning myofascial unit or pain along a myofascial sequence (Stecco and Day, 2010). The proponents of MFR approach further consider human body as a tensegrity structure where solid bones maintain its alignment through their elastic myofascial fibers connection (Stecco, 2004). Fascia is believed as one continuous piece of tissue working in connected "chains" to create tensegrity in the body (McKenney et al., 2013). Whenever external forces are applied to the tensegrity system, the entire system reacts with an adaptive redistribution of tension and the preexisting patterns of tension within the system are modified (Schwind, 2006). Tension within one part of myofascial element developed due to trauma or stress can produce symptoms in some distant unrelated structure either through direct mechanical effects or through its neural connections. This concept provides the basis for the global treatment of the musculoskeletal apparatus where the manipulation of fascia of unconnected body part may bring relive at a distant site (Schwind, 2006; Grant and Riggs, 2008).

The application of prolonged pressure with stretch can be transformed to the connective tissue fascia from a gel (thickened) state to a sol (liquid) state. In MFR literature, this concept is referred as thixotropy. The term release in osteopathic literature means the capacity of fascia and other tissues to lengthen when subjected to a constant tension load resulting in less resistance to a second load application (Grant and Riggs, 2008).

MFR approach uses a combination of manual traction and sustained gentle pressure maneuvers for stretching the fascia and breaking up the fascial adhesions. It is believed that a low load applied slowly would allow a viscoelastic fascia to elongate. The key feature of these group techniques is the detection of fascial restrictions through touch and application of the appropriate amount of sustained pressure guided entirely by feedback from the recipient's body to determine stretch direction, force, and duration to address specific soft tissue restrictions (Manheim, 2001). Treatment session is performed directly on skin usually without oils or lubricants.

Direct release and indirect release are the two categories of myofascial release techniques (Grant and Riggs, 2008). Direct release techniques—also known as "deep tissue work"—use force or weight, using tools, knuckles, or elbows to slowly stretch the fascia. Indirect release is a gentler method where the practitioner applies less pressure. During direct release techniques, the pressure to stretched tissue is applied in opposition to the direction that the fascia may freely allow movement whereas during indirect release the therapist applies slow, steady pressure to the stretched tissue in the direction where the fascia can be felt to allow greatest ease of movement (Barnes, 1997).

Any muscle or myofascial unit that allows the placement of two hands or two fingers can be stretched to release myofascial tightness or restrictions. One hand or finger acts as the anchor from which the stretch originates. The other is used to provide the stretching force. Stretches are described as horizontal stretch and vertical stretch. A vertical stretch is any stretch applied perpendicular to the fibers of the target muscle whereas the stretch applied parallel to muscle fibers is termed as horizontal stretch.

According to Manheim (2001), treatment using myofascial release begins with gross superficial stretches and feedback from the gross stretches leads to the next layer of tightness and restriction. Treatment continues layer-by-layer with frequent alterations between superficial and deeper tissues. A gross stretch is followed by large area stretches and ultimately a focused stretch of the muscles in the same body area is applied. The gross stretch involves either a large part of or an entire myofascial unit, or nonspecific stretching of a large body area. The focused stretch narrows the stretch to a very small area within a myofascial unit.

During MFR sessions, the therapist monitors tissue tightness through touch and detects subtle restrictions within myofascial unit. The initial stretch is applied to take up the available slack. The stretch is held until the release is felt and new slack appears under the stretching hands. The stretching force is increased to take up the new slack and held until the next release occurs. This sequence is repeated until no more slack is available and the end feel is reached. Responding to feedback, the next area of tightness or restriction is then addressed (Manheim, 2001).

In MFR concept, release is the tissue relaxation that feel like a smooth melting away of tightness and restriction under the therapist's hand. It is described that just before a release, a fluttering or "ratcheting" sensation or increase in muscle tension may be felt in the targeted area and after the release a reflex vasodilatation occurs during which the therapist may feel a vast column of heat originating from the patient. It is claimed that sometime the patient loses so much body heat that his core temperature drops, causing a severe chill and violent shivering which resolves with time (Manheim, 2001). Before starting the treatment, therapists monitor the pulse of various arteries. All patients are made to rest in a horizontal position for 10–15 minutes following treatment and made to drink enough water because it is believed that myofascial release consistently lowers blood pressure.

MFR techniques are utilized in a wide range of settings and diagnoses producing pain, movement, restriction, spasm, spasticity, and neurological dysfunction (Grant and Riggs, 2008). According to Barnes, complex, global, or specific pain complaint that does not follow dermatomes, myotomes, or visceral referral patterns, an underlying chronic condition that causes tightness and restrictions in the soft tissues (e.g. fibromyalgia and postpolio syndrome), painful complex postural asymmetries, asymmetrical muscle weakness due to an acute or chronic peripheral or central neuropathy, impaired respiration and inflexible ribcage due to chronic respiratory disease, frequent intense headache, impaired mouth closure, swallowing and phonation, tightness and restriction of hyoid and muscle of mastication, vertigo and dizziness, and performance enhancement by sports persons are some of the indications of MFR.

Manheim (2001) considers unstable medical condition, dermatitis, contagious or infectious disease, and patient under the influence of drugs or alcohol as contraindication. According to Manheim (2001), MFR should not be applied when patient does not tolerate close physical contact or touch, does not understand the concept of the "Good Hurt", does not trust the therapist, and also when therapist does not feel comfortable with the patient.

The term myofascial release as a technique was coined in 1981 by Robert Ward, an osteopath who along with a physical therapist John Barnes that are considered as the two primary founders of myofascial release. According to Ward, myofascial release originated from concepts used by Andrew Taylor Still, the founder of osteopathic medicine in the late nineteenth century (Grant and Riggs, 2008).

CHAPTER 10

Sports Massage

Sports massage is routinely recommended as an aid for speedy recovery from vigorous exercises. It is found useful, when an athlete has to participate in a series of events, where successive intense muscular activity is required. There are numerous massage techniques, which are used by sports physiotherapists and masseurs with the intention of enhancing functional recovery, promoting soft tissue healing, alleviating tension and stress as well as stimulating the muscles of the athletes.

The commonly employed massage techniques in the sports setups are effleurage, superficial stroking, kneading, petrissage, tapotement, and friction. While effleurage, kneading and petrissage are used for restorative effects, the superficial stroking and tapotement are used for stimulation and maintenance of an optimal arousal level. The role of friction/cross-fiber massage in the management of acute and chronic soft tissue injuries is now well-recognized. Apart from classical manual massage, specialized massage techniques, such as connective tissue massage, trigger point massage, and acupressure massage are also used by those therapists who are well-trained in these techniques. Other types of massage techniques used in athletic setting include mechanical vibratory massage and underwater massage.

It is clear that the techniques used in sports massage are not different from those used in therapeutic massage. In fact, the sports massage can be more appropriately defined as the skillful selection and application of various techniques of massage on a sports person with the aim of enhancing and prolonging the quality length of a person's career in the sports.

Even though the both groups utilize the essential techniques of classical massage along with few specialized techniques, the aims and objectives of these two setups are entirely different. Therapeutic massage primarily concerned with aiding the healing process after an injury or functional disorder, whereas in sports massage this aim becomes secondary. The primary objective of sports massage is to help improve performance in those individuals whose physical abilities are far above the average. By ensuring pain-free training and maintaining an appropriate arousal level, it not only prolongs the overall career of an athlete but also enhances the athletic performance. Apart from promoting quicker recovery from acute and chronic musculoskeletal injuries, sports massage also address the goal of injury prevention.

HISTORICAL PERSPECTIVE

The useful role of massage in conjunction with sports activities was well-known in all the ancient civilization and it had been very popular among all those interested in physical beauty and education. In Ancient Greek and Rome, it was practiced by medical practitioners, priest, slaves, and anointer, when main duty was to relieve pain, reduce swelling, and refresh the gladiators before and after their exercises. The use of massage for improving performance of the athlete had been mentioned in the writing of Hippocrates, Galen, and Epictetus. Preparatory and warm down massage were included in the Galen's 18 different variants of massage, which he distinguished by combining the three basic qualities of massage. In those times, the trainer adjusted his treatment to the needs of athletes. Paintings from ancient Greece show back rubs and chest massage of boxers, Achilles tendon massage for runners, and a self-massage for the calf muscles (Kuprian, 1981). In those days, massage was always used in conjunction with active and passive exercises and breathing exercises.

In India, the mention of massage as *Champan* and *Mardan* is found in *Ayurveda*, the medical part of *Atharvaveda*, supposed to have written around second millennium BC, where its restorative, rejuvenative, and soothing effects are described in detail. Massage was an inseparable part of Indian sports culture. This fact is reflected by the observation that the traditional masseurs in India are known as *Pehalwan* (wrestlers) and athletes massaging each other are still a common sight in all the traditional *akharas* (wrestling ground).

In modern times, also sports massage, otherwise also called apotherapy (Liston, 1995), has gained immense popularity and recognition as an important preventive, restorative, and therapeutic modalities. The athletes, coaches, and those concerned with sports throughout the world acknowledge that massage is an effective modality that can enhance the rate of recovery and reduce soreness and discomfort following intense physical activity.

Massage is an important part of Soviet system of athletic training. It is extensively practiced in European countries including those of the former Communist Bloc. Though not taken seriously, before, massage has also reclaimed its important place in United States Athletic World. It was included in 1984 Olympic as a service available to all athletes (Kresge, 1988). Statistics from Great Britain team in 1996 Olympic revealed that massage formed 47% of all treatment to the athletes from all sports (Callaghan, 1998).

Galloway and Watt (2004) examined the data recorded by the head team physiotherapist from 12 major national and international athletics events between 1987 and 1998, and observed that a significant proportion of physiotherapists' time was devoted to the delivery of massage treatment at athletics events which ranged from 24.0 to 52.2% of the total number of treatments made. The demand for massage treatment had been steady over the studied time period of 9 years, which indicated a consistent use of this treatment modality.

Many claims on the utility of massage in sports setup have not been conclusively proved. However, sports massage is among many of the methods that follow lack of experimental verification, yet they have been found to be helpful by clinicians and coaches who have tried them. The anecdotal evidences favor that it should continued to be used.

ROLE OF MASSAGE IN ATHLETIC WORLD

It is generally accepted that sports massage reduces exercise-induced muscle strength loss, reduces muscle soreness, decreases paracompetitive anxiety, and improves mood which ultimately may lead to rapid recovery and enhanced performance. By decreasing the detrimental effects of training, it also helps to improve training consistency. The value of massage in identification and correction of the silent (asymptomatic) areas of abnormal biomechanical stress, reflected in the form of exaggerated muscle tension, also makes it a powerful adjunct to the prevention programs of sports injuries **(Box 10.1)**.

The role of sports massage in the athletic setting can be discussed under the following headings:
- DOMS management
- Physiological fatigue and recovery
- Psychological recovery
- Prevention of injuries.

Box 10.1: Role of massage in sports.

- Facilitates recovery following intense exercise
- Relieves discomfort of DOMS
- Lessens fatigue
- Helps identify hidden soft tissue injuries
- Identify abnormal area of biomechanical stress
- Identify and treat old soft tissue lesion
- Enhances psychological recovery
- Modulates psychosomatic arousal during competition

DOMS Management and the Efficacy of Massage

The occurrence of delayed-onset muscle soreness (DOMS) can seriously handicap the athlete. Apart from causing considerable suffering, it can also temporarily impede the performance. It occurs in both trained and untrained individuals in response to the heavy unaccustomed exercise. In a typical sportsman, it arises when activity level is increased or when activity begins after a period of relative inactivity.

The pain and stiffness associated with DOMS generally appears between 8 hours and 24 hours postexercise, peaks around 48 hours, and dissipates over the course of a few days. The discomfort may range from slight stiffness to extremely disabling pain. The location of soreness is generally more prominent at the musculotendinous junction. However, in severe cases, pain might be felt throughout the entire muscle belly.

It is due to the associated reduction in the range of motion (ROM) of involved joints and the reduction in the force output; this condition not only interferes with immediate athletic performance, but also limits the activities of daily living. It also impedes adherence to exercise program, and may compromise with individual's willingness to perform therapeutic exercises during rehabilitation.

Sports massage is routinely recommended as an aid for speedy recovery from DOMS. No consensus exists about the treatment of this condition and several methods are being tried with variable results. For this purpose, massage is more effective if it is administered shortly within 1-2 hours after the strenuous effort (Kresge, 1988).

The exact cause of DOMS is not known and several hypotheses exist on its pathophysiology. Ernest (1998) precisely summarized these hypotheses as follows:

- Exercise leads to local accumulation of metabolic waste which in turn sensitize $A\delta$ and C fibers causing pain.
- Exercises cause muscle ischemia, which results in the production of pain substance. Pain in turn produces a reflex spasm which in a vicious cycle prolongs ischemia and pain.
- Exercise results in intramuscular edema, which activates nociceptors causing pain.
- Eccentric exercises lead to damage of the connective tissue in the area of muscle and this damage is responsible for the pain.
- Exercise leads to the release of inflammatory byproducts, which sensitize nerve fibers causing pain.
- Exercise leads to destruction within muscle fibers liberating creatine kinase, which is the cause of pain.

Massage may positively affect each of these processes by improving the circulation, as well as the lymph flow and relaxing the muscles. This in turn may reduce edema, ischemia, accumulation of waste substances, and enhance the regenerative processes. Application of a second sensation such as massage to a sore muscle could increase discharge from other low threshold sensory fibers and thereby temporarily could block soreness sensation (Tiidus, 1997). It is also plausible that massage disrupts the initial development of inflammatory process by preventing the accumulation of neutrophils at the site of microtrauma by increasing the blood flow and thereby diminishing the muscle damage and affects later developing muscle soreness (Smith et al., 1994). However, there is limited amount of research to substantiate these claims and uncertainly exists about the effectiveness of massage on DOMS.

Bale and James (1991) in their controlled clinical trial included 9 male athletes. After a maximum run, all participants were either rested, or asked to warm down by exercising at a moderate level or massaged manually for 17 minutes. They reported that DOMS was less in the massaged group who also showed a more rapid decline in the lactate level. On the other hand, Wenos et al. (1990) found no effect of massage on DOMS. They induced DOMS in untrained seated subjects by asking them to lower a weight of 75% of lean body mass from knee extension to knee flexion. Immediately after eccentric exercises, one side of the subjects was massaged while the other served as control. Soreness perception was evaluated 24, 48, and 72 hours after exercise. Ellison et al. (1992) and Drews et al. (1990) have also found no effect of massage on DOMS.

Tiidus and Shoemaker (1995) asked 9 volunteers to perform a bout of bilateral eccentric quadriceps work. For each volunteer, one leg only was randomized to receive treatment. Massage consisting of superficial and deep effleurage was carried only daily for 10 minutes. They found a small but significant tendency for massage to reduce DOMS sensation out after 48 hours postexercise. At other measuring points during the 96 hours follow-up, no such difference occurred.

In a well-designed experiment, Smith et al. (1994) examined that whether 30-minute massage performed within 2 hours after exercise affect the accumulation of neutrophils in the muscle. They made 14 healthy untrained males to perform eccentric isokinetic contraction of elbow flexors and extensor muscles on a kin-com muscle testing system. At 2 hours following exercise, half of the subjects were given 30 minutes management treatment consisting of effleurage, kneading, friction, and shaking, whereas the control group rested for 30 minutes. They observed that the massage group had consistently lower DOMS score as compared to the control group from 24 to 96 hours postexercises. Neutrophil count of massage group was approximately 15% above baseline at 8 and 24 hours after exercise while the same for the control group at these same times were approximately 4% above baseline. This they attributed to the reduced migration of neutrophil into the tissue space following the massage. In addition, the massage group also demonstrated a high cortisol level compared to the control. They suggested that the reduced migration of neutrophil would reduce intensity of the inflammatory event and reduce the pain and the soreness associated with DOMS.

The varying results observed with the use of massage may be attributed to the time of massage application and the type of massage technique used (Cheung et al., 2003). Zainuddin et al. (2005) using an arm-to-arm comparison model concluded that massage was effective in alleviating DOMS by approximately 30% and reducing swelling, but it had no effects on muscle function. In this study, ten healthy subjects (5 men and 5 women) with no history of upper arm injury and no experience in resistance training performed 10 sets of 6 maximal isokinetic eccentric actions of the elbow flexors with each arm on a dynamometer, separated by 2 weeks. One arm received 10 minutes of massage 3 hours after eccentric exercise while the contralateral arm received no treatment. Main outcome measures were maximal voluntary isometric and isokinetic elbow flexor strength, range of motion, upper arm circumference, plasma creatine kinase activity, and muscle soreness. It was observed that DOMS was significantly less for the massage condition for peak soreness in flexing and extending the elbow joint and palpating the brachioradialis and brachialis muscles. A significantly lower peak value of plasma creatine kinase activity was observed in the massage group at 4 days postexercise. However, significant effects of massage on recovery of muscle strength and ROM were not observed.

Investigating the physiological and psychological effects of massage on DOMS, Hilbert et al. (2003) concluded that massage administered 2 hours after exercise-induced muscle injury did reduce the intensity of soreness 48 hours after muscle insult but did not improve the function of exercising muscle. Eighteen volunteers were randomly assigned to either a massage or control group. DOMS was induced with six sets of eight maximal eccentric contractions of the right hamstring, which were followed 2 hours later by 20 minutes of massage or sham massage (control). Peak torque and mood were assessed at 2, 6, 24, and 48 hours postexercise. ROM and intensity and unpleasantness of soreness were assessed at 6, 24, and 48 hours postexercise. Neutrophil count was assessed at 6 and 24 hours postexercise. No significant differences for peak torque, ROM, neutrophils, unpleasantness of soreness, and mood were observed between massage and control groups. The intensity of soreness, however, was significantly lower in the massage group relative to the control group at 48 hours postexercise ($p < 0.05$).

Farr et al. (2002) investigated the effects of a 30-minute therapeutic massage on delayed-onset muscle soreness and muscle function following downhill walking. Eight male subjects performed a 40-minute downhill treadmill walk loaded with 10% of their body mass. A qualified masseur performed a 30-minute therapeutic massage to one limb 2 hours postwalk. Muscle soreness, tenderness, isometric strength, isokinetic strength, and single leg vertical jump height were measured on two occasions before and 1, 24, 72 and 120 hours postwalk for both limbs. Subjects showed significant ($p < 0.004$) increase in soreness and tenderness for the nonmassaged limb 24 hours postwalk with a significant ($p < 0.001$) difference between the two limbs. A significant reduction in isometric strength was recorded for both limbs compared to baseline 1 hour postwalk. Isokinetic strength at 60°/s and vertical jump height were significantly lower for the massaged limb at 1 and 24 hours postwalk. No significant differences were evident in the remaining testing variables. They suggested that therapeutic massage may attenuate soreness and tenderness associated with delayed-onset muscle soreness. However, it may not be beneficial in the treatment of strength and functional declines.

Imtiyaz et al. (2014) reported that both vibration and massage are equally effective in prevention of DOMS though massage was more effective in restoration of concentric strength. In this experimental study, 45 female nonathlete subjects randomly assigned to the three equal groups received vibration, massage, or no intervention just before the eccentric exercises of nondominant elbow flexor. Muscle soreness, ROM, maximum isometric force (MIF), repetition maximum (RM), lactate dehydrogenase (LDH), and creatine kinase (CK) level were recorded before and after intervention. They reported that in comparison to control group, muscle soreness was significantly less for experimental (vibration and massage) group at 24, 48, and 72 hours of postexercise. The experimental group also demonstrated lesser serum CK value. Both the groups did not show any significant difference in maximal isometric force but significant differences were observed in ROM at 48 and 72 hours of experimental group. Jay et al. (2014) reported that massage with a roller device reduces muscle soreness.

Few authors have strongly questioned the use of massage in sports setup (Tiidus, 1997) because of the existence of very little evidence which could support the efficacy of massage on various sports-specific problems. However, a consensus about massage is difficult to obtain from the literature because of wide variation in parameters, the techniques, time, and area of body selected (Callaghan, 1998). Ernest (1998) suggested that massage may be a promising intervention for reduction of DOMS and considering the paucity of well-designed studies on this topic, its effectiveness should be investigated in the vigorous trials with a sufficiently large sample size.

In the recent years, some systematic reviews and meta-analysis (Torres et al., 2012; **Guo** et al., 2017; Dupuy et al., 2018) of published randomized clinical trials have demonstrated the effectiveness of massage intervention in alleviating DOMS.

In a systematic review and meta-analysis of 35 studies, Torres et al. (2012) compared the efficacy of massage in treating the signs and symptoms of exercise-induced muscle damage with cryotherapy, stretching, and low-intensity exercise and reported that massage was the only intervention with positive effects in the relief of symptoms and signs but its mean effect was too small to be of clinical relevance. Massage was found reducing soreness at 24 hours, on average, 0.33 on 10 cm visual analog scale and increasing muscle recovery by 1.87%. However, the observation of Guo et al. (2017) and Dupuy et al. (2018) was in variance with this study.

Guo et al. (2017) in a meta-analysis held that current evidences support the use of massage for DOMS alleviation. They conducted a meta-analysis of 11 RCTs involving 504 participants and observed that massage intervention after strenuous exercise resulted in a significant reduction in muscle soreness rating as a total effect in comparison with no intervention. Massage intervention after exercise showed higher efficacy at 48 and 72 hours after exercise than at 24 hours. Further, their meta-analysis showed that massage therapy improved maximum isometric force and peak torque as total effects and produced reduction in the serum CK level. They concluded that massage is not only effective in reducing muscle pain after intense exercise, but also in increasing muscle performance and reducing the serum CK level.

Dupuy et al. (2018) found massage to be the most powerful technique for recovering from DOMS and fatigue. This meta-analysis compared the impacts of a single session of the most commonly used recovery techniques such as active recovery, stretching, massage, massage combined with stretching, the use of compression garments, electrostimulation, immersion, contrast water therapy, cryotherapy/cryostimulation and hyperbaric therapy/stimulation on muscle damage, DOMS, inflammation, and the perception of fatigue. They identified 1,693 potentially relevant publications spanning from 1958 to 2017, of which 99 studies were found suitable for inclusion in meta-analysis. Massage was found to be the most effective recovery technique not only for reducing DOMS and perceived fatigue, but also for reducing concentration of circulating CK and IL-6 in the blood after exercise. Reduction of blood CK concentration is considered as a marker for reduction in muscle damage and a faster recovery after exercise (Clarkson and Hubal, 2002; Sorichter et al., 2007; Bishop et al., 2008). A 20–30 minutes massage performed immediately following or up to 2 hours after exercise were shown to effectively reduce DOMS for 24 hours after exercise.

Some studies (Hou et al., 2012; Haas et al., 2013; Urakawa et al., 2015; Andrzejewski et al., 2015) have used animal models to study the possible mechanism of effectiveness of massage in exercise-induced damage.

Hou et al. (2012) explored the possible molecular mechanisms of massage in repair of quadriceps femoris muscle injury repair in a rabbit model. Quadriceps femoris injury induced by self-made beater and RT-N2 intelligent massage device was used for massage therapy at 8 days after injury, massage was given for 15 minutes at the rate of 3,000–3,100 r/min everyday for 7 days or for 14 days. Quadriceps femoris specimens were taken at 14 days and 21 days, and the effect of massage therapy was evaluated by the histomorphological change and desmin and alpha-actin expressions. They observed that the skeletal muscle morphology and muscle atrophy were improved with regenerated muscle fibers when compared with no massage condition. Massage group demonstrated significantly stronger desmin and α-actin expressions. The authors concluded that the histomorphology and cytoskeletal structure can be significantly improved after massage, which may help to repair muscle injury by upregulation of desmin and α-actin expressions.

Haas et al. (2013) conducted an experimental study using a rabbit model and found that immediate massage was more beneficial than delayed massage in restoring muscle function and in modulating inflammatory cell infiltration after eccentric exercise.

In an interesting study, Urakawa et al. (2015) developed an animal model of massage therapy in DOMS in order to gain insight of the physiological mechanisms of MT and investigated early effects of massage on the metabolite profiles of the muscle experiencing DOMS using capillary electrophoresis time-of-flight mass spectroscopy (CE-TOFMS). Lengthening contraction, which is known to induce DOMS, was applied to the rat gastrocnemius muscle under anesthesia, which induced mechanical hyperalgesia after 2–4 days. The rats were divided in three groups of which one received massage after lengthening contraction. Concentrations of eight metabolites, including branched-chain amino acids, carnitine, and malic acid, were found significantly different between those who received massage after lengthening contraction and those who did not. The observations of the study suggests that massage significantly altered metabolite profiles in DOMS and according to the authors, the ameliorative effects of massage might be mediated partly through alterations in metabolites associated with mitochondrial respiration.

In a study that has attempted to examine the role of massage in recovery using a rodent model, Andrzejewski et al. (2015) investigated whether muscle massage performed before and during running exercise affects the expression of VEGF-A in muscles. Vascular endothelial growth factor (VEGF) enhances blood vessel growth, and contributes to the regeneration of tissues. About 75 adult buffalo rats were subjected to running exercise training for 10 weeks. Rats were massaged prior (group PM) or during exercise (group M) or were not massaged (group C). The massage consisted of spiral movements along the plantar surface of flexor digitorum brevis muscle. After 1, 3, 5, 7, and 10 weeks of training, five rats from every group were anesthetized and immunohistochemistry, Western blot, and PCR analyzes were performed on obtained muscle tissue to determine VEGF-A expression. The authors reported that a significant increase of VEGF-A gene expression in muscle tissue was observed after the first week of training in the PM group whereas in the third week, the predominant growth of studied marker was seen in the M group. Increased VEGF-A expression on the protein level was observed in both massaged groups following the first week. The authors concluded that short-term repeated massage may contribute to processes of creation of new and development of already existing vascular networks in the skeletal muscle tissue during increased exercise.

The results of these studies point to a new dimension of massage research.

Efficacy of Massage on Fatigue and Recovery Following Intense Exercises

For a sportsperson, the recovery from intense physical exercises plays an important role for maximizing performance as skill acquisition, strength, speed, and endurance training. Post-event massage is widely used in world over to facilitate recovery from physical exertion.

A maximal or submaximal exercise session stresses the body to the maximum. The demands on cardiovascular, respiratory, and neuromuscular systems are very high and in order to meet that, several metabolic and hormonal adjustments occur in the internal milieu of the body. With increase in duration or intensity of exercise, the O_2 consumption, heart rate, and cardiac output demonstrate a progressive increase till a point where the system cannot cope up any further with the increasing demand. It is at this point that the subject begins to experience the symptom of general fatigue.

Fatigue is a complex concept, which involves both psychological and physiological factors. Physiological fatigue can be considered as a warning mechanism preventing overexertion of individual and as a rule it is always muscular in nature. Physical fatigue is defined as a state of disturbed homeostasis due to work and work environment (Christensen, 1960). It gives rise to subjective and objective symptoms. Subjective feelings may range from slight feeling of tiredness to complete exhaustion. Objectively, it is reflected in the form of decreased work output.

General physical fatigue is commonly seen in prolonged events, such as marathon, cross country, etc. In the intermittent and short duration of explosive sports, the local fatigue is commonly experienced. Local fatigue is defined as the failure to maintain the required expected power output from the muscles. It has been well-documented that intense unaccustomed exercise or exercises involving a significant eccentric component will result in reduced muscle strength which lasts up to 5–10 days after the exercises. Similarly, in heavy prolonged exercises, maintained for hours, the energy output during maximal effort gradually decreases. For example, after one hour of rest, a rate of exercise that normally could be tolerated for 6 minutes had to be terminated after 4 minutes because of exhaustion.

Therefore, the adequate and speedy recovery is paramount for those athletes who have to participate in a series of events over a scheduled timeframe because inadequate recovery during rest day will invariably affect the performance.

The ability of muscle fibers to maintain a high force and the subjective feeling of fatigue depends on the blood flow through the muscle. During contractions, the intramuscular pressure rises and at a point when it exceeds the arterial blood pressure it partially or completely occludes the blood flow. Decrease in muscle blood flow starts at 30% of maximum voluntary contraction and it completely arrests at about 70–80% of maximum voluntary contraction. This seriously interferes with the supply of O_2 and nutrients and the removal of CO_2 and metabolites resulting in disturbed homeostasis which affect the excitation-contraction coupling of muscle fibers. Short-term muscle fatigue seen in vigorous aerobic muscle work could be a combined effect of exercise-induced alteration in muscle homeostasis including H^+ ions accumulation, K^+ loss, depletion of high energy phosphates (ATP + CP) and glycogen, loss of calcium homeostasis, lactate accumulation, and local ischemia.

A restoration of internal environment after exercise necessitates an adequate blood supply. Massage by virtue of increasing blood and lymph flow may enhance the removal of H^+ ions and lactic acid from muscle. These substances are known to interfere with the ability of muscle contractile protein to generate force by either reduction of the total number of cross-bridges formed or by decreasing the amount of force generated per cross-bridge.

By improving oxygen and nutrient delivery, it may also have a positive effect on the recovery of lost K^+ ions and on the synthesis of ATP and CP.

Apart from affecting the homeostasis process, the intense exercises also cause excessively prolonged elevation of muscle tone both in resting and in contractile states (Brunker and Khan, 1993). This phenomenon of increased muscle tone impairs the delivery of nutrients and O_2 to the cell and slows down the removal of metabolites during the recovery. Massage can reduce excessive postexercise muscle tone, which in turn may enhance the blood flow and facilitate the restoration of muscle homeostasis.

Research on the effects of massage on physiological recovery following an exhaustive workout has been focused on two main areas—(a) recovery of muscle function and performance, and (b) lactate recovery.

Recovery of Muscle Function

Massage techniques (light after heavy activity and deeper for light activity and lasting for 30–60 minutes) have been claimed to be two to three times more likely to promote recovery than resting alone (Crompton and Fox, 1987). However, experimental results regarding effects of massage on this area have been contradictory (Kresge, 1988).

Muller et al. (1966) demonstrated that massage of muscles tired from running or bicycle riding reduces recovery time as shown by faster decline in pulse rate and quicker recovery of muscle efficiency.

Balke et al. (1989) examined the effects of massage treatment and reported that manual massage using percussion techniques has a positive effect on the postexercise work performance.

Viitasalo et al. (1995) examined the effects of 20 minutes underwater jet massage on the recovery from intense physical exercise on 14 junior field and tract athletes. Each subject spent, in a randomized order, two identical training weeks engaged in 5 strength/power training sessions lasting for 3 days. Underwater jet massage was used three times during the treatment week but not during the control week. They observed that during the treatment week, continuous jumping power decreased and ground contact time increased significantly less than the control week ($p < 0.05$) along with increase in serum myoglobin. They suggested that underwater-jet massage in connection with intense strength/power training increases the release of protein from muscle tissue into the blood and enhances the maintenance of neuromuscular performance capacity.

The hypothesis that expedite removal of fatigue causing metabolites by massage could improve athletic performance was examined by Zelikovski et al. (1993) using a pneumatic sequential intermittent device. They conducted trials with 11 men who exercised at a constant rate on a cycle ergometer until exhaustion. During 20 minutes recovery period, mechanical massage was applied to the subject's leg. The subjects then performed second constant load exercise. They observed that mechanical massage brought about a 45% improvement in subject's ability to perform subsequent exercise bout. However, they could not observe any significant difference in the blood level of some fatigue causing metabolites, i.e., pyruvate, ammonia, bicarbonate, and pH during passive recovery and massage-assisted recovery. They suggested that the disappearance of accumulated fluid in the interstitial space after exercise could be a possible explanation for this result along with the psychological effects.

Improved muscle function following massage has been reported in other studies also (Rinder and Sutherland, 1995; Lane and Wenger, 2004, Brooks et al., 2005). Rinder and Sutherland (1995) investigated the effects of massage on quadriceps performance after exercise fatigue. Sample consists of 13 males and 7 females. In this randomized, crossover study, the subject completed maximum number of leg extensions against a half-maximum load. Thereafter, they were exercised to fatigue using an ergometer to perform ski-squats and leg extensions. It was followed by either a 6 minutes massage or rest. Thereafter, they again completed the maximum number of leg extensions against half-maximum load. The process was repeated a few days later with the alternative condition (rest or massage). The result showed that massage after exercise fatigue significantly ($p < 0.001$) improved quadriceps performance compared to rest.

Lane and Wenger (2004) examined the effects of active recovery massage and cold water immersion (on performance of repeated bouts of high-intensity cycling separated by 24 hours). For each recovery condition, subjects were asked to take part in 2 intermittent cycling sessions separated by 24 hours; one of four 15-minute recovery conditions immediately followed the first session and included cycling at 30% VO_2 max; immersion of legs in a 15°C water bath; massage of the legs; and seated rest. A significant decline in the total work completed between the first and second exercise sessions was observed only in seated rest group.

Brooks et al. (2005) examined the effects of using manual massage to improve power-grip performance immediately after maximal exercise on a sample of 52 healthy adults. Subjects randomly received either a 5-minute forearm/hand massage of effleurage and friction, 5 minutes of passive shoulder and elbow range of motion, or 5 minutes of nonintervention rest following 3 minutes of maximal exercise that produced fatigue to 60% of baseline strength. They observed that manual massage to the forearm and hand after maximal exercise was associated with greater effects than no massage on postexercise grip performance.

However, several other investigations have found no effect of massage on the objective parameters related to the recovery of muscle function on performance enhancement following an exhaustive workout (Drews et al., 1990; Tiidus and Shoemaker, 1995; Cafarelli et al., 1990; Robertson et al., 2004; Hilbert et al., 2003; Tanaka et al., 2002; Hemmings et al., 2000; Jonhagen et al., 2004; Farr et al., 2002).

Tiidus and Shoemaker (1995) performed 4 days of daily 10 minutes superficial and deep effleurage on one leg of the subjects following intense eccentric quadriceps muscle contraction involving both the legs. They demonstrated that for up to 4 days postexercise, massage did not improve the rate of recovery of quadriceps isokinetic peak torque (at the speed of 0°, 60°, and 180° per second) over that of unmassaged leg.

Cafarelli et al. (1990) studied the effect of percussive vibratory massage on recovery from repeated submaximal contractions. 12 male subjects performed repeated static contractions of the quadriceps at 70% maximal voluntary contraction (MVC) with periodic MVC performed after every fourth one. This pattern was continued until the subject could no longer produce 70% MVC. The entire process was repeated 3 times with rest period between each series. In the control conditions, the subjects rested for 5 minutes between each of the three series of contractions. In the experimental condition, the subject received 4 minutes of percussive vibratory massage and 1 minute of rest. The result showed that there was no significant difference in rate of fatigue between control and experimental conditions. It was concluded that short-term recovery from intense muscular activity is not augmented by percussive vibratory massage.

The aim of the study of Hemmings et al. (2000) was to investigate the effects of massage on perceived recovery, blood lactate removal, and repeated boxing performance. Eight amateur boxers completed two performance bouts on a boxing ergometer on two occasions in a counter-balanced design. After initial completion of performance, the boxer received a massage or passive rest intervention for 20 minutes. Massage was applied by one sports massage therapist and consisted of effleurage (30 strokes/min) and petrissage (50-60 strokes/min) techniques, encompassing the major muscle groups of the legs (8 minutes), back (2 minutes), and shoulder and arms (10 minutes). Participants received treatment while lying in the prone position followed by supine position. After the intervention, participants had a further 35 minutes rest whereupon they completed another self-selected warm up and a second performance bout. Overall, there was one-hour period between two boxing performances. Each boxer had perceived recovery rating before completing a second performance. Heart rate, blood lactate, and glucose levels were assessed before, during, and after all the performances. No differences in performance, blood lactate, or glucose were found following massage or passive rest intervention, though massage intervention significantly increased the perception of recovery.

Tanaka et al. (2002) investigated the influence of massage application on localized back muscle fatigue. 29 healthy subjects participated in two experimental sessions of massage and rest. On each test day, subjects were asked to lie in prone position on a treatment table and performed sustained back extension for 90 seconds. Subjects then either received massage on the lumbar region or rested for 5 minutes duration, then repeated the back extension movement. The median frequency (MDF), mean frequency (MNF), and root mean square (RMS) amplitude of electromyographic signals during the 90 seconds sustained lumbar muscle contraction were analyzed. The subjective feeling of fatigue was then evaluated using the visual analog scale (VAS). MDF and MNF significantly declined with time under all conditions. There was no significant difference in MDF, MNF, or RMS value between, before, and after massage, or between rest and massage conditions. There was a significant difference in fatigue VAS change between massage and rest conditions. It was suggested that massage application helped subjects to overcome the subjective feeling of the fatigue.

In a prospective randomized clinical trial (Jonhagen et al., 2004), subjects ($n = 16$) performed 300 maximal eccentric contractions of the quadriceps muscle bilaterally. Massage was given to one leg, whereas the other leg served as control. Subjects were treated once daily for 3 days. Maximal strength was tested on a Kin-Com dynamometer, and functional tests were based on one-leg long jumps. Pain was evaluated using a visual analog scale. Marked loss of strength and function of the quadriceps directly after exercise and on the third day after exercise was observed. However, the massage treatment did not affect the level or duration of pain or the loss of strength or function following exercise.

The indicator of altered homeostasis, i.e. increased heart rate, lactic acid, alteration in serum enzyme, and stress hormone level are shown to be related to the subjective feeling in strenuous prolonged physical effort. However, very little is known about the nature of this disturbed homeostasis of fatigue (Åstrand and Rodahl, 1986). Therefore, it will be improper to assess the effectiveness of any modality on fatigue on the basis of one or two physiological parameters. Rather, the actual effect of the modality can best be assessed in the actual competitive situation where both physiological and psychological factors exert a cumulative effect on the individual.

Of late, some studies attempted to examine the effect of massage in real-life situation (Hoffman et al., 2016; Kargarfard et al., 2016).

Hoffman et al. (2016) in a randomized controlled trial examined the effectiveness of massage and pneumatic compression on recovery from a 161-km ultramarathon. About 72 runners who finished the marathon race were randomized to a 20-minute postrace intervention of massage, intermittent sequential pneumatic compression, or supine rest race. Speed to complete 400-m run, muscle pain and soreness rating, and overall muscle fatigue scores were the outcome measured before the race and on day 3 and day 5 after the race. Immediately after treatment, massage resulted in lower muscle pain and soreness ratings compared with the supine-rest control condition and both massage and pneumatic compression resulted in lower overall muscular fatigue scores compared with the control group. However, there was no significant group or interaction effect on 400-m run time. The authors concluded that massage and intermittent sequential pneumatic compression provide some immediate subjective benefits, but do not provide extended subjective or functional extended subjective or functional benefits of clinical importance.

On the other hand, Kargarfard et al. (2016) held that a postexercise massage session can improve the exercise performance and recovery rate in male bodybuilders after intensive exercise. They examine the effect of massage on the performance of 30 experienced body builders randomly assigned either to a massage group ($n = 15$) or to a control group ($n = 15$). Both groups performed five repetition sets at 75–77% of 1 RM of knee extensor and flexor muscle groups. The massage group then received a 30-minute massage after the exercise protocol while the control group maintained their normal passive recovery. Plasma creatine kinase (CK) level, agility test, vertical jump test, isometric torque test, and perception of soreness were the outcome measures recorded before and immediately after the exercise, right after the massage, and 24, 48, and 72 hours after the massage. They reported that massage group demonstrated lower perceived soreness scores and performed better than the control group in less than 72 hours after the massage. In comparison to control group, massage group demonstrated improved vertical jump displacement and maximal isometric torque 48 hours after the massage. In author's words—"*The functionality of the control group continued to deteriorate whereas the performance of the massage group returned to "normal" level 72 hours after the massage.*" In addition, the CK levels of the massage group were significantly lower than the control group 48 hours and 72 hours after the massage.

The research literature to date is insufficient to conclude whether massage facilitates recovery of muscle function from a fatiguing effort. In a review article, Moraska (2005) noted that most studies on massage have several methodological limitations including inadequate therapist training, insufficient duration of treatment, few subjects, or over under working of muscles that limit a practical conclusion. The effects of massage depend primarily on the execution of the technique, which is highly therapist dependent. Unless the execution of the various techniques is standardized, the reports on the efficacy of massage would likely to remain contradictory and the debate is inconclusive.

Massage and Lactate Removal

Sports massage is commonly used in an effort to facilitate lactate clearance. Specific massage techniques are thought to produce local increase in skeletal muscle blood flow which theoretically may accelerate the rate at which lactate is shuttled to the various sites of elimination, thereby promoting its clearance. It is widely believed that massage by virtue of increasing the blood flow and lymphatic drainage may enhance the removal of H^+ ions and lactate from muscle and facilitate the transport of lactate into systemic circulation (Lehn and Prentice, 1994). However, this notion does not derive its support from research. The only study, which supports the notion that massage facilitates lactate removal compared to passive rest, is that of Bale and James (1991). This study, conducted on 9 male athletes, showed lower blood lactate level following 17 minutes of manual massage compared with passive rest, though it was higher than that obtained following warm down procedures.

The observation of Bale and James is not in agreement with other studies (Gupta et al., 1996; Hemmings et al., 2000; Monedero and Donne, 2000; Zelikovski et al., 1993; Robertson et al., 2004). That explored the effect of massage on blood lactate removal. All these studies have reported that massage has no better effect than the passive rest as far as the blood lactate removal is concerned. Studies that have reported no effect of massage on lactate removal used different exercise protocol, duration, and techniques of massage.

Gupta et al. (1996) used 10 minutes of manual massage of lower limb in sitting position after exhaustive exercise on bicycle ergometer, and reported no effect on lactate removal. Martin et al. (1998) compared a 5-minute sports massage routine for each leg in both the supine and prone positions using the techniques of effleurage, petrissage, tapotement, (pounding and hacking), and compression with active recovery and passive rest condition and noted no significant difference between sports massage and rest for either absolute or relative changes in blood lactate concentration. In this study, the exercise resulted in a 59.38% decrease in blood lactate concentration, compared with 36.21% and 38.67% for the sports massage and rest conditions, respectively. Robertson et al. (2004) in an extensively controlled experiment that controlled even the daily routine and dietary practices of the participants reported that 20 minutes of leg massage consisting of stroking, effleurage, kneading, picking up, wringing, and rolling with all petrissage techniques interspersed with effleurage in a centripetal direction did not produce any better reduction in blood lactate concentration when compared with passive supine rest.

Monedero and Donne (2000) reported no effect of 20 minutes massage, after exhaustive exercise in bicycle ergometer, consisting of effleurage, tapotement, and stroking in supine position, on lactate removal. Hemmings et al. (2000) used 20 minutes whole body massage consisting of effleurage and petrissage after exhaustive bouts on boxing ergometer and reported no benefit of massage on lactate removal. Zelikovski et al. (1993) used 20 minutes of pneumatic massage device on lower limb after bicycle ergometer workouts and reported no effects on lactate removal. Sinha (2005) used 20 minutes of manual lower limb massage consisting of effleurage, kneading, and petrissage in supine position with leg slightly elevated, and confirmed the findings of above studies.

Wiltshire et al. (2010) reported that massage therapy after strenuous exercise mechanically impedes the blood flow of the exercising muscle and impairs the removal of blood lactate and H^+ concentration. In their study, massage resulted in severe impairment to blood flow during the massage stroke, and this impairment had a net effect of decreasing muscle blood flow early in the recovery period after strenuous exercise leading to a reduced lactic acid efflux during massage.

Cè et al. (2013) observed that stretching and deep and superficial massage did not alter blood lactate concentration kinetics as compared to passive recovery. They compared the influence of deep and superficial massage and passive stretching recovery on blood lactate concentration ($[La(-)]$) kinetics after a fatiguing exercise with active and passive recovery. 8-minute fatiguing exercise at 90% of maximum oxygen uptake was followed by interventions after 1 hour of recovery. They observed lower blood lactate concentration as well as higher metabolic and cardiorespiratory parameters with active recovery in comparison to the other modalities. Stretching and deep and superficial massage did not alter blood lactate kinetics as compared to passive recovery. The author concluded that passive maneuvers did not play a significant role on postexercise blood lactate concentration levels.

These evidences may permit generalization that irrespective of the type of strokes, duration of application, and the area of body treated, massage has no effect on lactate removal.

The failure of massage to facilitate lactate clearance may be attributed to the following two presumptions:

- Massage does not increase the muscular blood flow to the extent sufficient enough to facilitate translocation of the lactate (Hemmings et al., 2000; Gupta et al., 1996).
- Increases in blood flow alone have little or no effect on lactate clearance (Martin et al., 1998; Sinha, 2005).

The prevailing popular proposition that postevent sports massage promotes lactate clearance by increasing blood flow through the skeletal muscle bed is at best that can be described as based on conflicting experimental evidences. The effect of massage on blood flow has been investigated since 1931 yet the evidence that currently exist is equivocal. Studies performed by Ek et al. (1985), Linde (1986), Shoemaker et al. (1997), and Tiidus and Shoemaker (1995) could not demonstrate an increased blood flow of muscle or skin following massage. Though the enhanced clearance of isotopes, i.e., insulin (Linde, 1986) and Xe^{133} (Dubrovsky, 1982; Hovind and Neilsen, 1974) have been reported, which have been attributed to better venous emptying following massage rather than increase in the arterial or systemic circulation.

On the other hand, there also exists some evidence to suggest that some massage techniques increase regional blood flow through skeletal muscle. Studies of Wolfson (1931), Wakim et al. (1949), Bell (1964), Serveni and Venarando (1967), and Dubrovsky (1982) reported increased flow of blood following massage. Recently, Hinds et al. (2004) compared the effects of massage against a resting control condition upon femoral artery blood flow, skin blood flow, skin, and muscle temperature after dynamic quadriceps exercise and observed that following massage the skin blood flow and temperature were elevated but no significant increase in the femoral artery blood flow was not observed. They opined that without an increase in arterial blood flow, any increase in skin blood flow has the potential to divert the blood flow away from the recovering muscle which puts a question mark on the use of massage in postexercise recovery session.

In the opinion of the author of this book, the answer of the question, i.e., massage fails to facilitate lactate clearance lies in understanding the metabolism of lactate in proper perspective. The hypothesis that increases in skeletal muscle blood flow may accelerate the rate at which lactate is shuttled to various sites of elimination, thereby promoting its clearance is based on the circumstantial evidences that are mostly correlational in nature (Gladden, 2000). There have been only a couple of studies that attempted to directly evaluate the potential role of blood flow on lactate removal (Gladden et al., 1992; Watt et al., 1994). These studies suggest a minor role of blood flow in net lactate exchange in in vitro muscle preparations. Uncertainty has been expressed on whether these results could be extended to higher metabolic rates possible in tetanic contraction and asynchronous contraction of voluntary exercise (Gladden, 2000).

On the other hand, there emerge mounting evidences that suggest that activation of larger muscle mass during recovery would result in better lactate removal (Thiriet et al., 1993; Baker and King, 1991). Thiriet et al. (1993) obtained lowest blood lactate value in active leg recovery, intermediate value in active arm recovery, and highest value in passive recovery following exhaustive bout on bicycle ergometer. Baker and King (1991) also observed lowest blood lactate value with active leg recovery, intermediate value in active arm recovery, and highest value in passive recovery following exhaustive bout on canoeing ergometer. In all the studies that compared massage with active recovery, it was observed that the lactate reduction could be facilitated by the active recovery only and significant differences between massage and passive rest condition did not exist as far as removal of lactate was concerned.

The emphasis on the role of blood flow in lactate removal is probably derived from classical "O_2" debt theory which held lactate as a dead-end metabolite that can be removed only during recovery by reconversion into glucose via Cori cycle in liver. Classical "O_2 debt" and "anaerobic threshold" theories held that lactate is produced in muscle because of O_2 lack and it is a dead-end metabolite that could only be removed during recovery (Hill and Lupton, 1923). According to classical concept, about 20% of the lactate produced during exercise is reoxidized into pyruvate and then disseminated to CO_2 and H_2O. The remaining 80% of lactate is taken up by liver and turned into glucose, via "Cori cycle", which then can be reconverted into glycogen or delivered to blood. The muscles can then use this glucose in glycogenesis to restore their glycogen depot (Krebs, 1964). In the light of this theory, it was reasonable to assume that increasing the blood flow during recovery by massage or other means would enhance lactate availability to liver and its removal.

However, advances in the last two decades have challenged this theory. The isotope (^{13}C) tracer studies conducted by Brooks et al. (1984), Brooks and Gaesser (1980), Donovan and Brooks (1983) on rats, by Depocas et al. (1969), Issekutz (1984) on dogs, by Pagliassotti and Donovan (1990) on rabbit as well as the human studies of Hubbard (1973), Brooks and Gaesser (1980), and Gaesser and Brooks (1984), etc. consistently indicated that combustion of lactate in the aerobic pathway is the main route of the lactate removal during exercise and recovery.

Lactate is now not considered as dead-end metabolite but as a substrate, which can be used to generate ATP (Brooks, 2000). Most of the lactate produced during exercise is removed by direct oxidation (55–70%), whereas the balance amount is converted to glycogen (<20%), protein constituents (<10%), and other compounds (<10%) (Gaesser and Brooks, 1984). Further, it is established that reduced splanchnic blood flow and incompatible hormonal milieu, which persist for some time after strenuous exercise, grossly reduce the capacity of liver to utilize the lactate available in systemic circulation. The circulating lactate mostly perfuse the heart and active muscle bed, which can use lactate as substrate (Brooks, 1986; Stanley, 1991).

In this situation, theoretically, accelerated reduction of blood lactate would not be obtained if the muscle bed remains inactive as happens in case of massage. On the other hand, increased requirement of ATP during muscle activity would call for more substrate, which can be provided by the circulating lactate. Active recovery helps to maintain an elevated metabolic rate which serves to promote lactate clearance via an accelerated rate of lactate oxidation. Active recovery also promotes lactate clearance via an increased use of lactate as a fuel by the heart and contracting skeletal muscle. Lactate, which is produced in type IIb fibers, is transported into type I or IIa fibers, where it is oxidized. Therefore, glycolytic fibers within an exercising muscle bed can shuttle oxidizable substrate (in the form of lactate) to neighboring cells with higher respiratory rates. From the above discussion, it becomes clear that muscle activity might be the most essential component of accelerated lactate removal strategies. The very nature of lactate metabolism may not allow any recovery intervention that excludes the component of muscle activity, to succeed in achieving the accelerated lactate removal.

Role of Massage in Psychological Recovery

Massage is an important aid in combating some of the psychological problems of the athlete. It helps in promoting the psychological recovery after an intense physical exertion.

Most of the studies on the effect of massage on recovery accede that as far as subjective parameters are concerned massage does exert positive effect on the recovery process. Robertson et al. (2004) observed a significant ($p < 0.05$) lower fatigue index in the massage trial. Tanaka et al. (2002) reported significant difference in fatigue VAS change between massage and rest conditions. Hemmings et al. (2000) observed that massage intervention significantly increased the perception of recovery. Similar observations on the subjective parameters were also made by Farr et al. (2002).

Autonomic nervous system more specifically its sympathetic component increases its activity during exercises to cope with the increased demand. After cessation of the activity, this effect should be reversed to ensure better replenishment of energy stores. However, many a times, the stress of losing or winning the game and associated emotions does not allow the sympathetic arousal to subside down. This manifests as an increase in heart rate, poor appetite, muscle tiredness, and inability to sleep. If this condition is prolonged, the individual can become exhausted leading to diminished work capacity and psychological burn out.

Massage is one of the most important techniques, which is employed to achieve lower arousal level along with several other techniques, such as spa, warm bath, showers, floatation tanks, etc. The positive effect of massage on the reduction of anxiety and the improvement of mood is well-established and it is utilized in sports setup not only after exercises but also before and during competitions.

Anxiety and muscular tension are interdependent phenomenon. Conversely, adequate muscular tension is a prerequisite for optimum performance. Experiments have demonstrated the relation of muscle tension and muscle response to anxiety. It is found that highly anxious subjects not only perform with an excess of muscular tension compared to less anxious subject, but their coordination is also affected. Weinburg and Genuchi (1980) pointed out that anxiety has a disruptive effect as the precise neuromuscular patterning has involved in precision sports.

Excess level of anxiety tends to restrict the attentional field and the athlete may begin to attend to a limited number of cues. However, all anxieties are not disruptive. An optimal level is necessary to perform well.

Massage can effectively modulate the level of anxiety associated with sports competition if utilized in a proper manner. Psychophysiological parameters associated with the symptoms of tension and anxiety have been shown to decrease significantly with massage (McKechnie et al.,

1983). It not only reduces muscle tension and facilitates deep relaxation, but also provides a feedback to athlete about the muscle tension. This helps athlete learn to monitor the muscle tone.

Regarding promotion of psychological recovery of the athletes, Brunker and Khan (1993) have opined that it is always better to complement progressive relaxation technique with deep therapeutic massage, as these two techniques highly reinforce each other.

Massage can be a useful remedy in following sports-related psychological symptoms:
- Inconsistency in performance
- Poor performance while traveling
- Diminishing performance on a session as the tournament progresses.
- Persistent tiredness
- Recurrent illness or injury

Role of Massage in the Prevention of Injuries

Heavy training predisposes to the development of tight bands within entire muscle or group of muscles due to prolonged contraction of the active muscle. It occurs during the period of adaptation to increased volume and intensity of training. It places an excessive force either at the muscle insertion or at the musculotendinous junction. If this tightness is asymmetric, it contributes to the development of biomechanical abnormalities apart from compromising the ability of muscles to elongate and to absorb the shock. This predisposes the tissue to strain especially when any movement attempts to stretch the tight tissues and reduces the range of motion and excursion of muscle. Many of these abnormalities detected during massage session can be corrected by massage techniques or alternately the athlete can be referred to other members of sports medicine team as appropriate.

Massage can reduce the excessive postexercise muscle tone, as well as increase the muscle range of motion and thereby help reduce the tight band and its associated problems. Dubrovsky (1982) found that massage decreased the resting as well as contractile muscle tone.

Heavy training also predisposes to the development of trigger points, which not only impairs the training and competition performance but can also progress to frank injury if athlete continues to work, ignoring their presence. The role of massage in deactivating the trigger points is well-known.

Regular massage also provides an opportunity to identify any soft tissue abnormality that if left untreated may progress to injury. This is more important for those anxious athletes who tend to hide their injuries in an attempt to prevent the appearance of cowardliness and subsequent social insecurity that withdrawal from contest might entail. In these persons, massage plays an extremely important role of finding and alleviating problem area before it becomes serious.

Crosman et al. (1984) found that general massage significantly increased the range of motion of hamstring in normal female subjects. They further suggested that athlete may also benefit from massage treatment for prevention of injuries associated with hamstring limitations.

Nordschow and Bierman (1962) found that generalized massage in which no special attention was given to specific tension area, 4 out of 5 subjects were constantly found to relax muscle and increase their flexibility.

A number of studies since then have examined the issue of flexibility increase following massage, the result of these studies are equivocal. Some studies have reported that massage increases the flexibility (Hopper et al., 2005; Arabaci, 2008; Huang et al., 2010; Arazi et al., 2012; Forman et al., 2014; Iwamoto et al., 2016; Park et al., 2017) whereas others have reported contradictory observations (Barlow et al., 2004; Thompson et al., 2017).

In a single-blinded randomized control trial, Hopper et al. (2005) reported that dynamic soft tissue mobilization (STM)—a specific massage technique in which the therapist identifies a target area of muscle tightness and focuses the treatment on that specific area—significantly increased hamstring flexibility in healthy male subjects. However, the application of classical massage techniques of effleurage, kneading, picking up, and shaking did not result in significant alteration of range of motion in comparison with a control group where the subjects were positioned in a prone-lying position for a period of 5 minutes. They conducted this study on forty-five healthy male volunteers between the ages of 18 and 35 years who had a straight leg raise (SLR) between 40° and 70°.

Arabaci et al. (2008) examined the acute effects of preperformance lower limb massage after warm-up on explosive and high-speed motor capacities and flexibility on twenty-four male volunteers. In a randomized order, each of the subjects receive three intervention protocols of massage, stretching, and rest. They reported that although 10 minutes posterior and 5 minutes anterior lower limb Swedish massage had a positive effect on sit and reach test, it produced adverse effect on vertical jump, speed, and reaction time. The massage intervention included simultaneously massage of posterior thigh (10 minutes) and anterior thigh (5 minutes) of left and right lower limbs by two masseurs using baby oil using the techniques of effleurage, friction, petrissage, vibration, and tapotement.

Huang et al. (2010) in an experimental study reported that short-duration massage at the hamstrings musculotendinous junction induces greater range of motion of hip. They investigated the effectiveness of 3 massage conditions (no massage, 10-second massage, and 30-second massage) on hip flexion range of motion. The massage was focused on the musculotendinous junction of hamstring. Hip flexion angle, passive leg tension, and electromyography (EMG) were measured thrice before and within 10 seconds after the intervention. They reported a significant 7.2% and 5.9% increase in hip flexion ROM following 30-second massage and 10-second massage, respectively in comparison with the control group which received no massage. They suggested that musculotendinous massage may be used as an alternative or a complement to static stretching for increasing ROM.

The observations of Forman et al. (2014) suggest that deep stripping massage strokes (DSMS) increase hamstring length in less than 3 minutes. Participants were administered 15, 10-s longitudinal DSMS on hamstring of one limb while lying passive. On their other hamstring, longitudinal DSMS were applied during 15, 10-s bouts of eccentric resistance with an elastic resistance band. All massage strokes were performed at a depth of 7 out of 10 on a verbal pressure scale index. Improved ($p < 0.01$) hamstring flexibility following both DSMS with eccentric resistance (10.7%) and DSMS alone (6.3%) was observed. However, strength was not significantly affected by either treatment.

Iwamoto et al. (2016) examined the effects of friction massage of the popliteal fossa on ankle flexibility and dynamic changes in muscle oxygenation. About 12 healthy males were administered friction massage of popliteal fossa, and dynamic changes in muscle oxygenation and ankle flexibility were measured by near-infrared spectroscopy before and after the intervention. They observed that after massage, range of ankle dorsiflexion was increased and the oxygenated hemoglobin was significantly higher.

The purpose of the study of Park et al. (2017) was to examine the effect of calf muscle massage on ankle flexibility and balance. Study was conducted on 32 healthy college students, divided into two groups. Both groups received five minutes of massage to each calf. Group A received effleurage, tapotement, and pressure, whereas massage group B received effleurage, friction, and petrissage. The functional reaching test and the modified one-leg standing test before and after the massage application significant increases in flexibility and balance was observed in both groups however the intergroup differences were not significant. They suggested the use of calf massage for improving balancing ability in athletes.

On the other hand, Barlow et al. (2004) could not observe any significant change in the scores of sit and reach test after 15 minutes of effleurage and petrissage of the hamstring muscle group both legs in comparison to supine rest with no massage. They concluded that a single massage of the hamstring muscle group does not significantly alter sit and reach performance.

Thompson et al. (2017) investigated the effect of massage on the passive mechanical properties of the calf muscle complex using an instrumented footplate and observed that massage did not affect the passive mechanical characteristics of the calf muscle. In this study, calf muscle compliance and ankle joint dorsiflexion range of motion of twenty-nine healthy volunteers were measured using an instrumented footplate before, immediately, and 30 minutes after a ten minutes application of deep massage or superficial heating to the calf muscle complex. Massage consisted of petrissage (kneading) strokes, with linking effleurage, applied distal to proximal over the belly of the calf muscle complex. A custom-built, hinged, footplate, instrumented with a load cell and potentiometer was used to record the passive stiffness measures of torque and angular displacement. Significant change in calf muscle stiffness or ankle dorsiflexion range of motion with/without the application of calf massage was not observed. They opined that the use of massage to increase tissue flexibility prior to activity is not justified.

The effect of massage on flexibility is a controversial topic. The use of massage for increasing flexibility of muscle is based on a variety of assumptions. It is believed that an increased extensibility of soft tissues is a direct mechanical effect of massage (Crosman et al., 1984) that produces a stretching effect on tissues and helps break fibrous adhesions. Relaxation of the antagonistic muscle (Barlow et al., 2004), increased local tissue temperature (Huang et al., 2010; Crommert et al., 2014), an increased pain threshold, and stretch tolerance (Huang et al., 2010; Mostafaloo, 2012) following massage have also been implicated as plausible mechanism for increased flexibility. It is also postulated that massage may break the stable cross-bridges between actin and myosin leading to elongation of the muscle fibers causing lengthening of the muscle (Crommert et al., 2014; Arabaci, 2008).

In the recent years, foam roller massage or self-myofascial release massage has become popular among the athletes. The basic consideration of myofascial release is different from that of classical massage. A number of studies have examined the effects of this technique on flexibility and other parameters of physical fitness. In general, most of the studies have reported that foam roller massage increases the flexibility (Škarabot et al., 2015; Bradbury-Squires et al., 2015; Halperin et al., 2015; Junker and Stöggl, 2015; Kelly and Beardsley, 2016; Behara and Jacobson, 2017; Monteiro et al., 2017; Monteiro et al., 2018; de Souza et al., 2018).

In an interesting study, Grieve et al. (2015) investigated the immediate effect of a single application of self-myofascial release massage on the plantar aspect of the foot on hamstring and lumbar spine flexibility. They reported that self-myofascial release massage applied to the plantar aspect of the foot via a tennis ball produced significant increase with large effect in sit and reach scores of experimental group.

DeBruyne et al. (2017) in a review reported the existence of grade B evidence in support of the use of roller massagers and foam roller for increasing hamstrings flexibility in asymptomatic physically active adults, though they also noted that neither device has been shown to confer a therapeutic benefit superior to static stretching.

Previously unresolved soft tissue may be irritated further by intense physical training. Repeated microtrauma of these lesions may lead to laying down of excessive connective tissue which tends to adhere and reduce flexibility. Regular massage not only mobilizes the tissue and prevents them to become adherent, but it also breaks down the established adhesion and restores the flexibility of soft tissue.

CATEGORIES OF SPORTS MASSAGE

Athletes have different physical and psychological requirements during various phases of sports sessions. The massage techniques should be tailored to meet these requirements. Depending upon the needs and the physical status of the athletes, the practice of sports massage can be classified under the following categories **(Table 10.1)**:
- Pre-event massage
- Preparatory massage
- Intermediate massage
- Postevent massage
- Training massage/regular fine tuning
- Medical massage/massage for injury rehabilitation.

Pre-event Massage

This kind of massage is given before 8–12 hours of competition. The goals are to ensure optimal arousal, to dispel excessive precompetitive anxiety, and to keep the muscles, to be used for competition, prepared for executing the physical task. After massage, the athlete should remain loose, but not overtly relaxed, with an alert mind. Techniques used in this kind of session should be light, relaxing, and warming. The session must remain pleasant, pain-free, and simulating to the psyche of the athlete.

The massage should be given to only those parts of the body which are going to withstand greatest stress during the event. It is important to identify the anatomical areas, which will be maximally stressed in the event. The stress imposed on different body segment is very much dependent upon the nature of sports. Therefore, the body part approached during preevent massage may not be the same for athletes of two different sports.

For example, weightlifting stresses the spine and arms to the maximum whereas for throwers the maximally stressed areas are shoulder girdle and arm muscles. Runner and jumper should be massaged from foot to thigh whereas in throwers (discus, javelin, and shot put) the muscles of hand, arm, and shoulder girdle should be prime site of intervention. The muscles of arms and shoulder should be treated symmetrically for rowers and gymnast, whereas in tennis, badminton, fencer, and bowler, the unilateral dominant upper extremity would be the area of emphasis.

Procedure

Aims
1. To decrease the precompetition anxiety by inducing generalized relaxation.
2. To increase the circulation and warm up the prime muscles.
3. To identify and correct the area of excessive tension.

Table 10.1: Categories of sports massage.

Categories	Used during	Duration
Pre-event massage	8 hours before competition	20–30 minutes
Preparatory massage	30 minutes before competition	5–10 minutes
Intermediate massage	During interval and half times	2–3 minutes
Postevent massage	1–3 hours after competition	30–60 minutes
Training massage	During conditioning period	60–90 minutes
Medical massage	As and when required	–

Techniques
- Superficial stroking, effleurage, kneading, picking up, skin rolling, hacking, and pounding
- Limited use of friction and deep kneading.

Time and Duration
About 8–12 hours before competition, preferably before active warm up and stretching exercises. *Duration:* 20–30 minutes.

Sequence
The preevent massage should be administered in two phases:
1. Massage for relaxation
2. Massage to specific muscle group.

Massage for relaxation: First massage is given to invoke its sedative effects in order to calm down the athlete having preactivity excitement. Back massage is preferred in this phase. Following is the outline of the protocol to be followed in this phase:
- Client should lie prone in comfortable position.
- Superficial stroking consists of long strokes used several times until change in the tone of muscle occurs.
- Then effleurage is done starting with light strokes, gradually progressing to deeper strokes.
- Kneading for erector spinae, latissimus dorsi, levator scapulae, and rhomboideus followed by picking up for upper fibers of trapezius.
- Ironing and skin rolling.
- The area of tension and pain should be identified during the effleurage and friction and kneading can be applied to those areas.
- To end with, deep effleurage is practiced once again.

Massage to specific muscle group: After the sedative back massage, the muscle groups, which are to be used in the events, should be treated in the following order:
- Deep effleurage followed by kneading, picking up, and muscle shaking over the muscle belly.
- The speed and rhythm of massage should be increased gradually and each maneuver should be repeated several times.
- Friction to musculotendinous junctions and ligaments, and finger kneading to the insertion of muscle can also be used.
- This phase should end with the application of percussion techniques in the form of hacking, beating, and pounding along with very brisk superficial stroking over the whole length of muscle.

Caution: The friction and deep kneading should be used with caution. These maneuvers should not produce pain. The area of chronic injuries should be left untouched during preevent massage, otherwise the painful procedure over these lesions will adversely affect the psychology of the athlete. These areas can be treated after the event.

At the end of preactivity massage, athlete should feel warm and comfortable. He should rest for sometime before participating in active warm up and stretching exercise program.

Preparatory Massage

This is used 30–45 minutes before competition prior to warm up and stretching exercises. The purpose is to achieve the optimal arousal level of player. It must not be painful and should be used only for those muscles, which are going to be used maximally during the event. It should be short, light, and loosening.

Aim: To modulate the arousal level, i.e. to stimulate the relax athlete and to relax the excited athletes.
Techniques: Superficial stroking, both hands palmar kneading, muscle shaking, hacking, and beating or pounding.
Time and duration: 30 minutes prior to competition for 5–10 minutes.
Sequence: The superficial stroking, double hand palmar kneading, and hacking should be practiced over the muscles; the rhythm of technique should be brisk and depth should be light.

Intermediate Massage

It is employed during half-time or between individual games of long series, as in boxing during the short interval period between the round. It should be short, light, and loosening. The techniques, procedure, and aim are similar to preparatory massage. For better effects, ice cold towels can be used prior to massage over the muscle that are either in use or going to be used.

Postevent Massage

This kind of massage is used after hard training or tough competition as an aid for a speedy recovery of the athlete. The intent of this massage is restorative. It facilitates the athlete's recovery by decreasing fatigue, soreness, spasm, and by speeding the removal of metabolic waste. It may significantly reduce the intensity of DOMS by increasing the blood and lymph flow and relaxing the muscle.

For massage to be effective, the time period after exercise at which massage is administered is critical. Soviet sports therapists have suggested that to enhance the athletic performance, restorative massage should be administered between one to three hours after termination of strenuous exercise (Smith et al., 1994). The hypothesis is that the residue of metabolic waste is not get fixed in the tissue immediately after the physical exertion and thus can be excreted out easily. However, it can be given even up to eight hours after the events when light techniques are used and one to two days later for deeper techniques (Liston, 1995).

Aims

1. To facilitate drainage of metabolic waste product by increasing the circulation.
2. To enhance the feeling of well-being.
3. To promote deep muscle relaxation.

Techniques used

Effleurage, kneading, picking up, wringing, and muscle shaking.
Time and duration: 1–3 hours after the competition for 30–60 minutes.

Deep penetrating techniques that encourage venous and lymphatic drainage are recommended. Hard painful massage techniques are contraindicated considering the relative postexercise anoxia in the muscle tissues.

Procedure

- The athlete should take warm shower prior to massage.
- Before massage, the player has to be examined thoroughly in order to detect any injury that might have occurred during events. If any contraindication, such as hematoma, tendon tear, muscle rupture, blows, kicks, etc. is found, massage should not be administered. Rather, prime attention should be given to the treatment of that injury.

- Athlete should be placed in a position of comfort. Then, the muscle groups primarily used in the event should be approached in the following order:
  - To start with slow and firm, effleurage is given to the part. Depth of it should be increased gradually keeping the speed and rhythm constant throughout.
  - Slow kneading, picking up, and muscle shacking should be practiced then. As the muscles relax, the depth of manipulation should be increased. This helps to squeeze out the accumulated waste product from the muscles.
  - To the end, deep and slow effleurage should be practiced once again.
  - All these techniques should be repeated several times.

Caution

- The use of percussion technique and deep friction should be avoided over the painful area.
- In general fatigue and exhaustion, it is especially effective to massage the body segment having greater receptive field, such as spine, thigh, etc.
- When there is strong fatigue, the emphasis should be given to lessen the activity of excitatory process which was increased under the influence of physical and psychological load (Paikov, 1986). For this purpose, superficial stroking with slow rhythm and finger kneading to temporal region of face may be interspersed between the other techniques.

Training Massage

It is otherwise also called regular fine tuning massage. Administered during the regular training session as a part of total conditioning program of the athlete, these massage sessions are designed to search out the area of biomechanical stress and to relieve them before they become problematic. When an activity is commenced after a period of relative inactivity or when the training level is increased, a lot of soft tissue changes take place in the body. Many of these changes like formation of tight bands, activation of silent trigger point, stressing of the previous chronic injuries, etc. can seriously affect the training schedule and many a time may compel the athlete to abandon the conditioning sessions. The aim of this massage is to support and prepare the body for the considerable conditioning, which one must undergo to reach the top form.

Ideally, these massage sessions should be incorporated on a weekly or fortnightly basis in the overall training schedule. This session can help an athlete to maintain a balance between optimal training and overtraining.

Procedure: In addition to all elements of postevent massage, deep kneading, friction, and trigger point work are the techniques of emphasis. However, the techniques should be selected as per the individual's requirement and physical status.

- As a rule, session should begin with light techniques and gradually depth should be increased.
- Deactivation of trigger point and mobilization of adherent structure are best done in this phase.
- Unlike all other categories where the emphasis is on the area to be used, here the massage should be administered to the whole body.
- Athlete may receive a treatment cramp during friction and trigger point work. He may also become very relaxed. Therefore, after these sessions, he should not immediately undergo for vigorous physical activity rather his training intensity should be increased gradually.

Medical Massage/or Massage for the Rehabilitation of Injuries

Unlike the previous categories, the client here is an injured athlete. Therefore, massage technique should be used only as an adjunct to the total therapy plan.

The sessions are designed to speed up the healing process, prevent compensatory problems, maintain as well as increase the range of muscle excursion, and to create a scar which is stronger yet does not inhibit normal broadening out of the muscle upon contraction.

Acute Injuries and Massage

Minor sprains and strains (grade I and II), tenosynovitis, tendinitis, painful scar, tenovaginitis, and indurated subcutaneous tissue, etc. are the common acute sports injuries where massage has a role. The massage treatment's aims and protocol for these conditions are described in detail elsewhere in this book. However, it is essential to point out that all acute injuries are associated with acute inflammation where massage is an absolute contraindication. Therefore, in dealing with an acutely injured athlete, one should refrain from administering massage to the painful area till the real cause behind the pain is determined.

Many coaches, players, and dance *gurus* in India have extreme faith in the healing capability of massage and frequently they undertake massage treatment, either by themselves or by quacks, in the conditions where massage is actually contraindicated. This does not alleviate the symptoms, but rather complicates the case. Therefore, application of massage in acute injuries should not be encouraged and if at all required, it should be administered by qualified and experienced physiotherapists.

Chronic Injury and Massage

Delayed-onset muscle soreness causing generalized pain, 48 hours after unaccustomed work, trigger points, chronic scar adhesions, fibrositis, and various myofascial pain are the conditions where deep massage techniques are extremely useful. In chronic ligamentous sprain, muscle strain, tenoperiosteal injuries, etc. where there occurs adhesion formation, the deep transverse friction is the treatment of choice.

Medical massage sessions are painful especially when the aim is to break the adhesion, and athlete should refrain from heavy training during this period.

CHAPTER 11

Ancient Massage Systems

Touch was the first and most naturally available means available to mankind for alleviation of pain and suffering. Touching a painful part is a natural instinct not only for human but also for other creatures. Therefore, the history of massage is as old as the history of human civilization. The mention of the systematic use of touch and pressure, i.e. massage—as therapeutic modality is found in the recorded history of almost all the ancient civilizations. Archeological evidences of the use of massage have been found in many ancient civilizations including China, Japan, Thailand, Indonesia, and India. The first written record about the use of massage comes from China and Egypt, however massage as preventive and curative modality was known in India much before its recorded use come into existence.

Many ancient civilizations considered the knowledge related to health and massage as divine and sacred. Generations to generations, this knowledge has been passed down in a closely guarded manner. Sometimes, the technical know how was bestowed only among the blood relations. This poses a challenge in gathering the authenticated information about these systems.

Each civilization had peculiar believes about illness and health which influenced the therapeutic principles and techniques of a given civilization. Though theories of ancient civilizations and cultures differ greatly from each other, the elements of commonality can be traced. For example, a closer look at the ancient medicinal theories reveals that despite differences in nomenclature believe in the existence of an all permeating vital life force is common in all of the Eastern civilizations and at times similarity in the techniques of massage can also be seen. Cultural exchange and migration of population from one country to another can be postulated as one of the reasons for this.

It is commonly held that the techniques of Western Swedish massage have roots in ancient Eastern massage systems and many ancient massage systems can be considered as forerunners of the newly developed systems of massage. In recent times, the resurgent emergence of massage in therapeutics has generated an interest in the ancient massage systems worldwide. A number of publications have appeared in literature in recent times that attempts to scientifically examine the traditional uses of massage as depicted in these systems.

The present chapter presents a brief description of the ancient massage systems originated from India, China, Japan, and Thailand. The theoretical foundation and fundamentals of technical aspects of these systems are included. Though for detailed information, the reader is advised to refer the sources mentioned in References and Bibliography section of this book.

AYURVEDIC MASSAGE

The massage component of Ayurvedic system is referred as *Abhyanga*. In Ayurvedic texts, massage is invariably mentioned as *champan* and *mardhan*. When these maneuvers are performed with oil, it is called *Abhyanga*. It is considered as an important rejuvenation and purification therapy of Ayurveda. It is often administered as a preactivity (*Purva Karma*) part of *Panchakarma*—the five acts of detoxification that includes *Vamana* (therapeutic emesis), *Virechana* (therapeutic purgation), *Anuvasana* (medicated oil enema), *Asthapana* (medicated decoction enema), and *Nasya* (nasal administration of medicaments) (Lavekar, 2010). Two synonyms of *Abhyanga* are *Abhyanjana* and *Snehana (Sinha* et al., *2017)*.

Benefits of *Abhyanga* along with its contraindications are described in all the Ayurvedic classics however the exact description of the actual method of performing Abhyanga and details about its techniques is scarcely available (Madhukar et al., 2018). The only description about the technique is available in the commentary of *Acharya Dalhana*, who mentioned that *Abhyanga* should be applied in *anulom gati* (downward movement) (Madhukar et al., 2018) which implies that movement of hand over the body should be performed in the direction of hair root.

It is also believed by many that massage practices followed in Ayurveda were originated from the *Siddha* system (Banjare, 2009) which is now mostly practiced in Tamil Nadu and Kerala states of India. Preponderance of *Marma* or *Varma Chikitsa* [*Varma Kalai* = art of *Varmam*] is a distinctive feature of *Siddha* system—where massage to specific points is used for alleviation of symptoms (Arjunan, 2014). According to *Dalhan*, the *marm sthal* is the shelter places of *prana* (life force) where an injury could be fetal. According to the *Charaka Samhita*, injury to *marm sthal* elicits relatively much pain and discomfort in comparison to any other parts of body (Arjunan, 2014). Texts also describe the ailments that may arise following the strike on various *marm sthals*. But the Ayurvedic texts are silent on the method of manipulation of these points. Such description is available in *Siddha* system where *Marma* or *Varmam* therapy constitutes an important component of therapy. It is held that the original script was written in palm leaves and kept secret for generations and taught only to the blood relations. Therefore, the detailed and reliable description is not available in literature (Arjunan, 2014).

The [Charaka Samhita describes 107 points (Marmas) (Joseph et al., 2012) out of which eleven are present in each limbs, twenty six in trunk (three in abdomen, nine in thorax, fourteen in the back) and thirty seven in head neck region (Negi et,2018)]. It is said that touching these vital points can have both positive and negative results. Proper stimulation of these points through massage and yogic asanas helps dissolve stresses or remove blocks accumulated there (Banjare, 2009).

Some practitioners of late have attempted to link these *marm sthal* to the acupressure points (Banjare, 2009). It is also claimed that during Buddhist era, the techniques of Indian massage have migrated to China and Japan and evolved as acupressure and acupuncture therapy (Banjare, 2009; Salguero and Roylance, 2011).

Abhyanga means applying oil and lightly massaging the body (Madhukar et al., 2018). *Abhyanga* is used both as therapeutic procedure and also as a part of daily routine. Ayurvedic massage is generally divided in three main divisions, viz. (a) *Dhehamardhanam* or athletic massage for development of strength and formation of the body, (b) *Samvahanam* or medical massage which includes pressing of limbs comfortably in a soothing position, when the subject is retired to bed, and (c) *Keshamardhanam* or shampooing of the hair (Arjunan, 2014). It is believed that daily massage with oil before bath helps to preserve the healthy state of body. It is further held that if it is not possible to perform whole body Abhyanga daily, then at least massage of head, ear, and feet should be done on daily basis (Sinha et al., 2017).

The therapeutic effect of *Abhyanga* is attributed not to the technique of massage but to the pharmacological action of the oil (Madhukar et al., 2018). It is believed that the substances applied on the skin during *Abhyanga* are digested by the *Bhrajaka Pitta* located in the skin (Madhukar et al., 2018). It is believed that *Bhrajaka Pitta* imparts the characteristics of color and luster of the skin. The oils commonly used during Abhyanga range from simple oils, such as sesame oil, coconut oil, and mustard oil to the medicated oils, such as *Triphaladi taila*, *Bhringamalakadi taila, Chandanadi taila, Ksheerabala taila, Narayana taila*, etc. (Joseph et al., 2012). Each medicated oils has its own indications and contraindications. Lukewarm sesame oil is considered as the best oil for strength (Tonde et al., 2016).

The main deciding factor for the efficacy of Abhyanga is the selection of oil according to nature (*prakriti*) of the ailment and also of the person. According to Ayurvedic philosophy, the entire cosmos is the interplay of energy of five elements—ether, air, water, fire, and earth. These are grouped in three basic types of energy—*vata, pitta,* and *kapha*—collectively called *tridoshas*. Ether and air together constitute *vata*, fire and water constitute *pitta*, and water and earth constitute *kapha* (Pal, 1991). These doshas are present in every person in different permutations and combinations but in equilibrium with each other. This determines the constitution (prakriti) of an individual. The disturbance of any of these three *doshas* is the cause of disease and through various procedures and drugs, the Ayurvedic physician tries to correct three imbalances. The oil for Abhyanga is selected on the basis of the dosha present in the person. It is claimed that Abhyanga helps mostly during the predominance of *vata dosha* (Joseph et al., 2012).

Besides the selection of oil the other factor that is claimed to influence the effects of abhyang is the duration for which the oil is rubbed over the skin. It is held that duration of rubbing influence the depth of penetration and distribution of oil [Madhukar et al., 2018]. In *ayurvedic* texts the duration of massage for enabling the oil to reach the particular area is given in *matra* (the unit of time smaller than a second) . It is held that one *matra* equals to 19/60 seconds [Agnihotri et al., 2015] . According to *ayurvedic* texts, massage of duration 300 *matras* [approximately 95 sec] is required for the oil to reach *roma koopa* [hair follicale]. Similarly for twk[skin], *rakta* [blood], *mamsa* [flesh or muscle], *meda* [fat], *asthi* [bone] and *majja* [marrow or neural tissue] the duration recommended are 400, 500, 600,700, 800, and 900 *matras* respectively [Madhukar et al., 2018; Agnihotri et al., 2018].

Direct references are not available but scattered references can be seen according to which Abhyanga is indicated in *Bala* (children), *Vruddha* (old age), Krusha (emaciated), and *Rogi* (diseased person) (Sharma and Sharma, 2014). It is claimed that *Abhyanga* retards aging, overcomes fatigue, and annihilates effects of aggravated *vata* (Sinha et al., 2017). It indicated in all vata rogas, skin rogas, hair fall, premature graying of skin, and is also recommended as a part of daily routine (*dinacharya*) to maintain health (Kothainayagi and Gupta, 2017). It is recommended that the best time for *Abhyanga* is after performing physical exercise and just before commencing bath when the person starts to have a desire for food and drinks (Tonde et al., 2016).

Abhyanga is not ideal to practice in the some conditions like Kaphagrastha (suffering from Kaphaja disorders), Ajirna (suffering from indigestion), Krita samsudha (who are just subjected to Shodhana procedure), Samadosha (having vitiated dosha in Aama state), Navajwara (suffering from fever of short duration), Santarpana Samutha Roga (diseases caused by overnourishment), and Agnimandya (suffering from impaired digestive activity) (Madhukar et al., 2018).

Gua Sha

Gua sha is one of the many old empirical practices of the traditional Chinese medicine (TCM). This technique involves application of repeated strokes of deep pressure (scrapping) over a localized area of skin using any smooth edged hard object till the appearance of redness. This technique produces controllable tissue damage and low-scale inflammation in the skin tissue which is believed to have therapeutic effects (Nielsen et al., 2012). This ancient technique can be considered as forerunner of the newly advocated instrument-assisted soft tissue mobilization technique.

Tools for *Gua sha* include porcelain soup spoon, a smooth edge coin, to a jade stone (green stone), buffalo horn, Chinese soup spoon, a slice of water-buffalo horn, a cow rib, polished stick, etc. (Lee et al., 2010). The edge of the tool should be smooth, so that it does not break the skin or produce pain.

During the *Gua sha* treatment, a special oil containing camphor is placed over the region to be treated. The skin is scraped in one direction until slight discoloration of skin is produced on the stroke line. A stroke line is typically 4–6 inches long. Then, the stroking is applied at the next stroke line directly adjacent to the one before. This goes on until the area to be treated is covered (Nielsen et al., 2012). The patient does not feel pain during or after the treatment (Barbalho and Moraes, 2016) however the discoloration produced due to hyperemia may turn into ecchymosis and pigmentation which gradually gets resolve within 2–5 days (Chen et al., 2016). After treatment, the patient is advised to keep the area protected from wind, cold, and direct sun until the *sha* (discoloration) fades and drink plenty of water. It believed that Gua sha procedure helps expel the toxicant which cannot be cleared and excreted by physiological processes (Chen at al., 2016).

As a part of culture, *Gau sha* is used as a form of familial care in the home (Lee et al., 2010) in China and other Asian countries. *Cao Gio*, *Kerik* or *Kerokan*, *Kos Kyal*, or *Ga Sal* are the terms used in Vietnamese, Indonesian, and Cambodian languages, respectively to describe the procedure of *Gua sha*. In Western literature, this technique is invariably referred as coining, scraping, and spooning (Barbalho and Moraes, 2016).

Gua sha consists of two Chinese words. Literally, *gua* refers to the scratching of the skin, while *sha* refers to the petechiae and texture appearing after scratching (Odhav et al., 2013). However, the word *sha* has complex meaning. In common uses, *sha* means sand-like or coarse appearance but conceptually the term *sha* represents the dirt or impurity stagnated with body which is released after the scratch (Chen et al., 2016). When the *sha* ultimately fades, it indicates that the toxins have left the body. In traditional Chinese medicine, it is believed that many toxic influences such as cold wind, hot, or dampness produce stagnation of life force (*qi*) in some area of body and produce disturbance in the functioning of the body. It is believed by the practitioners of *Gua sha* that by scraping along meridian lines leads to removal of toxins and clears blockages in the energy pathways and restores the normal flow of *qi*. Therefore, the scraping is applied only along meridian channels.

Gua sha is commonly used for providing relief in any case of recurring musculoskeletal pain. It is also used for treating common cold, flu, heat stroke, respiratory problems, and functional internal organ problems and MS pain (Lee et al., 2010). Recently, some papers appear in the literature that link the proclaimed benefits of *Gau sha* to improved immunological functioning of skin (Chen et al., 2016).

Recent, trauma, fracture, contusion, burn, lacerations, moles, and pimples are the contraindications of *Gau sha*. It is not applied over genitals. People receiving heparin therapy or demonstrating hemorrhagic diathesis tendencies are also not suitable candidate for this procedure (Nielsen et al., 2012).

Tuina

Tuina (pronounced "*Twee Nah*") or Chinese medical massage is an important component of traditional Chinese medicine (TCM) which is often used in conjunction with acupuncture, moxibustion, fire cupping, Chinese herbalism, Tai chi, and qigong (Wikipedia). *Tuina* has been used in China for over 2,000 years (WHO, 2010). *Tuina* is not used for pleasure or relaxation rather it is a treatment technique to address specific patterns of disharmony in qi energy flow in the body (Al-Bedah et al., 2017).

In ancient times, *Tuina* was also called *"An Mo", "An Qiao",* or *"Qiao Mo"* (WHO, 2010). *Tui* means to "push" and *Na* means to "grasp" (Ilić et al., 2012). *Tuina* includes soft tissue massage techniques directed toward muscles and tendons, acupressure techniques to directly influence the flow of Qi, and manipulation techniques to realign the musculoskeletal system. These techniques can be divided into two categories: Reinforcing manipulations and reducing manipulations. Massage, using a light and slow touch covering a short distance along the meridians, is known as reinforcing manipulation. Massage, with a heavy and quick touch covering a long distance, is called reducing manipulation (Ilić et al., 2012). Scraping, pressure, patting, shaking, rolling, rotating, and wave techniques are the main *Tuina* techniques. In addition, combinations of the techniques called compound techniques and the techniques especially designed for children are also the part of practice. There are more than 110 diverse manipulations, though only 20–30 are commonly used in practice. These techniques are applied along the meridian movement or opposite to it, locally, or on acupunctural points (Ilić et al., 2012). Fingers, thumbs, hands, elbows, and feet are used to apply the manipulations on the body surface and stimulate the points. In addition, patients may be asked to perform prescribed exercises as supplementary therapies (WHO, 2010).

The diagnosis is based on the palpation of pulse and examination of tongue. The treatment is planned in accordance with the season, as well as mental and individual abilities (Ilić et al., 2012). *Tuina* is applied every second day, and for acute diseases every day or even twice a day. The therapy usually lasts for seven to fourteen days.

If one compares classical manual massage and *Tuina*, one can observe great similarities with regards to techniques, indications, and contraindications (Ilić et al., 2012). However, the philosophy of treatment is entirely different. The Western medicine treats the disorder of organs or organ systems, whereas TCM treats the energy balance disorder in the entire body (Ilić et al., 2012). It is claimed that classical massage of Ling has emerged from *Tuina* (Ilić et al., 2012). According to Singleton (2015), the work of PH Ling may have drawn inspiration from the Chinese body exercises.

The TCM principles that guide *Tuina* practice include *yin* and *yang*, five elements (wood, fire, earth, metal, and water), *qi*, blood and body fluids, and by the identification of syndromes and patterns (WHO, 2010). According to classic Chinese philosophy, *qi* is the primary state of the universe and the essential substances for life activities. Qi is commonly translated as bioenergy, a special vital energy. *Qi* flows constantly inside the body in the specified direction called meridians and collaterals which connect the upper and lower body, the exterior and the interior and different *visceral organs*. There are places where *qi* of organs, meridians, and collaterals infuses and gathers toward the surface of the body. These points are called acupoints. The majority of acupoints are found along the pathway of meridians and collaterals. According to traditional Chinese medicine, good physical health depends on the circulation of *qi* and blood. The common causes of pain are stagnation of *qi* and stasis of blood. It is believed that in diseases of visceral organs, there occurs imbalance of qi flow which makes these points sensitive and specific stimulation of these points using pressure or prick corrects the imbalances of *qi* flow and helps in the restoration of health (Wu et al., 2019).

Tuina treatment aims to unblock the meridians, promotes the circulation of *qi* and blood, regulates the functions of the *zang-fu* organs, and strengthens the body's resistance to pathogens (Ilić et al., 2012; Wu et al., 2019). *Tuina* tends to develop a balance in *qi* and to establish a more harmonious flow of *qi* through channels.

Tuina is commonly used for the treatment of neuromusculoskeletal conditions though it has now also been incorporated into the practice of other clinical disciplines, such as acupuncture, internal medicine, gynecology, and pediatrics (Ilić et al., 2012).

Main indications of *Tuina* are injuries; rheumatic, cardiac, gynecologic, otolaryngologic, ophthalmic, pediatric diseases; special entities such as insomnia, neurasthenia, headache, epigastric pain, diarrhea, constipation, hemiplegia, facial nerve palsy, stiff neck, shoulder pain (frozen shoulder), general obesity, muscular torticollis, etc. (Al-Bedah et al., 2017). Contraindication of *Tuina* includes acute infective diseases, fractures in early stages, malignant tumors, internal diseases, mental diseases, pregnancy and menstruation, hemorrhage and inclination to hemorrhage, etc. (Al-Bedah et al., 2017). Chinese massage should not be applied if the patient is too hungry, too full, or too tired (Ilić et al., 2012).

In 1956, the first *Tuina* school was established in Shanghai, China. Higher education for *Tuina* is now available in universities and colleges of TCM throughout China (WHO, 2010). It is used as an independent method and as an additional method to traditional and Western methods of treatment (Ilić et al., 2012).

Shiatsu

Shiatsu is recognized as an independent traditional method of treatment in Japan. The literal meaning of the word *Shiatsu* is finger pressure. It is a manual therapy of Japanese origin in which the practitioner applies pressure on certain points of the body in order to activate the body's own healing capacities (Cabo et al., 2018). The technique was developed in Japan by combining a Chinese type of massage, the *Anma* and Western physical therapy techniques. It is based on the same concepts as that utilized by Chinese acupuncture and traditional Chinese medicine (TCM) (Robinson et al., 2011). Therefore in the literature *Shiatsu* and acupressure are often used interchangeably (Robinson et al., 2011).

However, there are several key technical differences between the two, including the type of pressure applied, the way in which the thumb is positioned, and the way in which body weight is used (Cabo et al., 2018). Pressure used in *shiatsu* is always stationary and sustained whereas in acupressure, the pressure applied is often circular or may use a pumping action in which the thumb repeatedly presses and releases pressure quickly. In *Shiatsu*, the thumb is always in an extended position whereas in acupressure, the thumb is flexed at the metacarpophalangeal joint. *Shiatsu* uses the whole weight of one's body to apply pressure, whereas acupressure uses the strength of the arms or hands (Cabo et al., 2018). Though *Shiatsu* implies treatment using fingers but the practitioners use elbows, knees, and feet as well. When massage is performed using feet alone, it is called Ashiatsu (*Ashi* = foot, *atsu* = pressure).

One of the features that distinguishes *Shiatsu* from acupressure or traditional massage is that *Shiatsu* is given without undressing the body parts. *Shiatsu* is done with the recipient wearing light and comfortable cotton clothes, usually lying on a comfortable cotton or futon mattress on the floor (Oki et al., 2017). During application of techniques, no oil or cream is used.

Tokujiro Namikoshi (1905–2000) is often credited with inventing modern *Shiatsu*. He founded his *Shiatsu* college in the 1940s. Currently, there are many schools of *Shiatsu* which varies in styles, philosophical approaches, and theoretical bases (Robinson et al., 2011). Some of these schools are Zen *Shiatsu*, Macrobiotic *Shiatsu*, Healing *Shiatsu*, Tao *Shiatsu*, Seiki, Namikoshi *Shiatsu*, Hara *Shiatsu*, etc.

Shiatsu is a holistic discipline that approaches treatment by considering the whole body. *Shiatsu* diagnosis is primarily through touch. The *Shiatsu* techniques include stretching, grip, and inclination of therapist's body weight over many parts of the recipient's body. The treatment focuses mainly along meridians. *Shiatsu* practitioners are trained in the anatomical location, functions and uses over 150 pressure points on the body (Robinson et al., 2011).

The problems in which *Shiatsu* is claimed to offer benefit include headaches, migraine, stiff necks and shoulders, backaches, coughs, colds, menstrual problems, respiratory illnesses including asthma and bronchitis, sinus trouble and catarrh, insomnia, tension, anxiety and depression, fatigue and weakness, digestive disorders and bowel trouble, circulatory problems, rheumatic and arthritic complaints, sciatica, and conditions following sprains and injuries (Robinson et al., 2011). However, it is a holistic therapy that focuses on balancing the body's energy level and brings a harmony among mental, physical, emotional, and spiritual aspects.

TRADITIONAL THAI MASSAGE

Traditional Thai massage (TTM) can be described as a combination of acupressure, yoga, and massage. The principles and practices of Thai massage bear direct influence of Buddhism, Ayurveda, yogic practices, traditional Chinese medicine, and traditional Thai medicine (Salguero and Roylance, 2011).

Nuad phaen borarn, or ancient massage is one of the four main branches of traditional medicine of Thailand. The word *Bo'Rarn* is derived from the Sanskrit word *Puran*—the ancient religious text of India. This implies that *Nuad Borarn* or ancient Thai massage is derived from a body of teaching handed down over time from generation to generation (Gold, 2007).

Thai massage is directly related to yogic principles originating in India. It is also in many ways similar to Chinese massage techniques. In Thai medical theory, body is comprised of four primary elements (earth, water, fire, and air or wind) and every part of the body is linked to every other part through an infinite and intricate mesh of vital energy (*lom* in Thai). The equivalent term for this vital energy is *Prana-Vayu* in Sanskrit and *qi* in Chinese. This vital energy travels throughout the body on specified pathways called *Sen*. Thai massage uses the ten energy line system (*Sen Prathan Sip*). The *Sen* can be correlated to the meridians of Chinese medicine and also with the *nadi* of yogic system. Anatomically, the *Sen* lines do not correspond with the paths of the blood vessels or the lymph vessels (Ryan et al., 2003).

There are ten main *Sen* lines, i.e. *Sen Sumana (after Sushumna nadi* of yoga), *Sen Ittha (after Ida nadi), Sen Pingkhala (after Pingala nadi), Sen Kalathari, Sen Sahatsarangsi, Sen Tawari, Sen Lawusang, Sen Ulangka, Sen Nanthakrawat,* and *Sen Khitchanna* from which the rest of the 72,000 *Sen* branches out (Salguero and Roylance, 2011). All of the *Sen* lines originate from the naval and all have different exit points. Each Sen line is associated with different parts of the body and organ systems. The blockage or increase of wind flow through these lines will cause bodily pain or dysfunction. The 10 main lines have the center underneath and around the umbilicus and are orderly distributed in all parts of the body (Juntakarn et al., 2017). Acupressure points are found along these lines. Bodily disturbances manifest on these lines which a traditional healer identifies through touch, vision, or experience. It is believed that manipulating the energy manually on these lines and points releases the stagnated energy and clears energy blockages and restores the balance in the essence of life, earth, air, wind, and fire (Ryan et al., 2003) which promotes the natural healing process and influence the patient's mind and body (Gold, 2007).

A complete Thai massage session incorporates a combination of pressure techniques closely resembling acupressure and passive stretching by placing the body part in various yogic asanas. A classic Thai massage session consists of 108 steps consisting of various pressing and stretching techniques (Salguero and Roylance, 2011).

Pressing techniques utilizes thumb, finger, palm, forearm, elbow, and on occasion ankle, foot, and knee to apply either downward pressure (deep press) or pressure in circles (circular pressure) on selected points along the selected Sen lines. Some techniques—used over groin and axilla—intend to obstruct the superficial flow of the blood and direct the blood flow to deeper tissue areas. These are known as "stop-the-blood-flow techniques" during which the practitioner locates the pulse and exerts a deep downward pressure with the heel of the hand and maintain the pressure for up to 30 seconds. The palm pressing technique is considered as an integrative technique to be used before and after the detailed work out. Absence of long stroking techniques, such as effleurage is one of the main differentiating features of TTM. After a point has been treated directly with thumb or finger pressure, the practitioner works on the area in a circular motion using the techniques of thumb, finger, or palm circles. Deep pressing techniques are not used over the knees, joints, and along the bones. In these areas, circular motion techniques with the fingers, thumbs, or palms are used. The techniques of Thai massage are applied very slowly (Salguero and Roylance, 2011).

Another critical component of Thai massage is stretching of the limbs, torso, and neck. The therapists passively move the relaxed body of the clients in various postures in order to provide sustained stretch. Many of these stretch positions resemble the yogic asanas.

Massage sessions always start from the extremities and proceed toward the core of the body (medially), and then back to the extremities. The feet are approached first and therapists move gradually upward. The head and face massages are generally administered lastly to the patient (Ryan et al., 2003). In each part, *Sen* work (pressing around the points along the *Sen*) is perform first, thereafter the joint mobilization and stretches are applied. Steps performed on one side are always performed on the contralateral side in order to give a balanced massage. The entire body should be massaged in order to experience the health benefits of massage (Ryan et al., 2003). It is held that patients will remain tired if he received an unbalanced massage session. According to Thai medical theory, all of the vital Sen lines energy originates deep in the abdomen in the vicinity of the navel. Therefore, abdominal massage constitutes an important component of this system of treatment (Gold, 2007).

The classic Thai Massage routine lasts about an hour and a half during which the therapists move back and forth between acupressure and stretching with seamless fluidity (Salguero and Roylance, 2011).

Thai massage is practiced on a mat placed on the floor or on a low-standing futon. The client remains completely clothed throughout the session and no oil is used during massage session. The experience of traditional Thai massage is not altogether pleasant, and sometimes it can be quite painful (Ryan et al., 2003).

There are two styles of Thai massage, Southern style or Wat Pho style originated at Wat Pho in Bangkok and Northern style originated from the Old Medicine Hospital in Chiang Mai. Southern style focuses primarily on acupressure and energy lines and employs a much stronger pressure. Northern style is slower and gentler and focuses more on the yoga-like stretching (Salguero and Roylance, 2011).

Ailments where a traditional Thai massage may prove beneficial include asthma, bronchitis, heart disease, angina, nausea, nasal obstruction, eye problems, throat problems, shock, schizophrenia, hysteria, various mental disorders, manic depression, diseases of the urogenital system, appendicitis, deafness, ear diseases, frequent urination, impotence, precox ejaculation, irregular menstruation, uterine bleeding, facial paralysis, hypothermia, and diarrhea (Ryan et al., 2003).

Thai massage treatment is contraindicated in cancer, serious illness, state of profound weakness, high fever, osteoporosis, bleeding disorders, and acute spinal pain. Pregnancy women are not treated during menses due to cultural taboo (Salguero and Roylance, 2011). The procedures of "stopping the blood flow" are not used in the clients with a history of heart problems, diabetes, and vascular problems.

Thai traditional massage is an ancient form of healing that has evolved within the cultural context of Theravada Buddhism. Therefore, this massage has deep roots in spirituality. Buddhist monks performed Thai massage in the temples as part of their Vipassana meditation to assist them in attaining a clear and peaceful mind (Ryan et al., 2003).

The legendary founder of Thai medicine is a native of India known as *Jivaka Komarabaccha* (usually spelled in Thailand as "*Shivago Komarapat*" or "*Shivagakomarpaj*") (Salguero and Roylance, 2011). *Jivaka* was a close personal associate of the *Buddha* and was the head physician of the original *Sangha*. *Jivaka* is revered in Thailand as the progenitor of the traditional medical knowledge. Keeping a statue of *Jivak* and Buddha in their workplace is customary for the Thai healers. Thai massage is practiced within the ethical boundaries of "Five Precepts of Buddhism" (*panchsheel*). Before the commencement of massage session, the therapists kneel at their clients' feet with folded hands and closed eyes and say a silent prayer to *Jivakkumarbachcha* in order to prepare themselves to perform massage in most ethical manner.

Despite these high ethical considerations, it is unfortunate that Thai massage is often associated with the sex industry. There are many misconceptions about this ancient art of healing mostly because of the illegitimate Thai massage parlors operating throughout Thailand (Ryan et al., 2003) that serve as fronts for brothels (Salguero and Roylance, 2011). It is important to remember that traditional Thai massage is an ancient form of healing that has been practiced in Thailand for thousands of years and traditional Thai massage is an important aspect of the primary healthcare system in Thailand (Ryan et al., 2003). The effects of traditional Thai massage have been shown to enhance health and well-being (Juntakarn et al., 2017; Miyahara et al., 2017).

Outlines of the Lymphatic System

CHAPTER 12

In order to practice massage in a scientific manner, it is necessary to know the arrangement of lymphatic vessels and nodes in the body. The salient features of this arrangement are presented in this chapter. The text mainly deals with the course of lymphatic vessels. The location of lymphatic nodes and their respective area of drainage are presented schematically in the charts. The readers are advised to refer textbooks of anatomy for further reading.

GENERAL CONSIDERATIONS

Lymphatic system is an accessory route by which the larger molecules like protein, debris, and other matters from tissue space return back to the circulation. 10% of the fluid filtering from the arterial capillaries enters the lymphatic system. Lymphatics have valves at the very tip of the terminal lymphatic capillary and also along their larger vessels, up to the point where they empty into venous circulation.

Lymphatic capillaries form plexuses in the tissue space, which have much wider mesh than those of adjacent blood capillaries. They are generally permeable to colloidal material and larger particles, such as the cell debris and the microorganism.

Lymphatic capillaries join to form wider lymphatic vessels, which pass to the local lymph node. The lymph nodes are arranged in the form of regional groups and each group has its specific region of drainage. Nodes within a group are often interconnected to each other.

A normal young adult has some 400–450 lymph nodes. The arm and the superficial thoracoabdominal wall contain about 30 nodes. The leg, superficial buttock, infraumbilical abdominal wall, and perineum contain about 20 nodes. Head and neck carry some 60–70 nodes. Rest is divided between the thorax, abdomen, and pelvis.

All lymphatic vessels are divided into superficial and deep vessels according to their location in respect to the deep fascia. These vessels terminate ultimately into either the left thoracic duct or the right lymphatic duct which in turn open into left and right brachiocephalic veins, respectively. Therefore, the lymphatics from all parts of the body empty into the venous system.

The thoracic duct receives lymphatics from the lower limbs, abdomen and left side of head, part of chest, and the left upper limbs. The right lymphatic duct receives the lymphatics from the right side of the head and the right side of the chest.

The lymphatic capillaries are not present in the avascular structures, such as epidermis, hair, nails, cornea, articular cartilage, central nervous system, and bone marrow.

LYMPHATIC DRAINAGE OF THE UPPER LIMB

Most superficial and deep lymphatic vessels of the upper limb drain into lateral axillary lymph node. Therefore, each stroke of effleurage in the upper limb should be directed toward the axilla **(Flowchart 12.1)**.

Chapter 12: Outlines of the Lymphatic System

Flowchart 12.1: Lymph nodes of the upper limb.

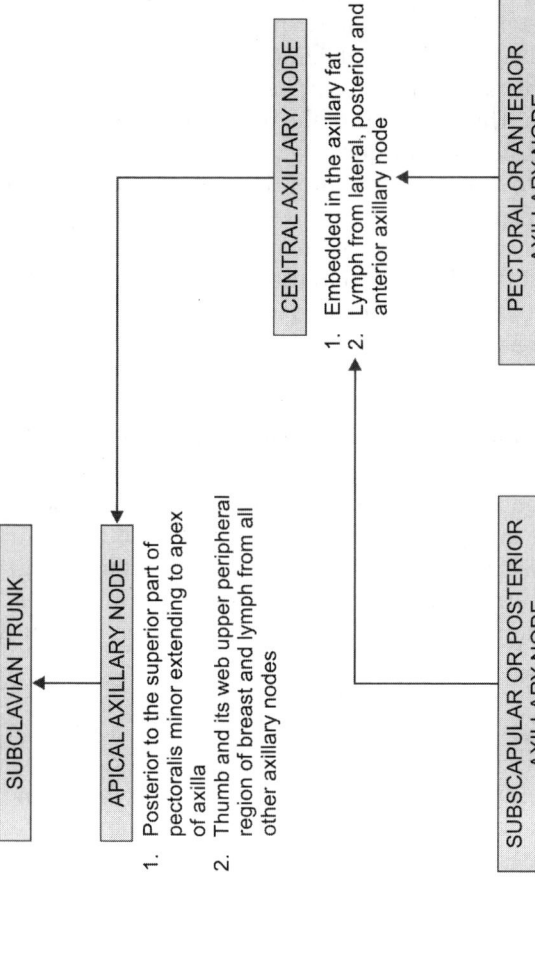

Superficial Drainage

Superficial lymph vessels of the upper limb drain the skin and subcutaneous tissues and end mostly at the lateral axillary node. They begin in the cutaneous plexus. Fingers are drained by the digital plexus along the medial and lateral borders of the fingers up to their web space. In the web space, the digital plexus joins the palmar vessels which pass back to the dorsum of hand and joins the dorsal vessels of the forearm. The lymphatic of the proximal palm drains toward the wrist medially along its ulnar border. Laterally, they join the vessels of the thumb.

The dorsal vessels after running proximally in parallel through the forearm curve successively around the borders of the limb to join the ventral vessels. Anterior carpal vessels run in the forearm parallel with the median vein of the forearm up to the level of elbow region, and then they follow the medial border of the biceps up to the anterior axillary fold. They then pierce the deep fascia at the anterior axillary fold and end into the lateral axillary lymph node. Vessels, which are lateral in the forearm, follow the cephalic vein up to the level of the tendon of the deltoid. Thereafter, most vessels incline medially to reach the lateral axillary nodes, whereas some vessels continue with the vein to the infraclavicular nodes. Vessels, which are medial in the forearm, follow the course of the basilic vein. They are joined by the vessels curving around the medial border of the limb. Some of these vessels end in the supratrochlear node, proximal to the elbow. The lymphatic vessels from the deltoid region (outer and upper arm) pass around the anterior and posterior axillary fold to end in the anterior and posterior axillary node, respectively. Overall lymphatic vessels from the forearm emerge on the medial side of the upper arm to reach the lateral axillary lymph nodes. The scapular skin drains either to the subscapular axillary lymph node or to the inferior deep cervical node (supraclavicular node).

Deep Drainage

The structures situated beneath the deep fascia, mainly muscles, are drained by the deep lymphatic vessels. Deep lymphatic vessels accompany the main neurovascular bundle of the upper limb (radial, ulnar, interosseous, and brachial) and drain into the lateral axillary lymph node.

The lymphatics of the scapular muscles empty themselves mainly into the subscapular axillary node whereas those of the pectoral muscles drain to the pectoral, central, and apical groups of axillary nodes.

LYMPHATIC DRAINAGE OF THE LOWER LIMB

The lower limb has a superficial and a deep set of lymphatic vessels. Unlike upper limb, they drain into two different sets of lymph nodes and there exists no communication between the superficial and deep lymphatic channel. However, this arrangement does not affect the direction of effleurage in the lower limb, because both the superficial and the deep inguinal nodes are situated at the groin (femoral triangle) **(Flowchart 12.2)**.

Superficial Drainage

Like upper limb, the superficial lymph vessels of the lower limb drain the skin and subcutaneous tissue. They are much more numerous than the deep vessels and take a direct course to the superficial inguinal lymph node.

The superficial lymph vessels begin in the subcutaneous plexus.

Superficial lymphatics from the medial side of foot and leg ascend with the long saphenous vein to the superficial inguinal node. Those from the lateral side of foot and leg ascend and cross in the region of knee to join the medial group of vessels.

Chapter 12: Outlines of the Lymphatic System

Flowchart 12.2: Lymph nodes of the lower limb.

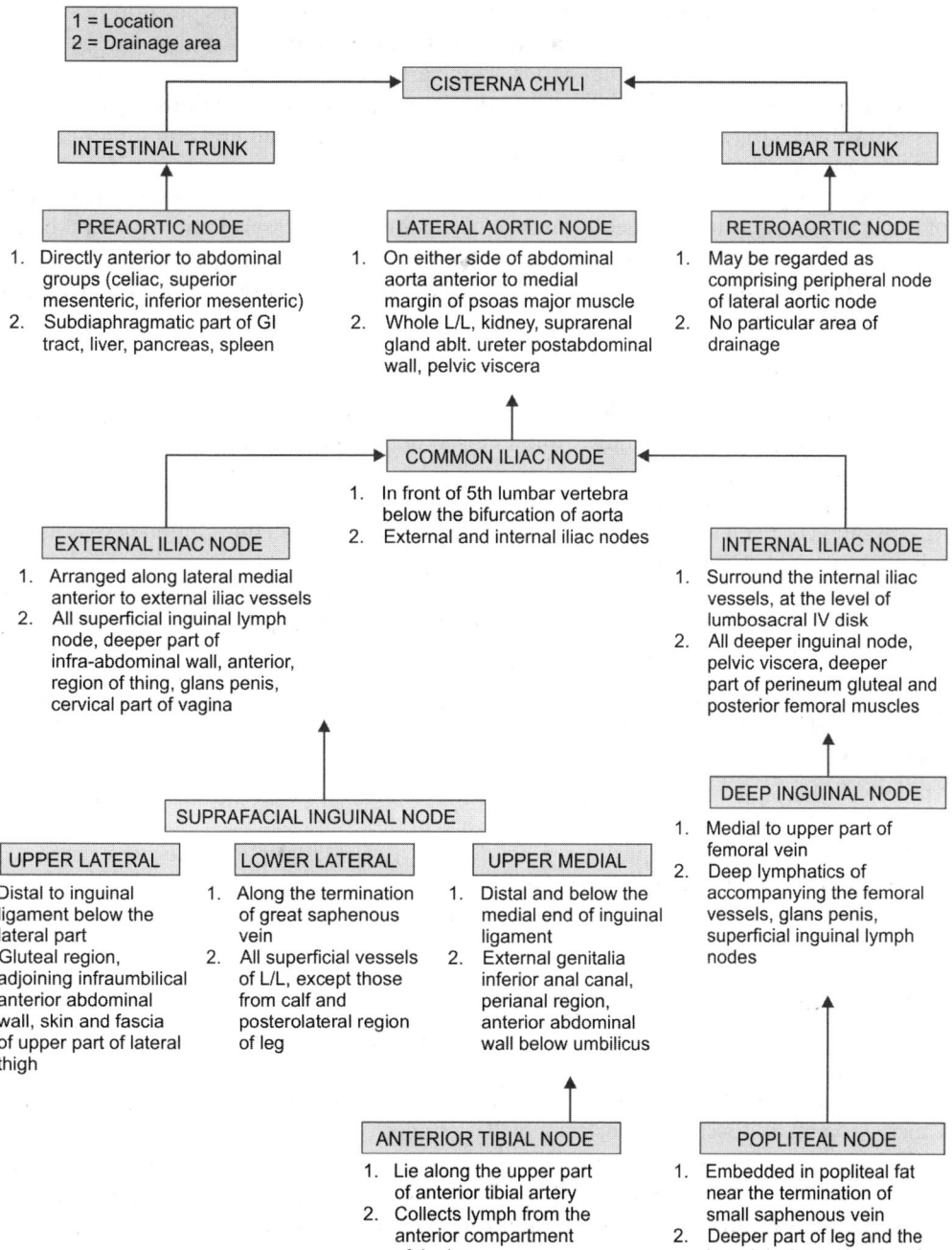

(GI: gastrointestinal; IV: intravenous; L/L: lower limb)

The medial vessels begin on the tibial side of the dorsum of foot. Around medial malleolus, they branch off. Some vessels pass anteriorly whereas the other passes posteriorly around the medial malleolus. They again join each other near the great saphenous vein and follow its course up to the distal superficial inguinal nodes, which are situated at the groin.

The lateral vessels begin on the fibular side. Some cross the leg anteriorly to join the medial vessels, whereas the others accompany the small saphenous vein and end into the popliteal lymph node situated at the back of knee.

There is a lymph shed, along the back of the lower limb. The vessels from the medial half of the limb pass around the medial surface of the limb. The vessels from the lateral half pass around the lateral surface of the limb to converge on the inguinal lymph nodes.

The superficial lymph vessels of the gluteal region drain anteriorly to the lateral superficial inguinal lymph node.

Deep Drainage

The deep lymph vessels of the lower limb accompany the main blood vessels (anterior and posterior tibial, peroneal, popliteal, and femoral) of the lower limb and terminate at the deep inguinal node situated at the groin.

The deep vessels from the foot and the leg enter into the popliteal node at the back of knee. This node is connected to the deep inguinal lymph node through the lymphatic vessels, which follow the course of the femoral vessels in the thigh.

The deep vessels from the gluteal and the ischial region drain along with the corresponding blood vessels (gluteal and internal pudendal) through the greater sciatic foramen into the internal iliac node situated in the pelvis.

LYMPHATIC DRAINAGE OF TRUNK (FLOWCHART 12.3)

Neck

The vessels draining the superficial cervical tissue pass along the margin of sternocleidomastoid muscle and drain into the superior deep cervical node.

The vessels from the superior region of the anterior triangle of the neck drain to the submandibular and the submental nodes.

The deep tissues of the head and the neck drain to the deep cervical nodes either directly or through the distant groups.

Thoracic Wall

The superficial lymphatic vessels of the thoracic wall branch off subcutaneously and converge on the axillary nodes.

The vessels superficial to the trapezius and the latissimus dorsi unite to form 10–12 trunks which end in the subscapular posterior axillary nodes.

The vessels in the pectoral region including those from the skin covering the periphery of mammary gland and its subareolar plexus drain into the pectoral (anterior) axillary node.

The vessels near the lateral sternal margin pass between the costal cartilage to the parasternal nodes.

A few vessels from the upper pectoral region ascend over the clavicle and drain into the inferior deep cervical nodes, which are arranged in a vertical chain.

The lymphatic vessels from the deeper tissues of the thoracic wall drain mainly to the parasternal, intercostal, and the diaphragmatic lymph node.

The parasternal nodes are situated at the anterior end of the intercostal space. They drain mammary glands, deeper structures of the supraumbilical anterior abdominal wall, and the

Flowchart 12.3: Lymphatic trunks.

1 = Location and formation
2 = Drainage area

JUGULAR TRUNK
1. Extends along the ventrolateral aspect of internal jugular vein, formed by the efferents from deep cervical lymph nodes
2. Drains head and neck

SUBCLAVIAN TRUNK
1. Extends along the axillary and subclavian vein, formed by terminal apical axillary nodes
2. Drains the L/L, and superficial tissue of thoracic abdominal wall down to umbilicus (anterior) and iliac crest (posterior)

BRONCHOMEDIASTINAL TRUNK
1. Formed by the efferents from brachiocephalic node and tracheobronchial nodes
2. Drains the lung, half of the mediastinum, part of anterior wall of abdomen and thorax

LYMPHATIC DUCT
1. Formed by the fusion of all three trunks, it inclines across the medial border of scalenius anterior muscle to the ventral aspect of venous junction
2. Drains right head and neck, thorax and its content superficial tissue of abdomen and trunk down to umbilicus (anterior) and iliac crest (posterior)

BRACHIOCEPHALIC VEIN

THORACIC DUCT
1. Begins in front of L2 vertebra from the upper end of cysterna chyli, traverses thorax, forms an arch at the level of the transverses process of C7 above clavicle
2. Drains right side of head, neck and chest left U/L, and entire body below ribs

RIGHT AURICLE

CISTERNA CHYLI
1. About 5–7 cm elongated lymphatic sac, formed between lumbar and intestinal trunk, situated in front of L1 and L2 vertebra, right to the abdominal aorta
2. Its upper end is continuous with the thoracic duct

INTESTINAL TRUNK
1. Formed by the efferents from preaortic nodes
2. Drain the stomach, intestine (to midrectal level), pancreas, spleen and anterior inferior part of liver

LUMBAR TRUNK
1. Formed by efferents from lateral aortic lymph nodes
2. Drain the L/L, full thickness of the pelvis, perineal and infraumbilical abdominal wall, deep tissue of most of supraumbilical abdominal wall, the pelvic viscera, testes, ovaries, kidney and suprarenal gland

(L/L: lower limb; U/L: upper limb)

deeper parts of the anterior thoracic wall. The vessels emerging from these nodes form the bronchomediastinal trunk.

The intercostal nodes are situated posteriorly in the intercostal space near the head and neck of the ribs. They drain the posterolateral aspect of the chest and the mammary gland. The lymphatics of the posterior muscles attached to the ribs, and end mostly in the axillary node. Some lymphatic vessels from the pectoralis major end in the parasternal nodes. The intercostal muscles of the anterior thoracic wall are drained by the intercostal lymphatic vessel to the parasternal node. The intercostal muscles of the posterior thoracic wall drained to the intercostal nodes.

Abdominal Wall

The umbilicus forms the "watershed" for the anterior abdominal wall as far as the lymphatic drainage is concerned.

Superficial lymphatics of the region above the umbilicus run obliquely upward to the pectoral and the subscapular axillary nodes whereas those from the region below the umbilicus drain downward to the superficial inguinal nodes.

The deep lymphatic vessels follow the course of the deep arteries. The posterior vessels run along with the lumbar arteries to the lateral aortic and the retroaortic nodes. The vessels from the upper anterior abdominal wall run along with the superior epigastric vessels to the parasternal node. The vessels from the lower part of abdominal wall end in the circumflex iliac, inferior epigastric, and the external iliac nodes. The vessels of the pelvic wall follow the course of the internal iliac artery and terminate in the iliac or the lateral aortic nodes.

LYMPHATIC DRAINAGE OF THE HEAD

The overall lymphatic drainage of the head can be divided into 4 territories, namely—upper, middle, lower, and the lateral **(Flowchart 12.4)**.

The upper territory, which includes the greater part of the forehead, the lateral halves of eyelid, the conjunctiva, the lateral part of the cheek and the parotid area, drains into the preauricular (parotid) node, which is situated just anterior to the tragus.

The middle territory, which includes a strip over the medial part of forehead, the external nose, the upper lip, the medial part of the lower lip, the medial halves of the eyelid, the medial part of the cheek, and the greater part of the lower jaw, drains into the submandibular node. The lower territory, which includes the central part of the lower lip and the chin, drains into the submental nodes situated below the chin. A strip of scalp above the auricle and the upper half of the auricle's cranial aspect and margin constitute the lateral strip, which drains into the upper deep cervical and the retroauricular nodes. The occipital scalp is drained partly to the occipital nodes, which are commonly superficial to the upper attachment of the trapezius.

Chapter 12: Outlines of the Lymphatic System

Flowchart 12.4: Lymph nodes of the head and neck.

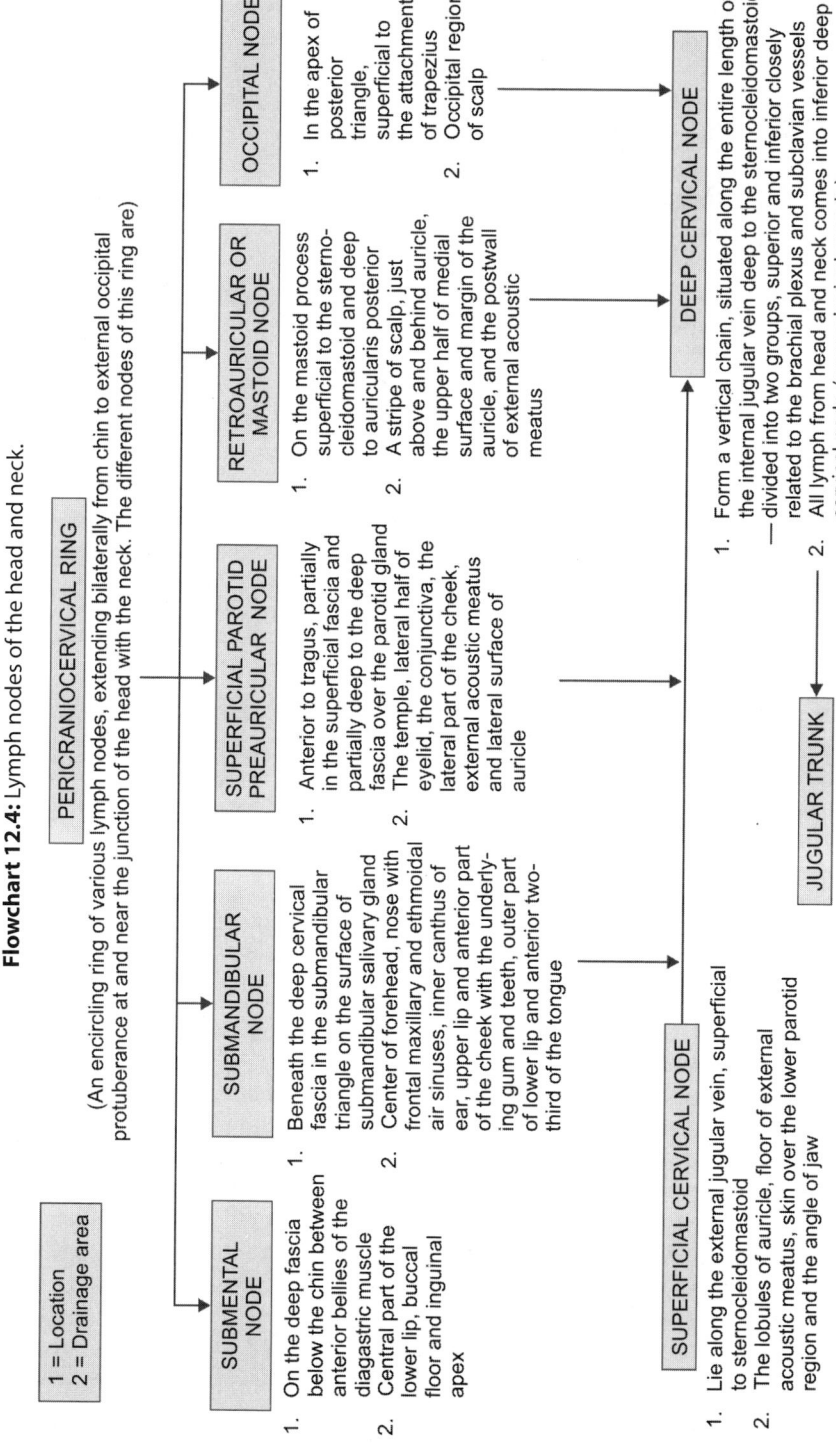

GLOSSARY

Abduction	:	A movement that takes a body part away from the midline of the body.
Adduction	:	A movement that brings a body part toward the midline of the body.
Adhesion	:	The result when two structures become attached, united, or struck together.
Adipose tissue	:	Tissue largely composed of fat cells.
Anterior	:	Front portion of the body.
Arousal	:	A psychological state of preparedness, willingness to execute a task.
Cardiac arrhythmia	:	Any variation in either the force or rate of heartbeat from the normal.
Centrifugal	:	Away from the center of circulation, i.e., heart.
Centripetal	:	Toward the center of circulation, i.e., heart.
Cocontraction	:	Simultaneous contraction of two opposing groups of muscles around joint/joints, so that tension develops in the part but no movement results.
Connective tissue	:	Supporting or framework tissue of body formed by collagenous and elastic fibers, basic cell type is fibroblast, derived from mesoderm.
Contractile unit	:	The structures having inherent property of contraction functionally related to muscles.
Contralateral	:	Opposite side.
Distal	:	Part farthest from a reference point, for example, in reference to shoulder elbow is distal.
Dorsiflexion	:	Act of moving the foot up toward the leg.
Embolism	:	Sudden blocking of a blood vessel by a blood clot or other foreign materials introduced into the circulation.
Erythema	:	Redness of skin due to increased blood flow.
Extension	:	A movement that brings two parts of a joint toward a straight line or movement that returns a segment from flexed position to neutral position.
Facilitation	:	The promotion of performance of function, the reinforcement of a reflex and neural activity.
Fascia	:	A sheet of fibrous tissue that envelops the body beneath the skin and also encloses the muscle or group of muscles and separates their several layers.
Flexion	:	A movement that brings the two parts of a joint into a bend position.
Hemoptysis	:	The spitting of bright red blood from lungs.
Homeostasis	:	A state of equilibrium between the opposing forces in the body with respect to various functions and to the chemical compositions of fluid and tissue.
Hypothenar eminence	:	Slightly elevated area of the palm near medial border of hand.
Inflammation	:	A reaction of living tissue to injury characterized by increased flow of blood and exudation of fluid from blood vessels with consequent redness, pain, heat, and swelling.
Inhibition	:	Putting restraint on an activity or function, so that a stimulus evokes no response.
Ipsilateral	:	Same side.
Ischemia	:	Insufficient blood supply to a part of body relative to local need.
Lateral	:	Outer side of a segment, the side away from the midline of body.

Lesion	:	The site of injury, pathological condition, or dysfunction.
Lordosis	:	Hollow of spine in neck and lower back, spinal curvature with convexity in the forward direction.
Medial	:	Inner side of a segment, the side closer to the midline of body.
Muscle tone	:	A state of slight tension, usually present in muscles even at rest, a state of preparedness of a muscle to resist the stretch, controlled by nervous system. In injuries involving brain and spinal cord, the tone of muscle increase (hypertonicity) whereas injuries to peripheral nerves or anterior horn cells or spinal nerve roots result in decrease of tone (hypotonicity).
Noncontractile unit	:	Structures having no inherent property to contract or relax, includes joint capsules, ligaments, bursa, fascia, etc.
Periosteum	:	The thick fibrous membrane covering the entire outer surface of bone except at the articular ends. It consists of an inner layer which forms new bone tissue and an outer layer containing blood vessels and nerves supplying the bones.
Placebo	:	A treatment which is known to have no physiological curative effects when given to a patient brings about favorable results mostly due to psychological factors.
Plantar flexion	:	Act of moving the foot downward away from the leg.
Posterior	:	Back portion of the body, dorsal.
Pronation	:	Act of turning the palm downward, performed by the medial rotation of forearm.
Prone	:	Lying on the tummy.
Proximal	:	Part closer to a reference point, for example, in reference to elbow shoulder is proximal.
Scar	:	A mark remaining after healing of the wound which consists of the fibrous tissue replacing the normal tissue destroyed by injury or by disease.
Sedation	:	The act of soothing or allying irritability, relief of pain, or production of calmness.
Stretch reflex	:	Involuntary contraction of muscle when it is suddenly stretched, due to stimulation of proprioceptors controlled by central nervous system.
Supination	:	Act of turning the palm upward, performed by lateral rotation of forearm.
Supine	:	Lying flat on the back.
Tender	:	Abnormal painful sensitivity to touch and pressure.
Thenar eminence	:	Small elevated area of the palm at the base of thumb.
Trigger point	:	A hyperirritable site on the external surface of body which is painful on pressure and gives rise to characteristic referred pain and autonomic responses to a distant area which is located away from the site of stimulation.

REFERENCES

1. Adcock D, Paulsen S, Jabour K, et al. Analysis of the effects of deep mechanical massage in the porcine model. Plast Reconstr Surg. 2001;108(1):233-40.
2. Agarwal KN, Gupta A, Pushkarna R, et al. Effects of massage and use of oil on growth, blood flow and sleep pattern in infants. Indian J Med Res. 2000;112:212-7.
3. Agnihotri Vk, Kumar V, Sharma R. Therapeutic significance of shiroabhyanga: a review.Int. J Ayurveda Pharma 2015;6(6):725-30.
4. Al-Bedah AM, Ali GI, Abushanab TS, et al. Tui Na (or Tuina) Massage: A Minireview of Pertinent Literature, 1970–2017. J Complement Altern Med Res. 2017;3(1):1-14.
5. Aourell M, Skoog M, Carleson J. Effects of Swedish massage on blood pressure. Complement Ther Clin Pract. 2005;11(4):242-6.
6. Arjunan S. (2014). Effect of South Indian ancient art of Varmam points and massage therapy to develop selected psychological variables for men athletes. PhD thesis of Manonmaniam Sundaranar University. Available at http://hdl.handle.net/10603/61592. Last acessed nov 2019 [online].
7. Arkko PJ, Pakarinen AJ, Kari-Koskinen O. Effects of whole body massage on serum protein, electrolyte and hormone concentrations, enzyme activities, and hematological parameters. Int J Sports Med. 1983;4(4):265-7.
8. Arora J, Kumar A, Ramji S. Effect of oil massage on growth and neurobehavior in very low birth weight preterm neonates. Indian Pediatr. 2005;42(11):1092-100.
9. Astrand PA, Rodahl K. Textbook of Work Physiology: Physiological Basis of Exercise. Singapore: McGraw Hill; 1986.
10. Atkinson HW. Principles of Treatment. In: Downie PA (Ed). Neurology for Physiotherapist. London: Wolfe Publishing Co.; 1992. pp. 148-217.
11. Ault P, Plaza A, Paratz J. Scar massage for hypertrophic burns scarring: a systematic review. 2018;44(1):24-38.
12. Backus D, Manella C, Bender A, et al. Impact of Massage Therapy on Fatigue, Pain, and Spasticity in People with Multiple Sclerosis: a Pilot Study. Int J Ther Massage Bodywork. 2016;9(4):4-13.
13. Bale P, James H. Massage, warmdown and rest as recuperative measures after short-term intense exercise. Physiother Sports. 1991;13:4-7.
14. Banjare Hiraman. Marm aek adhayayn aekyupeshar chikitsa pdhati ke vishesha shandrabha me. PhD thesis of Pt Ravishankar Shukla University, 2015. Available at http://hdl.handle.net/10603/41426. Last accessed on 28 novemebr 2019.
15. Barbalho MM, Moraes PH. The effects of the Gua Sha technique (western view) on the flexibility of the posterior chain: series of cases. MTP Rehab J. 2016;14(2):373.
16. Barnes MF. The basic science of myofascial release: morphologic change in connective tissue. J Bodywork Movement Ther. 1997;4(1):231-8.

17. Barr JS, Taslitz N. The influence of back massage on autonomic functions. Phys Ther. 1970;50(12):1679-91.
18. Basler AJ. Pilot study investigating the effects of Ayurvedic Abhyanga massage on subjective stress experience. J Altern Complement Med. 2011;17(5):435-40.
19. Basmajian JV, Hyberg R. Rational Manual Therapies. Baltimore: Williams and Wilkins; 1993.
20. Bateman JR, Daunt KM, Newman SP, et al. Regional lung clearance of excessive bronchial secretions during chest physiotherapy in patients with stable chronic airways obstruction. Lancet. 1979;313(8111):294-7.
21. Beard G. A history of massage technique. Phys Ther. 1952;32:613-24.
22. Behringer M, Jedlicka D, Mester J. Effects of lymphatic drainage and cryotherapy on indirect markers of muscle damage. J Sports Med Phys Fitness. 2018;58(6):903-9.
23. Bell AJ. Massage and the physiotherapist. Physiotherapy. 1964;50:406-8.
24. Birk TJ, McGrady A, MacArthur RD, et al. The effects of massage therapy alone and in combination with other complementary therapies on immune system measures and quality of life in human immunodeficiency virus. J Altern Complement Med. 2000;6(5):405-14.
25. Birukov AA. Training massage during contemporary sports loads. Soviet Sports Rev. 1987;22:42-4.
26. Bishop PA, Jones E, Woods AK. Recovery from training: a brief review: brief review. J Strength Cond Res. 2008;22(3):1015-24.
27. Blackman PG, Simmons LR, Crossley KM. Treatment of chronic exertional anterior compartment syndrome with massage: a pilot study. Clin J Sport Med. 1998;8(1):14-7.
28. Blake B, Anthony J, Wyatt F. The effects of massage treatment on exercise fatigue. Clin Sports Med. 1989;1:189-96.
29. Bodian M. Use of massage following lid surgery. Eye Ear Nose Throat Mon. 1969;48(9):542-7.
30. Boone T, Cooper R. The effect of massage on oxygen consumption at rest. Am J Clin Med. 1995;23(1):37-41.
31. Braun M, Schwickert M, Nielsen A, et al. Effectiveness of traditional Chinese "gua sha" therapy in patients with chronic neck pain: a randomized controlled trial. Pain Med. 2011;12(3):362-9.
32. Brooks GA, Donovan CM, White TP. Estimation of anaerobic energy production and efficiency in rats during exercise. J Appl Physiol Respir Environ Exerc Physiol. 1984;56(2):520-5.
33. Brooks GA, Gaesser GA. End points of lactate and glucose metabolism after exhausting exercise. J Appl Physiol Respir Environ Exerc Physiol. 1980;49(6):1057-69.
34. Brooks GA. Intra- and extra-cellular lactate shuttles. Med Sci Sports Exer. 2000;32(4):790-9.
35. Brunker P, Khan K. Clinical Sports Medicine. Sydney: McGraw Hill; 1993.
36. Cabo F, Baskwill A, Aguaristi I, et al. Shiatsu and Acupressure: Two Different and Distinct Techniques. Int J Ther Massage Bodywork. 2018;11(2):4-10.
37. Cafarelli E, Sim J, Carolan B, et al. Vibratory massage and short-term recovery from muscular fatigue. Int J Sports Med. 1990;11(6):474-8.
38. Callaghan M. Commentary. Br J Sports Med. 1998;32:214.
39. Callaghan MJ. The role of massage in the management of the athlete: a review. Br J Sports Med. 1993;27(1):28-33.
40. Cambron JA, Dexheimer J, Coe P. Changes in blood pressure after various forms of therapeutic massage: a preliminary study. J Altern Complement Med. 2006;12(1):65-70.
41. Campbell AH, O'Connell JM, Wilson F. The effect of chest physiotherapy upon the FEV1 in chronic bronchitis. Med J Aust. 1975;1(2):33-5.
42. Casley-Smith JR, Boris M, Weindorf S, et al. Treatment for lymphedema of the arm—the Casley-Smith method: a noninvasive method produces continued reduction. Cancer. 1998;83(12 Suppl American):2843-60.

43. Cassileth BR, Vickers AJ. Massage therapy for symptom control: outcome study at a major cancer center. J Pain Symptom Manage. 2004;28(3):244-9.
44. Chaitow L, Deleny J. Modern Neuromuscular Techniques. Elsevier: Churchill Livingstone; 1996.
45. Chamberlain GJ. Cyriax's Friction Massage: A Review. J Orthop Sports Phys Ther. 1982;4(1):16-22.
46. Chatterjee CC. Human Physiology. Calcutta: Medical Allied Agency; 1985. p. 1.
47. Chaudhuri SK. Concise Medical Physiology. Calcutta: New Central Book Agency (P) Ltd.; 1993.
48. Chaurasia BD. Human Anatomy. New Delhi: CBS Publishers and Distributors (P) Ltd.; 1985. pp. 1-4.
49. Cheatham SW, Kolber MJ, Cain M, et al. The effects of self-myofascial release using a foam roll or roller massager on joint range of motion, muscle recovery, and performance: a systematic review. Int J Sports Phys Ther. 2015;10(6):827-38.
50. Cheatham SW, Lee M, Cain M, et al. The efficacy of instrument assisted soft tissue mobilization: a systematic review. J Can Chiropr Assoc. 2016;60(3):200-11.
51. Cheatham SW, Stull KR. Roller massage: a commentary on clinical standards and survey of physical therapy Professionals—part 1. Int J Sports Phys Ther. 2018;13(4):763-72.
52. Chen T, Liu N, Liu J, et al. Gua Sha, a press-stroke treatment of the skin, boosts the immune response to intradermal vaccination. PeerJ. 2016;4:e2451.
53. Cheung K, Hume P, Maxwell L. Delayed onset muscle soreness: treatment strategies and performance factors. Sports Med. 2003;33(2):145-64.
54. Christensen EH. Muscular work and fatigue. In: Rodahl EH (Eds). Muscle as a Tissue. New York: McGraw Hill Book Co.; 1960.
55. Ciesla N, Klemic N, Imle PC. Chest physical therapy to the patient with multiple trauma. Two case studies. Phys Ther. 1981;61(2):202-5.
56. Clarkson PM, Hubal MJ. Exercise-induced muscle damage in humans. Am J Phys Med Rehabil. 2002;81(11):S52-69.
57. Corbin L. Safety and efficacy of massage therapy for patients with cancer. Cancer Control. 2005;12(3):158-64.
58. Crane JD, Ogborn DI, Cupido C, et al. Massage therapy attenuates inflammatory signaling after exercise-induced muscle damage. Sci Transl Med. 2012;4(119):119ra13.
59. Crompton J, Fox J. Regeneration vs. burnout: prevention is better than cure. Sports Coach. 1987;10(4):7-10.
60. Crosman LJ, Chateauvert SR, Weisberg J. The effects of massage to the hamstring muscle group on range of motion. J Orthop Sports Phys Ther. 1984;6(3):168-72.
61. Cunningham JE, Kelechi T, Sterba K, et al. Case report of a patient with chemotherapy-induced peripheral neuropathy treated with manual therapy (massage). Support Care Cancer. 2011;19(9):1473-6.
62. Cuthbertson DP. The Effect of Massage on Metabolism: A Survey. Glasgow Med J. 1933;120(6):200-13.
63. Cutshall SM, Mahapatra S, Hynes RS, et al. Hand Massage for Cancer Patients Undergoing Chemotherapy as Outpatients: A Pilot Study. Explore (NY). 2017;13(6):393-9.
64. Cyriax J. Textbook of Orthopedic Medicine: Treatment by Manipulation Massage and Injection. London: Bailliere Tindall Ltd.; 1998. p. 2.
65. Cè E, Limonta E, Maggioni MA, et al. Stretching and deep and superficial massage do not influence blood lactate levels after heavy-intensity cycle exercise. J Sports Sci. 2013;31(8):856-66.
66. Danneskiold-Samsøe B, Christiansen E, Lund B, et al. Regional muscle tension and pain ("fibrositis"). Effect of massage on myoglobin in plasma. Scand J Rehabil Med. 1983;15(1):17-20.
67. Darmstadt GL, Saha SK, Ahmed AS, et al. Effect of topical treatment with skin barrier-enhancing emollients on nosocomial infections in preterm infants in Bangladesh: a randomised controlled trial. Lancet. 2005;365(9464):1039-45.

68. Davidson CJ, Ganion LR, Gehlsen GM, et al. Rat tendon morphologic and functional changes resulting from soft tissue mobilization. Med Sci Sports Exerc. 1997;29(3):313-19.
69. Deng G, Cassileth BR. Integrative oncology: complementary therapies for pain, anxiety, and mood disturbance. CA Cancer J Clin. 2005;55(2):109-16.
70. Depocas F, Minaire Y, Chattonnet J. Rates of formation and oxidation of lactic acid in dogs at rest and during moderate exercise. Can J Physiol Pharmacol. 1969;47(7):603-10.
71. Doering TJ, Fieguth HG, Steuernagel B, et al. External stimuli in the form of vibratory massage after heart of lung transplantation. Am J Phys Med Rehabil. 1999;78(2):108-10.
72. Donovan CM, Brooks GA. Endurance training affects lactate clearance, not lactate production. Am J Physiol. 1983;244(1):E83-92.
73. Donovan CM, Pagliassotti MJ. Quantitative assessment of pathways for lactate disposal in skeletal muscle fiber types. Med Sci Sports Exerc. 2000;32(4):772-7.
74. Donoyama N, Wakuda T, Tanitsu T, et al. Washing hands before and after performing massages? Changes in bacterial survival count on skin of a massage therapist and a client during massage therapy. J Altern Complement Med. 2004;10(4):684-6.
75. Downey PA, Barbano T, Kapur-Wadhwa R, et al. Craniosacral Therapy: The Effects of Cranial Manipulation on Intracranial Pressure and Cranial Bone Movement. J Orthop Sports Phys Ther. 2006;36(11):845-53.
76. Downey PA. (2005). Craniosacral therapy: is there biology behind the theory? [online] Available from https://www.researchgate.net/publication/238621876_CRANIOSACRAL_THERAPY_IS_THERE_BIOLOGY_BEHIND_THE_THEORY. [Last accessed September, 2019].
77. Drews T, Kreider RB, Drinkard B, et al. Effects of post event massage therapy on muscle recovery and performance in repeated ultraendurance cycling. Int J Sports Med. 1990;11:407.
78. Dubrovsky VI. Changes in muscle and venous blood flow after massage. Tenoyaipraktika Fizichesti Kultury. 1982;4(2):56-7.
79. Dupuy O, Douzi W, Theurot D, et al. An Evidence-based Approach for Choosing Post-exercise Recovery Techniques to Reduce Markers of Muscle Damage, Soreness, Fatigue, and Inflammation: A Systematic Review With Meta-Analysis. Front Physiol. 2018;9:403.
80. Ebner M. Connective tissue massage. In: Huntington NY, Robert E (Eds). Theory and Therapeutic Application. USA: Krieger Publishing Co., Inc.; 1975. p. 2.
81. Ek AC, Gustavsson G, Lewis DH. The local skin blood flow in areas at risk for pressure sores treated with massage. Scand J Rehabil Med. 1985;17(2):81-6.
82. Ellison M, Goerhrs C, Hall L, et al. Effect of retrograde massage on muscle soreness and performance. Phys Ther. 1992;72(1):100.
83. Ernst E. Craniosacral therapy: a systematic review of the clinical evidence. Focus Altern Complement Ther. 2012;17(4):197-201.
84. Ernst E. Does post-exercise massage treatment reduce delayed onset muscle soreness? A systematic review. Br J Sports Med. 1998;32(3):212-4.
85. Ernst E. Massage therapy for low back pain: a systematic review. J Pain Symptom Manage. 1999;17(1):65-9.
86. Ernst E. The safety of massage therapy. Rheumatology (Oxford). 2003;42(9):1101-6.
87. Farr T, Nottle C, Nosaka K, et al. The effects of therapeutic massage on delayed onset muscle soreness and muscle function following downhill walking. J Sci Med Sport. 2002;5(4):297-306.
88. Field T, Diego MA, Hernandez-Reif M, et al. Massage therapy effects on depressed pregnant women. J Psychosom Obstet Gynaecol. 2004;25(2):115-22.
89. Field T, Henteleff T, Hernandez-Reif M, et al. Children with asthma have improved pulmonary functions after massage therapy. J Pediatr. 1998;132(5):854-8.

90. Field T, Hernandez-Reif M, Hart S, et al. Pregnant women benefit from massage therapy. J Psychosom Obset Gynaecol. 1999;20(1):31-8.
91. Field T, Peck M, Krugman S, et al. Burn injuries benefit from massage therapy. J Burn Care Rehabil. 1998;19(3):241-4.
92. Field T. Supplemental stimulation of preterm neonates. Early Human Dev. 1980;4(3):301-14.
93. Field TM, Quintino O, Hernandez-Reif M, et al. Adolescents with attention deficit hyperactivity disorder benefit from massage therapy. Adolescence. 1998;33(129):103-8.
94. Finer NN, Moriartey RR, Boyd J, et al. Postextubation atelectasis: a retrospective review and a prospective controlled study. J Pediatr. 1979;94(1):110-3.
95. Flore P, Obert P, Courteix D, et al. Influence of a biokinergia session on cardiorespiratory and metabolic adaptations of trained subjects. J Manipulative Physiol Ther. 1998;21(9):621-8.
96. Flynn TW, Cleland JA, Schaible P. Craniosacral Therapy and Professional Responsibility. J Orthop Sports Phys Ther. 2006;36(11):834-6.
97. Franklin NC, Ali MM, Robinson AT, et al. Massage therapy restores peripheral vascular function after exertion. Arch Phys Med Rehabil. 2014;95(6):1127-34.
98. Furlan AD, Giraldo M, Baskwill A, et al. Massage for low-back pain. Cochrane Database Syst Rev. 2015;(9):CD001929.
99. Gaesser GA, Brooks GA. Metabolic bases of excess post-exercise oxygen consumption: a review. Med Sci Sports Exerc. 1984;16(1):29-43.
100. Galloway SD, Watt JM. Massage provision by physiotherapists at major athletics events between 1987 and 1998. Br J Sports Med. 2004;38(2):235-6.
101. Gardiner D. Principles of Exercise Therapy, 1st edition. New Delhi: CBS Publishers and Distributors (P) Ltd; 1985.
102. Garradd J, Bullock M. The effect of respiratory therapy on intracranial pressure in ventilated neurosurgical patients. Aust J Physiother. 1986;32(2):107-11.
103. Gehlsen GM, Ganion LR, Helfst R. Fibroblast responses to variation in soft tissue mobilization pressure. Med Sci Sports Exerc. 1999;31(4):531-5.
104. Gensic ME, Smith BR, LaBarbera DM. The effects of effleurage hand massage on anxiety and pain in patients undergoing chemotherapy. JAAPA. 2017;30(2):36-8.
105. Givi M. Durability of effect of massage therapy on blood pressure. Int J Prev Med. 2013;4(5):511-6.
106. Gladden LB, Crawford RE, Webster MJ. Effect of blood flow on net lactate uptake during steady-level contractions in canine skeletal muscle. J Appl Physiol. 1992;72(5):1826-30
107. Gladden LB. Lactate metabolism: a new paradigm for the third millennium. J Physiol. 2004;558 (Pt 1):5-30.
108. Gladden LB. Muscle as a consumer of lactate. Med Sci Sport Exerc. 2000;32(4):764-71.
109. Glaser R, Rice J, Speicher CE, et al. Stress depresses interferon production by leukocytes concomitant with a decrease in natural killer cell activity. Behav Neurosci. 1986;100(5):675-8.
110. Goldberg J, Seaborne DE, Sullivan SJ, et al. The effect of therapeutic massage on H-reflex amplitude in persons with a spinal cord injury. Phys Ther. 1994;74(8):728-37.
111. Goldberg J, Sullivan SJ, Seaborne DE. The effect of two intensities of massage on H-reflex amplitude. Phys Ther. 1992;72:449-57.
112. Gold R. Thai Massage: A Traditional Medical Technique, 2nd edition. St. Louis: Mosby; 2007.
113. Goodfellow LM. The effects of therapeutic back massage on psychophysiologic variables and immune function in spouses of patients with cancer. Nurs Res. 2003;52(5):318-28.
114. Gore-Felton C, Vosvick M, Power R, et al. Alternative therapies: a common practice among men and women living with HIV. J Assoc Nurses AIDS Care. 2003;14(3):17-27.
115. Grant KE, Riggs A. Myofascial release. In: Stillerman E (Ed). Modalities for Massage and Bodywork, 1st edition. St. Louis: Mosby; 2008.

116. Green C, Martin CW, Bassett K, et al. A systematic review and critical appraisal of the scientific evidence on craniosacral therapy. Vancouver: University of British Columbia; 1999.
117. Green C, Martin CW, Bassett K, et al. A systematic review of craniosacral therapy: biological plausibility, assessment reliability and clinical effectiveness. Complement Ther Med. 1999;7(4):201-7.
118. Guo J, Li L, Gong Y, et al. Massage Alleviates Delayed Onset Muscle Soreness after Strenuous Exercise: A Systematic Review and Meta-Analysis. Front Physiol. 2017;8:747.
119. Gupta S, Goswami A, Sadhukaran AK, et al. Comparative study of lactate removal in short-term massage of extremities, active recovery and passive recovery period, after supramaximal exercise session. Int J Sports Med. 1992;17(2):106-10.
120. Haas C, Butterfield TA, Abshire S, et al. Massage timing affects postexercise muscle recovery and inflammation in a rabbit model. Med Sci Sports Exerc. 2013;45(6):1105-12.
121. Hansen MH. Manual Therapy Techniques in Lymphedema Treatment: A Case Report 2015. The Faculty of the College of Health Professions and Social Work Florida Gulf Coast University [online]. Available from https://fgcu.digital.flvc.org/islandora/object/fgcu%3A27384/datastream/OBJ/view/Manual_Therapy_Techniques_in_Lymphedema_Treatment.pdf. [Last accessed September, 2019].
122. Hansen TI, Kristensen JH. Effect of massage, shortwave diathermy and ultrasound upon 133Xe disappearance rate from muscle and subcutaneous tissue in the human calf. Scand J Rehabil Med. 1973;5(4):179-82.
123. Haralabidis T. Zen Shiatsu—the Japanese Way of Acupuncture without Needles. Int J Complement Alt Med. 2017;6(3):00187.
124. Harichaux P, Viel E. Dopplerography of the venous return of the foot in the healthy subject preliminary to a study of ambulation. Phlebologie. 1987;40(2):221-39.
125. Hartman SE. Cranial osteopathy: its fate seems clear. Chiropr Osteopat. 2006;14:10.
126. Hemmings B, Smith M, Graydon J, et al. Effects of massage on physiological restoration, perceived recovery, and repeated sports performance. Br J Sports Med. 2000;34(2):109-14.
127. Hernandez-Reif M, Field T, Hart S. Smoking cravings are reduced by self-massage. Prev Med. 1999;28(1):28-32.
128. Hernandez-Reif M, Field T, Ironson G, et al. Natural killer cells and lymphocytes increase in women with breast cancer following massage therapy. Int J Neurosci. 2005;115(4):495-510.
129. Hernandez-Reif M, Field T, Krasnegor J, et al. Children with cystic fibrosis benefit from massage therapy. J Pediatr Psychol. 1999;24(2):175-81.
130. Hernandez-Reif M, Ironson G, Field T, et al. Breast cancer patients have improved immune and neuroendocrine functions following massage therapy. J Psychosom Res. 2004;57(1):45-52.
131. Hilbert JE, Sforzo GA, Swensen T. The effects of massage on delayed onset muscle soreness. Br J Sports Med. 2003;37(1):72-5.
132. Hill AV, Lupton H. Muscular exercise, lactic acid and the supply and utilization of oxygen. Q J Med. 1923;16(62):135-71.
133. Hillier SL, Louw Q, Morris L, et al. Massage therapy for people with HIV/AIDS. Cochrane Database Syst Rev. 2010;(1):CD007502.
134. Hinds T, McEwan I, Perkes J, et al. Effects of massage on limb and skin blood flow after quadriceps exercise. Med Sci Sports Exerc. 2004;36(8):1308-13.
135. Holland B, Pokorny ME. Slow stroke back massage: its effect on patients in a rehabilitation setting. Rehabil Nurs. 2001;26(5):182-6.
136. Hollis M. Massage for Therapists. England: Blackwell Scientific Publications; 1987.
137. Hou Y, Liu M, Yu M, et al. Promoting effect of massage on quadriceps femoris repair of rabbit in vivo. Zhongguo Xiu Fu Chong Jian Wai Ke Za Zhi. 2012;26(3):346-51.
138. Hovind H, Nielsen SL. Effect of massage on blood flow in skeletal muscle. Scand J Rehabil Med. 1974;6(2):74-7.

139. Hubbard JL. The effects of exercise on lactate metabolism. J Physiol. 1973;231(1):1-18.
140. Ilić D, Djurović A, Brdareski Z, et al. The position of chinese massage (Tuina) in clinical medicine. Vojnosanit Pregl. 2012;69(11):999-1004.
141. Imle PC. Percussion and vibration. In: Mackenzie CF, Imle PC, Ciesla M (Eds). Chest Physiotherapy in the Intensive Care Unit. Baltimore: Williams and Wilkins; 1989. pp. 134-52.
142. Imtiyaz S, Veqar Z, Shareef MY. To Compare the Effect of Vibration Therapy and Massage in Prevention of Delayed Onset Muscle Soreness (DOMS). J Clin Diagn Res. 2014;8(1):133-6.
143. Ironson G, Field T, Scafidi F, et al. Massage therapy is associated with enhancement of the immune system's cytotoxic capacity. Int J Neurosci. 1996;84(1-4):205-17.
144. Issekutz B. Effects of beta-adrenergic blockade on lactate turnover in exercising dogs. J Appl Physiol Respir Environ Exerc Physiol. 1984;57(6):1754-9.
145. Jay K, Sundstrup E, Søndergaard SD, et al. Specific and cross over effects of massage for muscle soreness: randomized controlled trial. Int J Sports Phys Ther. 2014;9(1):82-91.
146. Johansson K, Albertsson M, Ingvar C, et al. Effects of compression bandaging with or without manual lymph drainage treatment in patients with postoperative arm lymphedema. Lymphology. 1999;32(3):103-10.
147. Johansson K, Lie E, Ekdahl C, et al. A randomized study comparing manual lymph drainage with sequential pneumatic compression for treatment of postoperative arm lymphedema. Lymphology. 1998;31(2):56-64.
148. Jonhagen S, Ackermann P, Eriksson T, et al. Sports massage after eccentric exercise. Am J Sports Med. 2004;32(6):1499-503.
149. Joseph RC, Cherian A, Joseph CT. Role of abhyanga (oil massage) to lead a healthy life. Ayurpharm Int J Ayur Alli Sci. 2012;1(7):163-7.
150. Juntakarn C, Prasartritha T, Petrakard P. The effectivness of Thai massage and joint mobilisation. Int J Ther Massage Bodywork. 2017; 10(2): 3-8.
151. Jäkel A, von Hauenschild P. A systematic review to evaluate the clinical benefits of craniosacral therapy. Complement Ther Med. 2012;20(6):456-65.
152. Kaada B, Torsteinbø O. Increase of plasma beta-endorphins in connective tissue massage. Gen Pharmacol. 1989;20(4):487-9.
153. Kalb SW. The fallacy of massage in the treatment of obesity. J Med Soc N J. 1944;41:406-7.
154. Kamenetz HL. History of massage. In: Basmajian JV (Ed). Manipulation Traction and Massage. Baltimore: Williams and Wilkins; 1985. p. 3.
155. Kargarfard M, Lam ET, Shariat A, et al. Efficacy of massage on muscle soreness, perceived recovery, physiological restoration and physical performance in male bodybuilders. J. Sports Sci. 2016;34(10):959-65.
156. Kasseroller RG. The Vodder School: the Vodder method. Cancer. 1998;83(12 Suppl American):2840-2.
157. Kellgren A. The Technique of Ling's System of Manual Treatment. London: Young J Pentland; 1890.
158. Kellogg JH. The art of massage. Battle Creek: Modern Medical Publishers; 1919. p. 190.
159. Kerr HD. Ureteral stent displacement associated with deep massage. WMJ. 1997;96(12):57-8.
160. Kiecolt-Glaser JK, Glaser R, Williger D, et al. Psychosocial enhancement of immunocompetence in a geriatric population. Health Psychol. 1985;4(1):25-41.
161. Kim J, Sung DJ, Lee J. Therapeutic effectiveness of instrument-assisted soft tissue mobilization for soft tissue injury: mechanisms and practical application. J Exerc Rehabil. 2017;13(1):12-22.
162. King RK. Performance Massage. Champaign: Human Kinetics; 1993.
163. Kisner CD, Taslibz N. Connective tissue massage: the influence of the introductory treatment on autonomic function. Phys Ther. 1968;48(2):107-19.
164. Knapp ME. Massage. In: Kohke FJ, Lehman JF (Eds). Krusen's Handbook of Physical Medicine and Rehabilitation. Philadelphia: Saunders; 1990. p. 4.

165. Korosec BJ. Manual lymphatic drainage therapy. Home Health Care Mang Pract. 2004;17(2):499–511.
166. Kothainayagi B, Gupta S. Conceptual and applied study on Abhyanga (Ayurvedic massage). Paripex Indian J Res. 2017;6(7):56-8.
167. Krebs H. The Croonian Lecture,1963. Gluconeogenesis. Proc R Soc Lond B Biol Sci. 1964;159:545-64.
168. Kresage C. Massage and sports. In Appanzellar O (Ed). Sports Medicine. Baltimore: Urban and Schwarzenberg; 1988. pp. 419-31.
169. Kumar J, Upadhyay A, Dwivedi AK, et al. Effect of oil massage on growth in preterm neonates less than 1800 g: a randomized control trial. Indian J Pediatr. 2013;80(6):465-9.
170. Kuprian W. Massage. In: Kuprian W (Ed). Physical Therapy for Sports. Philadelphia: Saunders; 1981. pp. 7-51.
171. Lavekar GS. A Practical Handbook of Panchakarma Procedures, 2nd edition. New Delhi: Central Council for Research in Ayurveda and Siddha, Department of Ayush, Ministry of Health and Family Welfare, Government of India; 2010.
172. Laws AK, McIntyre RW. Chest physiotherapy: a physiological assessment during intermittent positive pressure ventilation in respiratory failure. Can Anaesth Soc J. 1969;16(6):487-93.
173. Lee MS, Choi TY, Kim JI, et al. Using Guasha to treat musculoskeletal pain: a systematic review of controlled clinical trials. Chin Med. 2010;5:5.
174. Lehn C, Prentice WE. Massage. In: Prentice WE (Ed). Therapeutic Modalities in Sports Medicine. St. Louis: Mosby Year Book Inc., 1994. pp. 335-63.
175. Liao IC, Chen SL, Wang MY, et al. Effects of Massage on Blood Pressure in Patients with Hypertension and Prehypertension: A Meta-analysis of Randomized Controlled Trials. J Cardiovasc Nurs. 2016;31(1):73-83.
176. Linde B. Dissociation of insulin absorption and blood flow during massage of a subcutaneous site. Diabetes Care. 1986;9(6):570-4.
177. Liston BC. Massage. In: Zulanga M, Briggs C (Eds). Sports Physiotherapy: Applied Sciences and Practice. New York: Churchill Livingstone; 1995. pp. 223-32.
178. Loghmani MT, Warden SJ. Instrument-assisted cross-fiber massage accelerates knee ligament healing. J Orthop Sports Phys Ther. 2009;39(7):506-14.
179. Lucia SP, Rickard JF. Effects of massage on blood platelet production. Proc Soc Exper Biol Med. 1933;31(2):87.
180. Madhukar LS, Nivrutti BA, Bhatngar V, et al. Physio-Anatomical Explanation of Abhyanga: An Ayurvedic Massage Technique for Healthy Life. J Tradit Med Clin Natur. 2018;7(1):252.
181. Malila P, Seeda K, Machom S, et al. Effects of Thai Massage on Spasticity in Young People with Cerebral Palsy. J Med Assoc Thai. 2015;98(Suppl)5:S92-6.
182. Malone TR. Soft tissue mobilization. In: Malone TR (Ed). Sports Injury Management: A Quarterly Series. Baltimore: Williams and Wilkins; 1990.
183. Manheim CJ. The Myofascial Release Manual, 3rd edition. Thorofare: Slack; 2001.
184. Masson IF, de Oliveira BD, Machado AF, et al. Manual lymphatic drainage and therapeutic ultrasound in liposuction and lipoabdominoplasty post-operative period. Indian J Plast Surg. 2014;47(1):70-6.
185. Mayer VA, Mccue FC. Rehabilitation and protection of the hand and wrist. In: Nicholas JA, Hershman EB (Eds). The Upper Extremity in Sports Medicine; 1995. pp. 611-2.
186. McKechnie AA, Wilson F, Watson N, et al. Anxiety states: a preliminary report on the value of connective tissue massage. J Psychosom Res. 1983;27(2):125-9.
187. McKenney K, Elder AS, Elder C, et al. Myofascial release as a treatment for orthopaedic conditions: a systematic review. J Athl Train. 2013;48(4):522–7.

188. Mckenzie CF, Shin B. Cardiopulmonary function before and after chest physiotherapy in mechanically ventilated patients with post-traumatic respiratory failure. Crit Care Med. 1985;13(6):483-6.
189. Melzack R, Wall PD. Pain mechanisms: a new theory. Science. 1965;150(3699):971-9.
190. Mennell JB. Physical Treatment. Philadelphia: Blakiston Co; 1945. p. 5.
191. Mills E, Wu P, Ernst E. Complementary therapies for the treatment of HIV: in search of the evidence. Int J STD AIDS. 2005;16(6):395-403.
192. Miyahara Y, Jitkrisadakul O, Sringean J, et al.. Can therapeutic Thai massage improve upper limb muscle strength in Parkinson's disease? An objective randomized–controlled trial. J Tradit Complement Med.2018 :8(2):261-66.
193. Moeini M, Givi M, Ghasempour Z, et al. The effect of massage therapy on blood pressure of women with pre-hypertension. Iran J Nurs Midwifery Res. 2011;16(1):61-70.
194. Mohebbi Z, Moghadasi M, Homayouni K, et al. The effect of back massage on blood pressure in the patients with primary hypertension in 2012-2013: a randomized clinical trial. Int J Community Based Nurs Midwifery. 2014;2(4):251-8.
195. Monedero J, Donne B. Effect of recovery interventions on lactate removal and subsequent performance. Int J Sports Med. 2000;21(8):593-7.
196. Moraska A. Sports massage: a comprehensive review. J Sports Med Phys Fitness. 2005;45(3):370-80.
197. Morelli M, Seaborne DE, Sullivan SJ. Changes in H-reflex amplitude during massage of triceps surae in healthy subjects. J Orthop Sports Phys Ther. 1990;12(2):55-9.
198. Morelli M, Seaborne DE, Sullivan SJ. H-reflex modulation during manual muscle massage of human triceps surae. Arch Phys Med Rehabil. 1991;72(11):915-9.
199. Morelli M, Sullivan SJ, Chapman CE. Inhibitory influence of soleus massage onto the medial gastrocnemius H-reflex. Electromyogr Clin Neurophysiol. 1998;38(2):87-93.
200. Morhenn V, Beavin LE, Zak PJ. Massage increases oxytocin and reduces adrenocorticotropin hormone in humans. Altern Ther Health Med. 2012;18(6):11-8.
201. Mori H, Ohsawa H, Tanaka TH, et al. Effect of massage on blood flow and muscle fatigue following isometric lumbar exercise. Med Sci Monit. 2004;10(5):CR173-8.
202. Moyer CA, Rounds J, Hannum JW. A meta-analysis of massage therapy research. Psychol Bull. 2004;130(1):3-18.
203. Myers TW. Anatomy Trains: Myofascial Meridians for Manual and Movement Therapists. New York: Churchill Livingstone; 2009.
204. Müller-Oerlinghausen B, Berg C, Scherer P, et al. Effects of slow-stroke massage as complementary treatment of depressed hospitalized patients. Dtsch Med Wochenschr. 2004;129(24):1363-8.
205. Müller EA, Schulte AM, Esch J. The effect of massage on the efficiency of muscles. Int Z Angew Physiol. 1966;22(3):240-57.
206. Negahban H, Rezaie S, Goharpey S. Massage therapy and exercise therapy in patients with multiple sclerosis: a randomized controlled pilot study. Clin Rehabil. 2013;27(12):1126-36.
207. Nelson NL. Massage therapy: understanding the mechanisms of action on blood pressure. A scoping review. J Am Soc Hypertens. 2015;9(10):785-93.
208. Nielsen A, Kligler B, Koll BS. Safety protocols for gua sha (press-stroking) and baguan (cupping). Complement Ther Med. 2012;20(5):340-4.
209. Nielsen A. Gua sha research and the language of integrative medicine. J Bodyw Mov Ther. 2009;13(1):63-72.
210. Nordqvist H. Massages: a training must. Track Field News. 1979;32(5):50-1.
211. Nordschow M, Bierman W. Influence of manual massage on muscle relaxation: effect on trunk flexion. Phys Ther. 1962;42(10):653-57.

212. Odhav A, Patel D, Stanford CW, et al. Report of a case of Gua Sha and an awareness of folk remedies. Int J Dermatol. 2013;52(7):892-3.
213. Oki S, Ouchi K, Watanabe M, et al. Physical and Psychological Effects of the Shiatsu Stimulation in the Sitting Position. Health. 2017;9(8):1264-72.
214. Olney CM. The effect of therapeutic back massage in hypertensive persons: a preliminary study. Biol Res Nurs. 2005;7(2):98-105.
215. Ostrom KW. Massage and Original Swedish Movement. London: HK Lewis; 1909.
216. Pagliassotti MJ, Donovan CM. Glycogenesis from lactate in rabbit skeletal muscle fiber types. Am J Physiol. 1990;258(4 Pt 2):R903-11.
217. Paikov VB. Means of restoration in the training of speed skaters. Soviet Sports Rev. 1985;20:7-12.
218. Pal M. The tridosha theory. Anc Sci Life. 1991;10(3):144-55.
219. Patel KC, Gross A, Graham N, et al. Massage for mechanical neck disorders. Cochrane Database Syst Rev. 2012;(9):CD004871.
220. Patino O, Novick C, Merlo A, et al. Massage in hypertrophic scars. J Burn Care Rehabil. 1999;20(3):268-71.
221. Peshkov VF. The effect of 10-minute restorative point massage on the functional state of young gymnasts. Teonya I Praktika Fizicheskoi Kultury. 1981;12:35.
222. Priyanka S, Prashant S. Abhyanga—Way To Health. World J Pharma Pharmaceut Sci. 2014;3(9):970-7.
223. Rapaport MH, Schettler P, Breese C. A preliminary study of the effects of a single session of Swedish massage on hypothalamic-pituitary-adrenal and immune function in normal individuals. J Altern Complement Med. 2010;16(10):1079-88.
224. Resnick PB. Comparing the Effects of Rest and Massage on Return to Homeostasis Following Submaximal Aerobic Exercise: A Case Study. Int J Ther Massage Bodywork. 2016;9(1):4-10.
225. Reychler G, Caty G, Arcq A, et al. Effects of massage therapy on anxiety, depression, hyperventilation and quality of life in HIV-infected patients: A randomized controlled trial. Complement Ther Med. 2017;32:109-14.
226. Richards KC. Effect of a back massage and relaxation on sleep in critically ill patients. Am J Crit Care. 1998;7(4):288-99.
227. Robbins SL, Kumar V. Basic Pathology. Philadelphia: Saunders Company; 1987. p. 277.
228. Robinson N, Lorenc A, Xing Liao X. The evidence for Shiatsu: a systematic review of Shiatsu and acupressure. BMC Complementary and Alternative Medicine. 2011.
229. Rodenburg JB, Steenbeek D, Schiereck P, et al. Warm-up, stretching and massage diminish harmful effect of eccentric exercise. Int J Sports Med. 1994;15(7):414-9.
230. Ryan C, Keiwkarnka B, Khan MI. Traditional Thai massage: unveiling the misconceptions and revealing the health benefits. J Public Health Development. 2003;1(2):69–75.
231. Salguero P, Roylance D. Encyclopedia of Thai Massage. 2nd edition. Findhorn Press. United Kingdom; 2011.
232. Sankaranarayanan K, Mondkar JA, Chauhan MM, et al. Oil massage in neonates: an open randomized controlled study of coconut versus mineral oil. Indian Pediatr. 2005;42(9):877-84.
233. Sankaran R, Kamath R, Nambiar V, et al. A prospective study on the effects of Ayurvedic massage in post-stroke patients. J Ayurveda Integr Med. 2019;10(2):126-30.
234. Schneider EC, Havens LC. Changes in the blood flow after muscular activity and during training. Am J Physiol. 1915;36:259.
235. Schneider V. Infant Massage. New York: Bantam; 1982.
236. Schwind P. Fascial and Membrane Technique: A Manual for Comprehensive Treatment of the Connective Tissue System. New York: Churchill Livingstone; 2006.
237. Severini V, Venerando A. Effect on the peripheral circulation of substances producing hyperemia in combination with massage. Europa Medicophys. 1967;3:184-98.

238. Severini V, Venerando A. The physiological effects of massage on the cardiovascular system. Europa Medicophys. 1967;3:165-83.
239. Shin ES, Seo KH, Lee SH, et al. Massage with or without aromatherapy for symptom relief in people with cancer. Cochrane Database Syst Rev. 2016;(6):CD009873.
240. Shoemaker JK, Tiidus PM, Mader R. Failure of manual massage to alter limb blood flow measures by Doppler ultrasound. Med Sci Sports Exerc. 1997;29(5):610-4.
241. Shor-Posner G, Hernandez-Reif M, Miguez MJ, et al. Impact of a massage therapy clinical trial on immune status in young Dominican children infected with HIV-1. J Altern Complement Med. 2006;12(6):511-6.
242. Siegel K, Brown-Bradley CJ, Lekas HM. Strategies for coping with fatigue among HIV-positive individuals fifty years and older. AIDS Patient Care STDS. 2004;18(5):275-88.
243. Singleton M. (2015). Preface to the Serbian edition of Yoga Body: The Origins of Modern Posture Practice. [online] Available from https://www.academia.edu/17411279/Preface_to_the_2016_Serbian_edition_of_Yoga_Body_The_Origins_of_Modern_Posture_Practice_. [Last accessed October, 2019].
244. Sinha AG. A study on the relative efficacy of physiotherapeutic modalities on recovery pattern following high intensity intermittent exercise with special reference to lactate removal. [unpublished PhD thesis, Guru Nanak Dev University, Amritsar, India, 2005]
245. Sinha K, Lohith BA, Ashvini MK. Abhyanga: Different contemporary massage technique and its importance in Ayurveda. J Ayurveda Integr Med Sci. 2017;2(3):245-51.
246. Smith LL, Keating MN, Holbert D, et al. The effects of athletic massage on delayed onset muscle soreness, creatine kinase, and neutrophil count: a preliminary report. J Orthop Sports Phys Ther. 1994;19(2):93-9.
247. Smith MC, Kemp J, Hemphill L, et al. Outcomes of therapeutic massage for hospitalized cancer patients. J Nurs Scholarsh. 2002;34(3):257-62.
248. Solanki K, Matnani M, Kale M, et al. Transcutaneous absorption of topically massaged oil in neonates. Indian Pediatr. 2005;42(10):998-1005.
249. Soriano CR, Martinez FE, Jorge SM. Cutaneous application of vegetable oil as a coadjutant in the nutritional management of preterm infants. J Pediatr Gastroenterol Nutr. 2000;31(4):387-90.
250. Sorichter S, Koller A, Haid CH, et al. Light concentric exercise and heavy eccentric muscle loading: effects on CK, MRI and markers of inflammation. Int J Sports Med. 2007;16(5):288-92.
251. Stanborough M. Direct Release Myofascial Technique. New York: Churchill Livingstone; 2004.
252. Stecco C, Day JA. The Fascial Manipulation Technique and Its Biomechanical Model: A Guide to the Human Fascial System. Int J Ther Massage Bodywork. 2010;3(1):38-40.
253. Stecco L, Stecco A. Fascial Manipulation for Musculoskeletal Pain: Theoretical Part, 2nd edition. Italy: Piccin Nuova Libraria; 2017.
254. Steward B, Woodman R, Hurlburt D. Fabricating a splint for deep friction massage. J Orthop Sports Phys Ther. 1995;21(3):172-5.
255. Stow R. Instrument-Assisted Soft Tissue Mobilization. Int J Athlet Ther Train. 2011;16(3):5-8.
256. Sullivan SJ, Seguin S, Seaborne D, et al. Reduction of H-reflex amplitude during the application of effleurage to the triceps surae in neurologically healthy subjects. Physiother Theory Pract. 1992;9(1):25-31.
257. Sullivan SJ, Williams LR, Seaborne DE, et al. Effects of massage on alpha motoneuron excitability. Phys Ther. 1991;71(8):555-60.
258. Supa'at I, Zakaria Z, Maskon O, et al. Effects of Swedish massage therapy on blood pressure, heart rate, and inflammatory markers in hypertensive women. Evid Based Complement Alternat Med. 2013;2013:171852.

259. Tappan FM. Healing Massage Techniques: A Study of Eastern and Western Methods. Reston: Reston Publishing Company Inc; 1978.
260. Thanakiatpinyo T, Suwannatrai S, Suwannatrai U, et al. The efficacy of traditional Thai massage in decreasing spasticity in elderly stroke patients. Clin Interv Aging. 2014;9:1311-9.
261. Thiriet P, Gozal D, Wouassi D, et al. The effect of various recovery modalities on subsequent performance, in consecutive supramaximal exercises. J Sports Med Phys Fitness. 1993;33(2):118-29.
262. Thompson A, Skinner A, Piercy J. Tidy's Physiotherapy. Oxford: Butterworth-Heinemann Ltd.; 1991. p. 12.
263. Thompson WR. Worldwide Survey of Fitness Trends for 2018. ACSMs Health Fitness J. 2017; 21(6):10-9.
264. Tiidus PM, Shoemaker JK. Effleurage massage, muscle blood flow and long-term post-exercise strength recovery. Int J Sports Med. 1995;16(7):478-83.
265. Tiidus PM. Manual massage and recovery of muscle function following exercise: a literature review. J Orthop Sports Phys Ther. 1997;25(2):107-12.
266. Tonde S, Deshpande S, Kolarkar R. Abhyanga maacharet Nityam in Preventive Perspective. Int J Ayu Pharm Chem. 2016;4(3):149-54.
267. Torres R, Ribeiro F, Alberto-Duarte J, et al. Evidence of the physiotherapeutic interventions used currently after exercise-induced muscle damage: systematic review and meta-analysis. Phys Ther Sport. 2012;13(2):101-14.
268. Toups DM. A healing touch: massage therapy and HIV/AIDS. STEP Perspect. 1999;99(3):13-4.
269. Urakawa S, Takamoto K, Nakamura T, et al. Manual therapy ameliorates delayed-onset muscle soreness and alters muscle metabolites in rats. Physiol Rep. 2015;3(2):e12279.
270. Vaivre-Douret L, Oriot D, Blossier P, et al. The effect of multimodal stimulation and cutaneous application of vegetable oils on neonatal development in preterm infants: a randomized controlled trial. Child Care Health Dev. 2009;35(1):96-105.
271. Ventegodt S, Thegler S, Andreasen T, et al. A review and integrative analysis of ancient holistic character medicine systems. ScientificWorldJournal. 2007;7:1821-31.
272. Viitasalo JT, Niemelä AK, Kaappola R, et al. Warm underwater water-jet massage improves recovery from intense physical exercise. Eur J Appl Physiol Occup Physiol. 1995;71(5):431-8.
273. Wakim KG, Martin GM, Terrier JC, et al. The effects of massage on the circulation in normal and paralyzed extremities. Arch Phys Med Rehabil. 1949;30(3):135-44.
274. Wakim KG. Physiologic effects of massage. In: Basmajian JV (Ed). Manipulations, Traction, and Massage. Baltimore: Williams and Wilkins; 1985. p. 3.
275. Walaszek R. Impact of classic massage on blood pressure in patients with clinically diagnosed hypertension. J Tradit Chin Med. 2015;35(4):396-401.
276. Wale JO. Tidy's Massage and Remedial Exercises. UK: Johnbright and Sons; 1968.
277. Watt PW, Gladden LB, Hundal HS, et al. Effects of flow and contraction on lactate transport in the perfused rat hindlimb. Am J Physiol. 1994;267(1 Pt 1):E7-13.
278. Weiger WA, Smith M, Boon H, et al. Advising patients who seek complementary and alternative medical therapies for cancer. Ann Intern Med. 2002;137(11):889-903.
279. Weinberg RS, Genuchi M. Relationship between competitive trait anxiety, state anxiety, and golf performance: a field study. J Sport Psychol. 1980;2(2):148-54.
280. Weinberg RS, Jackson AJ, Kolodny K. The relationship of massage and exercise to mood enhancement. Sport Psychol. 1988;2(3):202-11.
281. Weiss JM. Treatment of leg edema and wounds in a patient with severe musculoskeletal injuries. Phys Ther. 1998;78(10):1104-13.
282. Wenos JZ, Brilla IR, Morrison MZ. Effect of massage in delayed onset muscle soreness. Med Sci Sports Exerc. 1990;22(1):534.

283. Wikipedia. (2019). Tui na. [online] Available from https://en.wikipedia.org/wiki/Tui_na. [Last accessed October, 2019].
284. Williams A. Manual lymphatic drainage: exploring the history and evidence base. Br J Community Nurs. 2010;15(4):S18-24.
285. Williams AL, Selwyn PA, Liberti L, et al. A randomized controlled trial of meditation and massage effects on quality of life in people with late-stage disease: a pilot study. J Palliat Med. 2005;8(5):939-52.
286. Williams PL, Dyson M. Gray's Anatomy. Edinburgh: Churchill Livingstone; 1993. p. 37.
287. Wiltshire EV, Poitras V, Pak M, et al. Massage impairs postexercise muscle blood flow and "lactic acid" removal. Med Sci Sports Exerc. 2010;42(6):1062-71.
288. Wiltshire EV, Poitras V, Pak M, et al. Massage therapy for essential hypertension: a systematic review. J Hum Hypertens. 2015;29(3):143-51.
289. Wittlinger H, Wittlinger D, Wittlinger A, et al. Dr. Vodder's Manual Lymph Drainage. Germany: Thieme Medical Publishers; 2011.
290. Wolfson H. Studies on the effects of physical therapeutic procedures on function and structure. JAMA. 1931;96(2):2019-21.
291. Wood EC, Becker PD. Beard's Massage. Philadelphia: Saunders; 1981.p. 3.
292. World Health Organization (WHO). (2010). Benchmarks for training in traditional/complementary and alternative medicine: Benchmarks for training in Tuina. [online] Available from https://www.who.int/medicines/areas/traditional/BenchmarksforTraininginTuina.pdf. [Last accessed October, 2019].
293. Wright J. The prescription of physical therapy. Phys Ther Rev. 1946;26(3):168-9.
294. Wu Z, Kong L, Zhu Q, et al. Efficacy of tuina in patients with chronic neck pain: study protocol for a randomized controlled trial. Trials. 2019;20(1):59.
295. Xiong XJ, Li SJ, Zhang YQ. Massage therapy for essential hypertension: a systematic review. J Hum Hypertens. 2015;29(3):143-51.
296. Yang YJ, Zhang J, Hou Y, et al. Effectiveness and safety of Chinese massage therapy (Tui Na) on post-stroke spasticity: a prospective multicenter randomized controlled trial. Clin Rehabil. 2017;31(7):904-12.
297. Zainuddin Z, Newton M, Sacco P, et al. Effects of massage on delayed-onset muscle soreness, swelling, and recovery of muscle function. J Athl Train. 2005;40(3):174-80.
298. Zane T. A Review of Craniosacral Therapy: Science, Fads, and Applied Behavior Analysis. The Current Repertoire, Fall 2011, Newsletter of the Cambridge Center for Behavioral Studies [online]. Available from http://www.behavior.org/resources/589.pdf. [Last accessed September, 2019].
299. Zeitlin D, Keller SE, Shiflett SC, et al. Immunological effects of massage therapy during academic stress. Psychosom Med. 2000;62(1):83-4.
300. Zelikovski A, Kaye CL, Fink G, et al. The effects of the modified intermittent sequential pneumatic device (MISPD) on exercise performance following an exhaustive exercise bout. Br J Sports Med. 1993;27(4):255-9.

BIBLIOGRAPHY

1. Aksenova AM, Teslenko OI, Boganskaia OA. Changes in the immune status of peptic ulcer patients after combined treatment including deep massage. Vopr Kurortol Fizioter Lech Fiz Kult. 1999;2:19-20.
2. Anderson SK. The Practice of Shiatsu. St. Louis: Mosby Elsevier; 2008.
3. Arkko PJ, Pakarinen AJ, Kari-Koskinen O. Effects of whole body massage on serum protein, electrolyte and hormone concentrations, enzyme activities, and hematological parameters. Int J Sports Med. 1983;4:265-7.
4. Armstrong RB. Mechanisms of exercise-induced delayed onset muscular soreness: a brief review. Med Sci Sports Exerc. 1984;16:529-38.
5. Baldry PE. Acupuncture, trigger points and musculoskeletal pain. London: Churchill Livingstone; 1993.
6. Balke B, Anthony J, Wyatt F. The effects of massage treatment on exercise fatigue. Clin Sports Med. 1989;1:189-96.
7. Bell GW. Aquatic sports massage therapy. Clin Sports Med. 1999;18:427-35.
8. Beresford-Cooke C. Shiatsu Theory and Practice, 3rd edition. London/Philadelphia: Singing Dragon; 2016.
9. Bernau-Eigen M, Rolfing A. A systematic approach to the integration of human structures. Nurse Pract Forum. 1998;9:235-42.
10. Bork K, Karling GW, Faust G. Serum enzyme levels after "whole body massage". Arch Dermatol Forsch. 1971;240:342-8.
11. Bredin M. Mastectomy: Body image and therapeutic massage: A qualitative study of women's experience. J Adv Nurs. 1999;29:1113-20.
12. Burovykh AN, Samtsova IA, Manuilov IA. An investigation of the effect of individual variants of sports massage on muscular blood circulation. Soviet Sports Rev. 1989;24:197-200.
13. Cafarellie E, Flint F. The role of massage in preparation for and recovery from exercise. Sports Med. 1992;14:1-9.
14. Casley-Smith JR. Modern Treatment for Lymphoedema, 5th edition. Adelaide: University of Adelaide; 1997.
15. Cinque C. Massage for cyclist: the winning touch. Phys Sports Med. 1989;17:167-70.
16. Cooper B. Massage of the forearms for male gymnasts. Sports Sci Med Quart. 1986;2:4-6.
17. Day JA, Mason RR, Chesrown SE. Effect of massage on serum level of beta-endorphin and beta-lipotropin in healthy adults. Phys Ther. 1987;67:926-30.
18. Dicke E, Schliach H, Wolff A, et al. A Manual of Reflexive Therapy of the Connective Tissue: "Bindege Webs Massage" (Connective Tissues Massage). New York: Simon and Schuster; 1978.
19. Ebel A, Wisham LH. Effect of massage on muscle temperature and radiosodium clearance. Arch Phys Med Rehabil. 1952;33:399-405.
20. Ebner M. Connective tissue massage. Physiotherapy. 1978;64:208-10.

21. Ebner M. Connective Tissue Massage: Theory and Therapeutic Application. Edinburgh: Churchill Livingstone; 1962.
22. Ernst E, Fialka V. The clinical effectiveness of massage therapy: a critical review. Forsch Komplementmed. 1994;1:226-32.
23. Ernst E, Matra A, Magyarosy J. Massage cause changes in blood fluidity. Physiotherapy. 1987;73:43-5.
24. Ernst E. Massage therapy for low back pain: a systematic review. J Pain Symptom Manage. 1999;17:65-9.
25. Ernst E. Massage: safe and effective. Eur J Phys Med Rehabil. 1997;7:101.
26. Földi M, Strossenreuther R. Foundations of Manual Lymph Drainage, 3rd edition. St. Louis: Elsevier; 2003.
27. Gam AN, Warming S, Larsen LH, et al. Treatment of myofascial trigger-points with ultrasound combined with massage and exercise—a randomised controlled trial. Pain. 1998;77:73-9.
28. Garcia RM, Horta AL, Farias F. The effect of effect massage before venipuncture on the reaction of preschool and school children. Rey Esc Entern Vsp. 1997;31:119-28.
29. Goats GC. Massage—the scientific basis of an ancient art: Part 1. The techniques. Br J Sports Med. 1994;28:149-52.
30. Goats GC. Massage—the scientific basis of an ancient art: Part 2. Physiological and therapeutic effects. Br J Sports Med. 1994;28:153-6.
31. Graham D. Massage, Manual Treatment and Remedial Movements. Philadelphia: Lippincott; 1913.
32. Graham D. Treatise on Massage: Its History, Mode of Application, and Effects. Philadelphia: Lippincott; 1902.
33. Greenman P. Principles of Manual Medicine, 2nd edition. Baltimore: Williams and Wilkins; 1996.
34. Hall D. A practical guide to the art of massage. Runner's World. 1979;14:55-9.
35. Harmer PA. The effect of pre-performance massage on stride frequency in sprinters. Ath Train. 1991;26:55-9.
36. Hoffa AJ. Technik der Massage, Atuttgart. Germany: Ferdinand Enke Verlag; 1909. p. 14.
37. Huebscher R. An overview of massage. Part I: History, types of massage, credentialing, and literature. Nurse Pract Forum. 1998;9:197-9.
38. Jacobs M. Massage for the relief of pain: anatomical and physiological considerations. Phys Ther Rev. 1960;40:93-8.
39. Kopysov VS. Use of vibrational massage in regulating the pre-competition condition of weight lifters. Soviet Sports Rev. 1979;14:82-4.
40. Krilov VN, Talishev FM, Burovikh AN. The use of restorative massage in the training of high level basketball players. Soviet Sports Rev. 1985;20:7-9.
41. Ladd MP, Kottke FJ, Blanchard RS. Studies of the effect of massage on the flow of lymph from the foreleg of the dog. Arch Phys Med Rehabil. 1952;33:604-12.
42. MacDonald G. Massage as a respite intervention for primary caregivers. Am J Hosp Palliat Care. 1998;15:43-7.
43. Meagher J, Boughton P. Sports Massage. New York: Doubleday and Company, Inc; 1980.
44. Melham TJ, Sevier TL, Malnofski MJ, et al. Chronic ankle pain and fibrosis successfully treated with a new noninvasive augmented soft tissue mobilization technique (ASTM): a case report. Med Sci Sports Exerc. 1998;30:801-4.
45. Mennell JB. Physical Treatment. Philadelphia: Blakiston and Company; 1945. p. 5.
46. Nielsen A. Gua Sha: A Traditional Technique for Modern Practice, 2nd edition. Edinburgh: Elsevier; 2012.
47. Phaigh R, Perry P. Athletic Massage. New York: Simon and Schuster; 1984.
48. Stamford B. Massage for Athletes. Phys Sports Med. 1985;13:178.
49. Stillerman E. Modalities for Massage and Bodywork, 1st edition. St. Louis: Mosby; 2008.
50. Tappan FM. Healing Massage Techniques: Holistic, Classic, and Emerging Methods. East Norwalk: Appleton and Lange; 1988. p. 2.

51. Tappan FM. Massage Techniques: A Case Method Approach. New York: Macmillan Company; 1961.
52. Upledger JE, Vredevoogt J. Craniosacral Therapy. Seattle: Eastland Press; 1983.
53. Upledger JE. Craniosacral therapy. In: Novey DW (Ed). Clinician's Complete Reference to Complementary and Alternative Medicine. St. Louis: Mosby; 2000. pp. 381-92.
54. Wakim KG, Martin GM, Krusen FH. Influence of centripetal rhythmic compression on localized edema of an extremity. Arch Phys Med Rehabil. 1955;36:98-103.
55. Wittlinger H, Wittlinger D, Wittlinger A, et al. Dr. Vodder's Manual Lymph Drainage. Germany: Thieme Medical Publishers; 2011.
56. Xinrong Y, Bingyi F, Fang S, et al. Tuina xue (Tuina therapy). In: Encyclopedia Editorial Committee of Traditional Chinese Medicine (Ed). Encyclopedia of Traditional Chinese Medicine. Shanghai: Shanghai Science and Technology Press; 1987.
57. Yackzan L, Adams C, Francis KT. The effects of ice massage on delayed muscle soreness. Am J Sports Med. 1984;12:159-65.
58. Zhang EQ. Chinese Massage: A Practical English-Chinese Library of Traditional Chinese Medicine. Shanghai: Publishing House of Shanghai University of Traditional Chinese Medicine; 1990.
59. Zuther J. Lymphedema Management: The Comprehensive Guide for Practitioners, 3rd edition. Germany: Thieme Medical Publishers; 2013.

INDEX

Page numbers followed by *b* refer to box, *f* refer to figure, *fc* refer to flowchart, and *t* refer to table.

A

Abdominal massage 35
Abdominal wall 156
Abdominoplasty 111
Abduction 158
Accessories 78, 78*f*
Acupressure 97
    massage 106
Adduction 158
Adherent skin
    burns 91
    techniques 91
Adhesion 158
    breakers 113
    formation 25, 140
Adipose tissue 8, 158
    effects on 22
Adrenocorticotropin hormone 15
Agitation 100
AIDS infection 30
Airways
    larger 21
    smaller 21
Amenorrhea 100
American Heart Association 107
Amino acids 124
Ammonia 126
Ankle sprain 112
Anomalous tension 115
Antihypertensive drugs 33
Anus 109
Anxiety 30, 100, 112, 132
    excess level of 132
Arachidonic acid 77
Arm muscles 136
Aromatherapy and massage 31
Arousal 158
Arterial blood flow 24
Arterial blood, oxygen in 64
Arterial pulsation adjacent 8
Arteriosclerosis 40
Assisted roller massage 114
Asthapana 142
Asthma 29
Asthmatic children 29
Asymmetrical muscle weakness 117
Atherosclerosis 36, 37
Athletes, muscles of 118
Attention deficit hyperactivity disorder 29
Autistic symptomology 112
Autonomic nervous system 7, 20, 99
Autonomic response, modulate 24
Axon reflex 9*f*
    activation of 9
Ayurvedic massage 18, 141, 142

B

Babies massage, saturated fats in 77
Baby massage 14
Back 81
    direction of effleurage strokes 81
    gluteal region 81
Back pain
    chronic 112
    unspecified 27
Bacterial infection 59
Balance
    dynamic 19
    left and right 102
    sagittal plane 102
    throughout system 102
    under body 102
Barthel index scores 18
Beating 5, 15, 33, 62*f*
    and pounding 60, 62
Bedsheet 78
Behavioral
    anxiety 29
    problems 112

Bell's palsy 28, 83, 86
  aims of treatment 86
  caution 87
  position 87
  sequence 87
  techniques 87
Beta-endorphin level 15
Bicarbonate 126
Biceps brachii 79
Bioenergy, constant flow of 19
Biokingeriga 13
Biomechanical stress 120
Bleeding tendencies 32
Blood
  cells 11
  effects on 7, 11
  flow, increased 27
  lactate concentration 130
  of babies massage 77
  oxygenation of 12
  pressure 32, 33
    loss of 107
  samples 23
  vessels 8
Body
  cavities of 60
  fascia 102
  muscle of 90
  structure and function practice 35
Bodybuilder, performance of 13
Bodyweight, self-roller massage 114
Bone disease 37
Bone mass, amount of 37
Bowel movements 14
Brachial artery 11
  blood velocity 10
Brachioradialis 79
Brain pulsates 112
Breast in female 69
Bronchospasm 64
Bulbous swelling 91
Bursitis 59

C

Calcium homeostasis, loss of 125
Calf muscle complex 135
Cancer, experience pain 30
Capillary
  and venules 37
  electrophoresis time-of-flight mass
    spectroscopy 124

Cardiac
  ailments 111
  arrhythmia 158
    onset of 37, 64
  diseases, severe 36, 37
  failure 37
  massage, external 106
    common errors 108
    complication of 108
    mouth-to-mouth breathing 107
    procedure 107
    technique 107
  output 64
Cardiopulmonary resuscitation program 106
Cardiovascular system 110
Carnitine 124
Carotid and pulmonary pulses, loss of 107
Carpal tunnel syndrome 112
CD25P lymphocytes 12, 24
Central nervous system 112
Central venous pressure 28
Centrifugal 158
Cerebral palsy 38
Cerebrospinal fluid 111, 112
Cervical magnetic resonance imaging 35
Chest
  cardiac massage 106
  percussion 37
  physiotherapy 94
Chest wall, vibration 66
Chinese massage therapy 18
Chinese medicine 143, 146
Circulating lymphocytes, number of 24
Cisplatin 31
Clapping 5, 28, 60, 60f
Classical massage, basic techniques of 41
  pressure manipulation 41
  stroking 41
  tapotement 41
  vibration 41
Classical massage, features of
    various techniques of 5t
Coconut oil group 77
Communication difficulties 112
Compression devices 103
Connective tissue 158
  fascia 115
  layers of 100
  massage 20, 97, 99, 118
    stroking 100
    termination of 15, 100
Consciousness, loss of 107
Constipation 146

Contact
　and continuity 75
　heel percussion 60, 63
Contractile unit 158
Contraindications 35, 67
　general 36
　local 36, 38
　massage 36, 36t
Cori cycle in liver 131
Cortisol 24
Couch 78
Coughing
　techniques to clear lungs 66
　removed 28
Cranial bones 112
Craniosacral mobility, component of 112
Craniosacral system 112
Craniosacral techniques 111
Craniosacral therapy 111
Cream 78
Creatine kinase 13
　level 122
Cryostimulation 123
Cryotherapy 13, 123
Culture, part of 144
Cupping 33
Cyriax 59
Cystic fibrosis 29, 94, 66

D

Dead cells, removal of 24, 47
Deep connective tissue 100
Deep drainage 152
Deep lymphatic vessels 150, 152, 154
Deep massage techniques 140
Deep muscular fasciae 115
Deep stripping massage strokes 134
Deep tissue work 116
Deep transverse friction 140
Deep X-ray therapy 36, 37
Delayed-onset muscle soreness 13, 120
Depression 112
Dermatome 100
Diarrhea 146
Digestive problems 112
Digital ischemic pressure 104
Digital kneading 49, 50
Disk herniation 35
Distal interphalangeal 51
Docetaxel 31
Dorsiflexion 158
Drainage, superficial 152

Draping 72
　during massage therapy 73t
　for back massage 73f
　for lower limb massage 73f
　for upper limb massage 73f
Dries up 28
Dyslexia 112
Dysmenorrhea 100
Dyspepsia 35

E

Ear infections 112
Eccentric exercise 121
Eccentric quadriceps work, bilateral 121
Edema 83
　cause of 37
　gravitational 37
　paralytic 37
　premenstrual 111
　reduce 25, 27, 46
Edible oils 77
Effleurage 4, 5, 15, 33, 103
　of back finish 45f
　produces squeezing 46
　to knee 47f
Elastic bandages 27
Elbow
　collateral ligament of 59
　movement 61
Electrodermal response 20
Electromyography 134
Endofascial fibers 115
Energy, basic types of 143
　kapha 143
　pitta 143
　vata 143
Engorged breast 83, 92
　aims of treatment 92
　sequence 92
　techniques 92
Enzyme collagenase 26
Epidural hematoma, acute 35
Epigastric pain 146
Erythema 158
Essential fatty acids 77
Exercise
　muscle bed 132
　therapy 19
Exocrine glands of skin 22
Extracellular signal-regulated kinase 11
Eyelid 25

F

Face 82
   gentle massage of 14
Facial massage 72f
Facial muscles, paralysis of 86
Facial nerve 82, 86
   palsy 146
Facilitates recovery 120
Fallout standing 74, 74f
Fascia 100, 115
Fascial abrasion technique 113
Fatigue
   index scale, modified 19
   chronic 100
Fatty acid 77
Female breast 109
Femoral artery
   blood flow 130
   blood velocity 76
Femoral pulses 107
Fever, high 36
Fibromyalgia 100, 111, 117
Fibrosis 57
Fibrositis 26, 27, 83, 90
   aims of treatment 90
   nodules 58
   position 91
   sequence 91
   techniques 91
Finger kneading 50
   over mandible 50f
Finger pad kneading 50
   over paraspinal area 51f
Finger, pulp of 42
Fingertip
   in particular locations 112
   kneading 51, 79
      over interosseous space 51f
Flaccid paralyses, type of 28
Flatulence 83, 93
   aim of treatment 93
   position 93
   technique 93
Flexible granulation tissues 39
Flexion
   attitude of spine 74
   left elbow 42
Flow-mediated dilation 11
Fluid in tissue space 24
Fluoroscopy-guided manual lymphatic drainage 110
Focal adhesion kinase 11

Forearm
   blood flow, measured 10
   effleurage 46f
   pronated 79
   single-handed picking 54
Fracture 37, 39
   rib 67
   unstable 113
Fragile 37
French chalk 77
Friction 4, 5, 48
   circular 4, 57
   transverse 4, 58
Fugl-Meyer assessment 18
Functional independence measure 19
Functional internal organ problems 144

G

Galvanic skin response 20
Gamma motor neuron fibers 17
Gaseous exchange 24, 28
Genitals 109
Glycogen 11, 125
Golgi tendon organ 57
Granulation tissue 39
Graston technique 113
Gravity, force of 8
Gua sha 143
   tools for 144
   treatment 144
Guillain-Barré syndrome 28

H

Hacking 5, 15, 33, 60-62f
   advances 61
Hair follicle 38
Hairy skin 38
Half lying, positioning in 71f
Hamstring, junction of 134
Hand
   edge of 42
   effleurage 45f
   linear movements of 5
   oscillatory movement of 5
   palm of 42
   palmar kneading 49f
   picking up 55f
   self-roller massage 114
   therapist 43
   use of heel of 42
Head, lymphatic drainage of 156
Headache 112

Healer local 35
Health, perception of 19
Heart beat, loss of 107
Heart rate 33
Heat
   dissipation 22
   shock protein 27 11
   stroke 144, 106
Hematoma 40, 111
Hemiplegia 38, 146
Hemoptysis 64, 158
   severe 67
Hepatitis 100
Hip flexion angle 134
HIV infection 23
Hoffa massage 102
Homeostasis 158
Homonymous motor neuron pool 17
Human embryo 99
Human ills, treatment for 25
Hyoid, restriction of 117
Hyperactive peristalsis 112
Hyperbaric therapy 123
Hyperemia 59
Hyperinflation 21
Hyperkeratotic scars 111
Hypertension
   causative factor for 32
   pharmacologic treatment of 34
   reduction of 32
   uncontrolled 113
Hypertrophic burns scarring 26
Hypothalamic-pituitary-adrenal 23
Hypothenar eminence 158
Hypotonic muscle 24

I

Illness, recurrent 133
Immune suppression 22
Immune system 8
Imperfecta 38
Inconsistency in performance 133
Indian medicine system 95
Infections, acute 111
Inflammation 59, 158
   acute 36, 39
   chronic 57
   systemic manifestations of 36
Inflammatory cytokines 11
Inflammatory products 48
Inflammatory response 25
Infraorbital foramina nerve 82
Inguinal lymph nodes 154

Injury and massage
   acute 140
   chronic 140
Injury prevention, goal of 118
Instrument-assisted soft tissue mobilization 113
Intellectual abnormalities 112
Intense exercises 124
Intercostal muscles 59
Interfascial planes 115
Intermittent compression devices 104
Interphalangeal joint, ligaments of 51
Interstitial pressures 110
Intestinal disorders 100
Intestinal obstruction 96
Intracellular adhesion molecule 33
Intracranial
   bleeding 112
   pressure 111, 112
Intrafibrillary adhesions 89
Intramuscular edema 120
Irritability 112
Ischemia 158
Isokinetic strength 122

J

Javelin 136
Joint capsule 59
Just touch no pressure 42

K

Karpasasthyadi oil 18
Keloid formation 25
Kidney, distal tubules of 37
Kinesitherapy 97
Kneading 4, 5, 33, 48
   circular movement of 49f
   digital 4
   palmar 4
   reinforced kneading 4
   techniques, variation of 52
Knee, collateral ligaments of 58f
Knuckles 43, 116

L

Labor and postnatal period 29
Lactate 11
   dehydrogenase 13, 122
   recovery 125
Lanolin 78
Lanolin-based creams 78
Legs, immersion of 126

Ligament sprain 26
Linolenic acid 77
Liquid paraffin 77
Locomotor apparatus 99
Lordosis 159
Lower limb 73
    massage, preparation of patient for 80
    over calf muscles 80
    over foot 81
    over knee 80
    over leg 80
    over thigh 80
    over tibial and peroneal muscles 80
Lower motor neuron lesion 83, 86
    cautions 86
    procedure 86
    sequence 86
    techniques 86
Lubricant 76
Lung disease, chronic 63, 94
Lung, mobilize secretions in 25, 28
Lymph drainage 31
Lymph moving 8
Lymph nodes of 150
    head and neck 157*fc*
    lower limb 153*fc*
    upper limb 151*fc*
Lymph vessels 111
    superficial 152
Lymphangions 111
Lymphatic capillary 150
Lymphatic drainage 46
    increased 11
    of lower limb 152
    of trunk 154
    of upper limb 150
    type of massage 13
Lymphatic fluids 46
Lymphatic pathways 111
Lymphatic system 111
    outlines of 150
Lymphatic trunks 155*fc*
Lymphatic vessels, course of 150
Lymphedema 31, 111
    adjunct therapy for 32
Lymphocyte 31
    phenotypic markers 24

M

Magnitude of applied force 2
Malic acid 124
Malignancy 36, 40
Malignant tumors 111

Manipulative massage 97
Manual lymph drainage 13, 110
Manual traction, combination of 115
Massage 29, 30
    acts 8
    and aids 29
    and hypertension 32
    and lactate removal 129
    application of 35, 127
    assisted recovery 126
    circulatory, effects of 9
    classic back 33
    classification of 1, 3*f*
    contraindications of 36
    exacerbates 39
    for injury rehabilitation 136, 139
    for relaxation 137
    healing art 1
    histological effect of 97
    history of 95
    imparts, different maneuvers of 15
    in prevention of injuries, role of 133
    in psychological recovery, role of 132
    intermediate 138
    kind of 101, 118, 136, 138
    main complications of 35
    maneuvers 10
        different 21
        stretch 16
    mechanical
        action of 8
        devices of 103
    new systems of 99
    on circulatory system 8
    on fatigue and recovery 124
    on lymphatic flow 97
    on motor system 16
        inhibitory effects of 17
    physiological effects of 7, 24*b*, 97
    postevent 138
    practical aspects of 68
    pre-event 136
    preparatory 137
    procedures 27
    promotes 12
    respiratory technique of 94
    role of 29
    sequence of 79
    session 33
    speeds 12
    stretches, mechanical movement of 26
    systems 105
        ancient 141

technique 2, 17, 118, 126
  classical 99
  classification of 2, 3
  deep 6
  features of 2
  in sports setups 118
  light 6
  specialized 118
  therapy
    applications of 83
    in spasticity 19
    on fatigue 19
    success of 68
    value of 7
  to specific muscle group 137
  training 139
  treatment 68
    steps of 69fc
  upper limb 71f
Maximal voluntary contraction 127
Mean frequency 127
Median frequency 127
Medical massage 136, 139, 140
Medicated oil enema 142
Medicinal oils 77
Menstrual disturbances 100
Mental health inventory 19
Mental state 63
Mesoderm 99
Metabolic rate 36
Metabolic waste products, removal of 24, 27, 48
Metabolism, effects on 7, 12
Metabolite
  exchange of 12
  quantification 12
Metacarpophalangeal joint 60
Metastasis 40
Metastatic deposition in 64
  ribs 64
  spine 64
Mind-body techniques 30
Mineral oil 77
Mitochondrial biogenesis signaling 11
Mitogen-induced lymphocyte stimulation 23
Mitogen-stimulated
  interferon-C 24
  levels 24
Mobilize adhesion 57
Mood, improving 29
Motion, active range of 18
Motor nervous system 7
Motor neuron excitability 16, 17
Motor system 16

Movement, restricted 7
Muscle
  activity, component of 132
  atrophy 100
  attachments 58
  belly of brachialis 59
  blood flow 125
  contraction 16
  fiber 16, 111
  function, recovery of 125, 126
  hypertrophy 100
  injury 83, 89
    aims of treatment 89
    position 89
    procedure 89
    techniques 89
  ischemia 120
  rolling to calf 56f
  soreness 122
    management of delayed-onset 11
  spasm 47
    and pain 25, 26
  spindle, activity of 16
  sprain 7
  strength 21
  temperature 130
  tension 57
  tone 159
  weakness 47
Muscular blood flow, increase 130
Muscular enzymes 13
Muscular injury 26
Muscular rheumatism
  acute 90
  chronic 90
Muscular torticollis 146
Musculoskeletal injuries
  acute 118
  chronic 118
Mustard and coconut oil 77
Myocardial dysfunction 100
Myofascial release 115
Myoglobin 13
Myositis ossificans 36, 40, 113

N

Nasal administration 142
Natural killer cell 23
  activity 23
Neck 154
Neck massage (posterior), positioning for 72f
Neonatal jaundice 14
Neonatal respiratory distress 66

Nephrotic syndrome 37
Nervous system, effects on 7, 15
Neurologic compromise 35
Neurological dysfunction 116
Neurological healthy person 24
Neurological signs, unstable 112
Neuroma, painful 83, 91
Neuromuscular excitability 16
Neurotmesis 28
Neutrophil count 11
Nitric oxide 15
Nonarticular rheumatism 90
Noncontractile unit 159
Nuad phaen borarn 147
Nuclear factor-kappa beta p65 12
Numbness and pain 31
Nutritive elements, exchange of 7, 27

O

Obesity 29
  reduction program 22
Oblique abdominal muscles 59
Obstructive pulmonary diseases, chronic 66, 94
Oil, composition of 77
Olive oil 33, 77
Oncology population 32
Osmotic pressure 37
Osseous deformity 100
Osteoblasts 40
Osteogenesis 38
Osteomalacia 38
Osteoporosis 36, 37, 64, 67, 113
  suspected cases of 38
Ovary, inflammation of 100
Oxygen
  consumption 13
  saturation, percutaneous 28
Oxytocin, effect of touch on 15

P

Paget's diseases 38
Pain 19
  neurotransmitter of 15
  reduction 15, 19
  relief 7, 15
Pain-spasm-pain, cycle of 26
Palm, circular movement of 50
Palmar
  and digital kneading 52
  kneading 49, 79, 81
Panic attack 40
Paralyzed muscle 28

Partial pressure 64
Passive leg tension 134
Percussion 5, 21, 60
  manipulations 5
  technique 61
    physiological effects of 63
Periaqueductal gray 15
Periosteal massage 97, 101
Periosteal membrane 90
Periosteum 159
  painful thickening of 90
Peripheral blood levels 23
Peripheral edema 37
Peripheral embolization, incidence of 35
Peripheral sensory receptors 27
Peroneal muscles 59
Persistent tiredness 133
Petrissage 4, 5, 33, 48, 53, 102
  picking up 4
  skin rolling 4
  wringing 4
Phlebitis 39
Phosphorylation 11
Physiotherapy 18, 19, 21
  chest 21
  examination subject of 64
  passive procedures of 38
  respiratory technique of 67
Picking up 53
  technique 53
  variation 54
Pillows 78
Pinda thailam oil 18
Placebo 159
Plantar flexion 159
Plasma creatine kinase
  activity 121
  level 128
Plaster cast 77
Plastic container 79
Plethysmography 98
Pleuritic pain 64
  acute 67
Pliability 26
Poisonous foci 36, 40
Poliomyelitis 28
  acute stage of 36
Popliteal fossa 109, 134
Postburn contracture 26
Postexercise muscle soreness 27
Postpolio syndrome 117
Pounding 5, 63f
Powder 77
Prakriti Dhanwantharam 18

Prana, spiritual terminology 106
Prehypertensive women 32
Pressure manipulations 48
Prone lying 69t
Prone lying, rationale of pillow placement 70t
Protein signaling analysis 12
Proximal interphalangeal joints 51
Proximal phalanges 54, 110
Proximal to distal 4
Pseudoscientific 112
Psoas 102
Psychiatric disturbances 100
Psychological disorders 40
Psychological effects 22
Psychophysiological parameters 132
Psychosomatic arousal, modulate 24
Psychosomatic origin 100
Pulmonary
    conditions 83
    dysfunctions 100
    embolism 37
    function 28
    mechanism 28
    tuberculosis
        active 67
        acute 64
Pumping 111
Pyruvate 126

Q

Qi flows 145
Quadriceps exercise
    concentric 10
    dynamic 10, 130
Quadriceps femoris specimens 123
Quality of life 19
Quasi-experimental design 31

R

Radiation therapy 32
Radical mastectomy 47, 83
    aims of treatment 84
    position 84
    sequence 84
    techniques 84
Radioactive isotope 98
Ratcheting 116
Raynaud's disease 100
Reconstructive surgery 26
Rectus abdominis 102
Reflex massage 97
Reflex sympathetic dystrophy 111

Reflex zone massage, type of 106
Region massage, basis of
    general massage 6
    local massage 6
Regional pain syndrome, chronic 113
Reinforced kneading 49, 52, 52f, 53
Relaxation 83, 93
    facilitation of 109
    general and local 28
    response 32
Renal disease, severe 36, 37
Respiration 102
    loss of 107
Respiratory disease, chronic 61, 117
Respiratory percussion technique 64
    specific contraindications of 64
Respiratory problems 144
Respiratory system, effects on 21
Rheumatoid arthritis 59, 113
Rhythmic compression 107
Rhythmic retrograde 10
Rib fracture 64, 66
Rolfing 102
Roller massage 114
    technique of 114
Root mean square 127
Rubbing 33

S

Sacrum 102, 112
Scar
    adhesions, chronic 140
    height 26
    mobilization of 78
    postsurgical 26
Sclerosis, multiple 19, 38
Scrotum in male 69
Sebaceous gland 24
Sebaceous secretions 22
Secretion, removal of 94
Sedation 159
Seizure disorder 112
Sensory nerve, stimulation of 26
Sensory nervous system 7
Sensory system 15
Sequential compression devices 104
Shaking 5, 28, 66
    on lateral chest wall 66f
    physiological effects 66
    technique 66
    therapeutic use 67
Shear stress 33
Shiatsu 146

Shoulder girdle muscle 103, 136
Siddha system of medicine 95, 142
Side lying
    positioning in 71f
    rationale of pillow placement 71t
Sinusitis 112
Skeletal muscle
    pump 8
    compresses 8
Skin blood flow 130
Skin, bruising of 115
Skin conductance 20
Skin diseases 36, 39
Skin, effects on 22
Skin grafting 92
Skin rolling 33, 53, 55f
    technique 54
    variations 56
Skin, temperature of 20
    investigation of 20
Sleep disturbances 100
Sleep, quality of 29
Soap, nonperfumed 79
Social relationships, poor 112
Soft tissue 40
    adhesions 24
    chest wall 61
    circular movements of 5
    effects on 20
    forming hematoma 40
    healing 118
    lesions, type of 98
    mobility of 7, 26
    mobilization 113, 133
    trauma 35
Soreness 47
    sensation, block 121
Soviet system of athletic training 119
Spasm associated with pain 57
Spasticity 19
    severe 36, 38
Spinal column 100
Spinal cord
    anterior 35
    compressing 35
    injury 35, 38
Spinal nerve root 90
Spine of scapula 103
Spinous processes 109
Sports massage 97, 118
    categories of 136, 136t
    historical perspective 118
    role of 119, 120b
        in athletic 119

Sports rehabilitation 113
Sports-related
    psychological symptoms 133
    soft tissue injury, management of 113
Sports-specific conditions 28
Sprain 83, 87
    aims of treatment 87
    caution 88
    position 87
    procedure 87
    techniques 87
Sputum retention 66
Squeezing 36
Stagnates 28
Standing, modification of 74
Sternum 107
Stimulating percussion technique 64
Straight leg raise 134
Strain 89
Stress 22
    incidence of 98
    related symptoms 22
Stress urinary incontinence 112
Stretch reflex 159
Stride standing 74, 74f
Stripping massage 101
Stroke 41
Stroke techniques
    pump 110
    rotary 110
    scoop 110
    stationary circle 110
Stroke, type of 130
Stroking 5, 15, 33
    back massage 32
    deep 41, 44
    effleurage 41
    group of manipulation 41
    manipulations 4
    superficial 4, 36, 41, 42f, 43f
Stylomastoid foramina 82
Stylus massage 105
Submandibular lymph nodes 82
Subscapular axillary lymph node 152
Sunflower oil 77
Supine lying
    patient's positioning in 70f
    rationale of pillow placement 70t
Supraorbital submental nerve 82
Supraspinatus tendon 59
Sweat gland 20, 24
Swedish massage therapy 23, 24, 33, 35, 134
Swelling 7

Index

T

Talcum powders 77
Tapotement 5, 33, 60
Tapping 5, 15, 60, 62
Technique
  in different conditions, use of 76t
  of thousand hands 43
  selection of 76
Temporomandibular dysfunction 112
Tenacious sputum 63
Tenderness 122
Tendinitis 26, 83
Tendonitis 88
  aims of treatment 89
  procedure 89
  techniques 89
Tendons, inflammation of 88
Tenosynovitis 26, 83, 88
  aims of treatment 88
  position 88
  procedure 88
  technique 88
Tension headache 57
Tenting 60, 63
  position of fingers 63f
Thai massage, traditional 147, 148
  treatment 148
Thenar eminence 159
Therapeutic
  applications of massage
    half lying 70
    prone lying 69
    side lying 71
    sitting 71
    supine lying 70
  modality 7
  uses 25
Therapist
  attitude of 75
  fingers tip of 105
  stance of 73
Thoracic duct 150
Thoracic pump 8
Thoracic wall 154
Thoracolumbar region 81
Thromboangiitis 100
Thromboembolism 111
Thrombophlebitis 100
Thrombosis 36, 40
Thrombus, presence of 40
Thumb
  ball of 42, 43
  kneading 50, 51, 79
  of right hand joints 55f
  pad kneading 51
    over hypothenar eminence 52f
  tip kneading 51
    over interosseous space of foot 52f
  tip side of 51
Tibial muscles, posterior 59
Tingling, resolution of 31
Tissue
  approached 6
  drawn in bands of 100
  flattened area of 100
  softening 111
  trauma 97
Tongue, examination of 145
Torque, measures of 135
Torticollis 112
Tortuous 39
Towel 78
Transcription-polymerase chain reaction 12
Transverse friction
  ankle with thumb 58f
  caution 60
  physiological effects 59
  specific contraindications 59
  technique 59
  uses 59
Traumatic arthritis 59
Traumatic brain injury 112
Traumatic periostitis 83, 90
  aim of treatment 90
  caution 90
  sequence 90
  techniques 90
Tread massage 101
Triceps 79
Tridoshas 143
Trigeminal nerve 82
Trigger point 47, 159
Tuina 144
  contraindication of 146
  critical component of 148
  practice 145
Tumor necrosis factor-α 24

U

Ulnar border 61
Ultrasound Dopplerography 10
Underwater massage 108, 109f
  equipment 108f
  technique 109
United States for chemotherapy 31

Upper limb 73, 79
  effleurage 46f
  limb forearm 79
    midpronated 79
    pronated 79
    supinated 79
  massage, preparation of patient 79f
Upper motor neuron lesion, feature of 38
Uterus, inflammation of 100

V

Vacuum cupping 105
Vagus nerve, stimulation of 14
Valves, incompetency of 39
Vamana 142
Variation 43, 45
Varicose ulcer
  gravitational 47
  mild 47
Varicose vein 39, 100, 113
  severe 36
Vascular changes 39
Vascular disorders like thrombosis 37
Vascular endothelial
  adhesion molecule-1 33
  growth factor 124
Vascular papillae 22
Vascular permeability 39
Vascularity 26
Vasodilators, release of 8
Veins 39, 46
Venous and lymphatic flow 8, 24
Venous congestion, decrease of 9
Venous ulcer 83, 85
  aims of treatment 85
  cautions 85
  procedure 85
  sequence 85
  techniques 85
Vertebra 35
Vertebral arteries 35
Vertigo 117
Vibration 5, 28, 33
  cautions 66
  circulatory effect of 97
  devices 103
  loosening 21
  physiological effects 65
  technique 65
  therapeutic uses 65
  to upper chest wall 65f
Vibratory manipulations 5, 64
Vibratory massage 104f
  principles of 29
Visceral organ 20, 145
Viscid secretions 28
Visual analog scale 128
Visual disturbances 112
Vital energy 18
Vital organs 107
  circulation of 40
Voluntary contraction 10, 131

W

Walk standing 74, 74f
Walking speed 19
Warmth, feeling of 15
Water, running 79
Weight gain, advantage of 77
Weight transfer from head to feet 102
Western physical therapy techniques 146
Western Swedish massage, techniques of 141
Wounds, open 36, 40
Wrestling ground 119
Wringing 53, 81
  physiological effects of 57
  technique 56
  therapeutic uses 57
  to thigh 56f

Y

Young gymnasts 20

Z

Zang-fu organs 145
Zenith 98